Occupational Science
The Evolving Discipline

Edited by

Ruth Zemke, PhD, OTR, FAOTA
Professor and Graduate Programs Coordinator
Department of Occupational Therapy
University of Southern California
Los Angeles, California

Florence Clark, PhD, OTR, FAOTA
Professor and Department Chairperson
Department of Occupational Therapy
University of Southern California
Los Angeles, California

 F.A. DAVIS COMPANY • Philadelphia

F. A. Davis Company
1915 Arch Street
Philadelphia, PA 19103

Printed in the United States of America

Last digit indicates print number: 10 9 8 7 6 5 4

Publisher: Jean-François Vilain
Senior Acquisitions Editor: Lynn Borders Caldwell
Developmental Editor: Crystal Spraggins
Production Editors: Marianne Fithian; Nancee A. Morelli
Cover Designer: Steven Ross Morrone

As new scientific information becomes available through basic and clinical research, recommended treatments undergo changes. The authors and publisher have done everything possible to make this book accurate, up to date, and in accord with accepted standards at the time of publication. The authors, editors, and publisher are not responsible for errors or omissions or for consequences from application of the book, and make no warranty, expressed or implied, in regard to the contents of the book. Any practice described in this book should be applied by the reader in accordance with professional standards of care used in regard to the unique circumstances that may apply in each situation.

Library of Congress Cataloging-in-Publication Data

Occupational science : the evolving discipline / [edited by] Ruth
    Zemke, Florence Clark.
        p.   cm.
    Includes bibliographical references and index.
    ISBN 0-8036-0138-7 (hardcover)
    1. Occupational therapy   2. Occupations.   I. Zemke, Ruth, 1943– .
    II. Clark, Florence, 1946– .
    [DNLM: 1. Occupational Therapy.   2. Work, WB 555 01403 1996]
    RM736.027   1996
    615.8′515—dc20
    DNLM/DLC
    for Library of Congress   96-10611
                                                              CIP

Dedication

This book is dedicated to Distinguished Professor Emerita Elizabeth J. Yerxa, whose vision, courage, and leadership stimulated the University of Southern California Occupational Therapy faculty to take on the awesome task of establishing a new academic discipline—Occupational Science.

Preface

Occupational science is an academic discipline, the purpose of which is to generate knowledge about the form, the function, and the meaning of human occupation. Occupations are defined in the science as chunks of daily activity that can be named in the lexicon of the culture.[1,2] Fishing, grooming, weaving, and dining are all occupations. When we come to understand these occupations within the framework of a human life, we can say "People are shaped by what they have done, by their daily patterns of occupation." Should disease or disability strike, individuals will be able to reconstruct meaningful lives—drawing on threads of their past selves to create a sense of continuity in their new situation.[3] One way they do this is through commitment to action—to occupation. Thus a person's history of occupation, to some extent, shapes what he or she will become in the future. Occupational science is apt to create changes in the way that therapists perceive and approach their work because of what they will have learned about occupation from occupational scientists, about occupation's role as the mortar and bricks in the construction of a new life—or in "getting a life" as common parlance would have it. After a tornado has leveled a house, the owners will either buy or construct a new dwelling. When catastrophe or illness strikes our minds or bodies we may desperately attempt to salvage our sense of self through a return to the chunks of daily activity that filled our time in the past and the forging of new activities in which to engage in the future.

What Kind of a Science Is Occupational Science?

Is it really a science? Founded in 1989 when the University of Southern California's (USC)[4] doctoral program was launched, occupational science today seems to have a life of its own. Its development reminds us of that of a child. We think of the belief a mother may have when her infant is born—she may envision that the child, for example, will be popular, athletic, and a star in every class play. But as the child matures, she discovers he or she is shy, unpopular, scholarly not athletic, and not at all interested in drama. What the mother learns is that the development of this child is to a considerable extent out of her control; what we have learned is that occupational science similarly is developing in ways that we could have never imagined or predicted—its shape and character are being formed by the scholars who embrace it and the students who earn doctoral degrees in the discipline.

Fortunately, it has remained identifiable as a science, the focus of which is on occupation. However, it is not developing as a science in the traditional sense, that is, it is not constrained by a positivistic view. Such a positivistic view would mean it would categorically (1) employ experimental and objective means of theory testing, (2) use a mathematical and statistical language to make knowledge claims, and (3) require that systematic procedures subject to public scrutiny are employed.[5]

Occupational science is quite open to forms of inquiry that are nonmathematical and subjective, although they would have systematic procedures subject to public scrutiny. In fact, Elizabeth J. Yerxa, who is credited with founding occupational science, believes that subjective, qualitative approaches to inquiry are more suited than experimental methods for the study of occupation because of occupation's richness in symbolic meanings and the science's ethical roots in occupational therapy.[6] Suppose, for example, we wished to study co-occupations of mothers and their infants. One approach might be to observe objectively what mothers do all day long with their infants and indicate the time spent in each occupation. This would represent a purely quantitative approach and would allow us, for example, to identify variation across mothers in time spent on certain activities. However, such a study would leave us wondering whether the quality of the bathing activity was comparable from mother to mother. In contrast one could use a research strategy, as did Gallimore and colleagues,[7] that probes symbolic meaning to gather narratives, the stories that mothers tell about the meaning they attribute to the routine activities in which they participate with their children. These researchers found that families used particular themes to guide the implementation of routine activities. One mother might see bathing as an opportunity to bombard the child with enrichment activities; another as an opportunity for natural normal contact between mother and child; and a third, burdened with six other children, as simply a chance to clean the baby efficiently and then get on with other chores. Here the methodology begins to generate knowledge by unpacking the storied nature of occupation that would have lost its richness if quantified.

Finally, an inquiry could be framed using a philosophical framework such as Ruddick's[8] ideas on the nature of maternal thinking. Ruddick believes that a unity of thought, judgment, and emotion emanates from everyday practices. For example, she believes that mothers, out of the experience of caring for a child, begin to conceive of their personal achievement as rooted in their ability, first, to keep their child alive; second, to nurture his or her growth; and third, to produce a child who is socially acceptable in the cultural world in which he or she lives. Ruddick then proposes that the practice of mothering produces notions in the mother about preservation, protection, and social conformity that may affect an overall life philosophy.

Mothers who view achievement as rooted in preserving the life of a child may want to preserve the rain forests; their experience of nurturing others may make them nurturing administrators; and their concern with social fit may render them sensitive to diversity. How, then, might an occupational scientist systematically study the relationship of bathing the baby and other areas of everyday occupation to the long-term development of political and philosophical views that shape the individual and his or her commitment to action? Research that seeks to identify this kind of longitudinal effect of participation in occupation on patterns of thought might employ methods such as the life history method used by Langness[9] and Langness and Frank.[10] Such inquiry requires the use of methods that can explain complexity when numbers are inadequate. Yet such research is capable of being systematic, replicable to some extent, and subject to public scrutiny, and, thus, is scientific.

The current direction of occupational science is consistent with the definition of science provided recently by Chalmers.[11] He defined science on the basis of its purpose—that is, science is seen as the means by which knowledge is produced. Its methods must be systematic and follow routine procedures; both the methods and the findings must be replicable by others. According to Chalmers, science has both a cognitive and a noncognitive dimension. The cognitive dimension involves the procedures used to generate knowledge; the noncognitive dimension is sociological and involves the politics used to promote the science. This definition echoes one formulated by Carlson and Clark[12] in which science is defined as a method of inquiry that is rule based, empirically based, and undertaken by a community of scholars. These definitions leave open the possibility of employing a multitude of research methodologies. So, to the extent that work in occupational science is rule based (or systematic), subject to public scrutiny, and undertaken by a community of scholars, it may be called scientific.

Why Is Occupational Science a Legitimate Discipline?

If one accepts our definition of occupation as chunks of daily activity that can be named in the lexicon of the culture,[1,2] occupation is ubiquitous—it seems to be everywhere and everything. Because of this, the prospect of developing an academic discipline that focuses on occupation can appear overwhelming.

There may be concerns that occupational science overlaps with other disciplines and is therefore not sufficiently unique to justify its establishment as a scholarly discipline. However, it is our view that occupational science, because of its unique subject matter and emphasis, "constitutes a conceptually distinct field of inquiry."[13] Historically, the social sciences establish their distinctiveness not by their formal description but by their emphases and traditions. The unique traditional base of occupational science "lies in the practice of occupational therapy, with its concern with the adaptation, by way of engagement in occupation, of persons with disabilities."[13]

Occupational science is distinct because it demands a fresh synthesis of interdisciplinary perspectives to provide a coherent corpus of knowledge about occupation. Although it is true that in the traditional disciplines, a researcher occasionally addresses issues of relevance to occupation, such efforts are interpreted in ways that do not ultimately place the focus on occupation. In the past, we have cited the research on television viewing as an example.[1] Studies on television viewing tend to regard the television viewer as a passive recipient of external stimulation and emphasize the specific effects of particular kinds of content (e.g., the portrayal of violence). These studies have not addressed topics more directly of concern to occupational scientists such as the long-term consequences of television viewing on achievement motivation or on the development of skill.[1]

Ultimately, we believe that the emergence of occupational science represents a timely and necessary evolution. Its existence should be catalytic in spawning scholarly efforts that will provide creative syntheses of extant knowledge on occupation. Moreover, it should inspire new research that pointedly addresses occupation and its centrality within the framework of human lives.

What About the Relationship of Occupational Science to Occupational Therapy?

Originally, occupational science was conceived of as a basic science.[2] As such, it was described as dealing "with universal issues about occupation without concern for their immediate application in occupational therapy."[14] In contrast, an applied science of occupational therapy would address treatment efficacy and methods. The perceived advantage of developing a basic science was to free scientists to focus on general questions about occupation without concern for its practical application in therapy. However, the first publications on occupational science produced by the USC faculty did include applied content.[15] Similarly, a second major paper was titled "Occupational Science: Academic Innovation in the Service of Occupational Therapy's Future."[1] Thus, from its inception, there was a natural inclination on the part of occupational scientists to make inferences to therapy, thereby demonstrating that the boundaries between the basic science and its application were fluid.

Recently, Mosey[16] has called for a complete partitioning of occupational science from occupational therapy, a position with which we take issue on several counts. Mosey argues that the advantage of such a partitioning includes (1) clarifying the focus and the form of each and (2) enabling each to focus on its own work. If Mosey's recommendations were followed, occupational scientists would make no inferences to therapy, and therapists would not focus on the study of occupation apart from its therapeutic impact. However, in reading Mosey's paper, one becomes aware of several problems.

In the discipline of psychology, Hoshmand and Polkinghorne[5] have provided an impressive critique of the very position Mosey advocates. They argue that the strict separation of applied from basic inquiry in psychology has resulted in a fragmentation of knowledge, thereby generating tensions and divisions between theorists and practitioners. In addition, the generation of knowledge that does not inform practice leaves practitioners without a knowledge base and creates obstacles to practitioners' contributions to knowledge development. These problems, they argue, can be diminished by embracing a postmodernistic perspective in which research and practice are not framed "as separate activities based on disparate modes of inquiry" but as "a unified interactive system of purposeful activity and action."[17] We are convinced that it would serve occupational therapists and occupational scientists well to think of occupational science as interlinked with practice. Occupational science may, in this sense, be thought of as focusing on the form, function, and meaning of human occupation, in all contexts, including the therapeutic context. We believe that the ramifications of a strict partitioning would be egregious, the net effect of which would be fragmentation, division between practitioners and theorists, and the production of poorer or irrelevant research.

In our response to Mosey's article,[18] we have argued that the claim that the field of occupational science is better served by applied than by basic research is unsubstantiated.[18] Just as Ayres' basic research on the sensorimotor foundations of academic abilities led to the development of sensory integration therapeutic procedures,[19] so too do we expect that basic knowledge about occupation will reshape practice.

The Concept of Occupation: Examples of How Basic Science Can Inform Practice

Having discussed occupational science's classification as a science and its relationship to occupational therapy, we now turn our attention to the concept of occupation and how expanding our understanding of occupation may enhance practice. One of the most thrilling aspects inherent in the development of the academic discipline of occupational science has been untangling the complexity of occupation and gaining a sense of its centrality in the framework of human lives. As already stated, occupational science encourages a view of people as becoming what they have done, or as being what they are doing. Each day each of us makes choices about what we will and will not do. Just as we optimally regulate our diet, we optimally balance our occupations. On the surface, engagement in occupation seems quite simple, but actually it is quite complex. The study of occupation entails syntheses of interdisciplinary perspectives.

Occupations are embedded in the lives of people and take on different nuances depending on their context. Daily participation in occupation accrues across time and is culture-laden. Sociological studies of occupation enable us to connect occupations to the societies in which they occur. Consider, for example, Schor's findings in *The Overworked American: The Unexpected Decline of Leisure*.[20] She reported that in the past two decades, Americans have had to extend their work day just to stay even in the "work and spend" cycle in which they find themselves. More and more products are produced, and individuals continue to buy products they think will bring them happiness but which are unnecessary. To pay the bills, longer hours must be worked, and personal debt inevitably accrues, resulting in stress. However, the happiness experienced by the purchase of a new product is fleeting, and soon the typical American is off to the mall for yet another product. To exacerbate matters, the main leisure activity of Americans is mall shopping, reinforced by television watching, which encourages Americans to continue in their get-and-spend pattern. Schor pointed out that time-honored leisure activities are no longer options because most Americans simply do not have the time or money to invest in them. In today's world, the most popular leisure activities are those that require little time and effort. For example, TV watching and mall shopping are relatively passive leisure pursuits involving quick fixes and little discipline.

Schor's work illuminates a causal chain in which increased consumption leads to more time at work, and less investment in active leisure, the kinds of occupations through which skill, competence, and discipline are developed. The popularity of occupations such as participating in community theater, singing in a chorus, developing a musical talent, or fishing is waning, and with it, a dramatic shift in the texture and rhythms of American life has surfaced. Schor's work is fascinating because she has gone beyond the simple description of a get-and-spend pattern to analyze how economic pressures, tied to a decision in favor of consumption, flatten the activity cycles of Americans. Because of the latter analysis, her work is particularly important to those seeking to understand occupation.

To gain control of this situation, Americans need to think carefully about the relationship of occupation to happiness and become more conscious of their impulsive choices and their long-term consequences on activities. Americans should deliberately reflect upon the most potent sources of happiness in their lives. Going to the mall to buy an unneeded product may not seem as enticing when one considers its long-range effects—debt, more work to pay off the debt, less time for active leisure and family.

Giddens,[21] another sociologist, saw lifestyle choice as a fundamental aspect of day-to-day activity in the modern world. He pointed out that the notion of lifestyle is not as applicable in traditional cultures, where few options were possible. In contemporary culture, self-identity can be made and remade in a multiple of fashions. "Each of the small decisions a person makes every day—what to wear, what to eat, how to conduct himself at work, whom to meet with later in the evening" contributes to the routines that become our self-chosen lifestyles. "All such choices . . . are decisions not only about how to act but who to be."[22] Individuals, Giddens suggests, forge their self-identities by a reflexive process in which they make choices of occupation and construct daily routines.

In this book, Bateson, an anthropologist and linguist, calls occupation the "web and woof of the human being," not a component inserted here and there. The improvisational process of composing a life rests on combining and weaving together activities. When discontinuities occur, such as traumatic injury, one enters a new phase in which old themes and activities can be recycled, in order to recover the self.

By embracing and gaining interdisciplinary knowledge about occupation, therapists could create a new understanding of their work. They would experience heightened concern with those activities in which their patients invest their energies and time, with how participation in occupation shapes self-identity, with identifying the fueling participation in occupation, and with how, through a reflexive process, patients can enhance their life opportunities.

Heidegger,[23] a German, philosopher, is cited by Calhoun and Solomon[24] as having implied that "to be human is to be 'there,' caught up in the world, taking a stand on one's life, active and engaged in ordinary situations, with some overview of what is at stake in living." Occupation, which embraces these elements, is key to helping individuals with disability reclaim their personhood.

If the primary role of the occupational therapist was to help his or her patients "be there" in the Heideggerian sense "caught up in the world, taking stances and position, and being active and engaged," what would he or she have to know? To begin with, the therapist would have to have a feel for how to nurture the human spirit to act, a notion which comes from Reilly's[25] Eleanor Clarke Slagle lecture. Murphy,[26] a renowned anthropologist who was diagnosed as having a progressive tumor of the spinal cord that eventually caused severe paralysis and death, writes about the "profound and deepening sense of tiredness—total draining weariness" that he felt, which was accompanied by "a desire to withdraw from the world, to crawl into a hole and pull the lid over his head." He speaks of the anger he felt at having a disability that was further aggravated by his interactions in the world of able-bodied people. Here he suffered snobbery, avoidance, patronization, and even cruelty. From his own experience and research, he identified the following as the most profound changes in the consciousness of people with disability: "lowered self-esteem; the invasion and occupation of thought by physical deficits; a strong undercurrent of anger and the acquisition of a new, total, and undesirable identity." Further, in addition to his own desire to withdraw from the world, Murphy[27] felt that American society tended to "wall him off."

If it is true that people with disabilities feel a need to withdraw from the able-bodied world, and if society, in a sense, gives them the message that they should become isolated, passive, and should also adopt a disabled role, then the proposed goals of occupational therapy will collide with both the individual's natural protective instincts and with the social order. We believe that occupational therapists should help the person with a disability reconstruct an active and meaningful life, when the person may feel too weary to leave his or her house. Entry back into society and into the world of activity is valued as being in the patient's best interest, and yet the able-bodied world possesses no etiquette through which to make the person with a disability feel comfortable and welcomed. The challenge confronting occupational therapists is formidable, and what we expect of patients requires heroism.

Sarbin[28] has recently identified some useful distinctions in the intensity with which people engage themselves in activity. These distinctions may assist therapists in tapping their patients' motivation to get on with the project of crafting a life for themselves. Lowest in intensity is casual involvement such as that which might be manifested during the act of paying for tickets at a movie theater. Next, he identified "uninvolved ritual acting" in which we "go through the motions," which might occur in completing our morning self-care routines. At a more intense level is "heated or engrossed" activity such as that which we may experience during a tennis match. Finally, there is ecstasy, at the upper end of the continuum. Participation in a religious experience, crafting a sublime work of art, or connecting spiritually with another person are examples of activities that might evoke ecstasy. If our patients are to fight the urge to withdraw and be passive, their lives will need to be filled not simply with an abundance of activity, but with a range of activities, including some about which they feel passionately.

Is it possible that a person with a disability might withdraw to the point that he or she would experience few occupations and only go through the motions when engaged in them? Joe Allston, the elderly protagonist in Wallace Stegner's novel *The Spectator Bird* describes his life in retirement as "just killing time, until time gets around to killing me."[29] Even at age 50, after a bout with myocarditis, he felt inside "adjacent to or below the ailing heart, a hungry, thirsty, empty, sore, haunted sensation of being unfinished, random, and unattached, as if, even if the heart were working perfectly, there was nothing there for it to run."[30] Joe Allston has the feeling at age 69 that "nothing is building, everything is running down," and that "there are no more chances for improvement."[31] His perspective may be shared by a segment of the patient population that is discharged from rehabilitation because medical staff believe they have plateaued.

This brings us back full circle to the question of how occupational therapists can nurture the human spirit to act. Sarbin's work[28] suggests that to understand why patients choose to engage in one pattern of activity versus another, the narratives through which they make sense of their experience must be accessed. Just as historians try to understand the choices made by war heroes through the construction of coherent narratives, so, too, can occupational therapists grasp what motivates patients by drawing out their stories in an effort to make sense of their traumatic experiences and subsequent commitment, or lack of commitment, to action. Sarbin sees choices to act, especially those that are significant, as "emplotted." That is to say, rather than being random events, choices to act are expressions of social and moral identities organized by use into a coherent narrative.[28] In a sense, in Sarbin's view, each person is creating a drama that will become his or her life history. In this drama, people enact social roles tied to their social identity and moral roles through which they assert their moral identity. When engaged in occupations like courtship, warfare, playing cards, or teaching, people perform a social role that expresses their social identity. Social roles, according to Sarbin, maintain the stability of the culture and address the question "Who am I?" In contrast, identity roles are expressed in acts that are in the service of the question: How do I fare in relation to the "good"? Acts that we think of as impelled by anger, grief, jealousy, and joy are performed to preserve or enhance moral identity, and are those about which we feel passionately. When the actor is asked to attach a narrative to the meaning of these acts, inevitably such a narrative will be organized around themes reflecting the moral aspects of human interaction such as "duty and obligation, wisdom and folly, pride and shame, honor and dishonor."[32] Finally, according to Sarbin, the moral codes that guide performance of identity roles are absorbed in childhood experience through only vaguely remembered morality plays, myths, novels, and folk songs. Sarbin[28] argues that the acts that are passionately performed by the actor represent solutions to moral problems.

Sarbin's ideas suggest that one key to nurturing our patients' desires to act is to tap that which undergirds their moral identity. The occupational behavior literature focused on the importance of occupational roles, which seems to fall within the genre of social roles as described by Sarbin.[28] Occupational science broadens the focus on occupational roles because, through it, we become concerned with the interface of moral identity with the full round of daily activity, and can ask the more general question of how occupational therapists are most apt to ignite our patients' intense engagement in a world of productivity and activity. The clue we can extract from Sarbin's work is that our patients will be most engrossed and passionate about those activities that preserve or enhance their moral identities. Nurturing the human spirit to act may involve, then, eliciting narratives from patients about how they understand their historical and future commitment to occupations within the overall framework of their lives, mining of the moral structures that they believe represent the "good," acquiring a blueprint of their social roles, and gaining a sense of their place and position within the cultural milieu to which they will return.

In summary, occupational science, although originally conceived of as a basic science, is inextricably tied to practice. Although its emphasis is broad, its concerns are distinct enough to warrant the establishment of a new scientific discipline. Finally, interdisciplinary work on the concept of occupation can forge new approaches to therapy. This book essentially elaborates on this idea.

The papers in this book reflect an extensive range of perspectives. The majority come from presentations at the Occupational Science Symposia. Since 1986, the USC Department of Occupational Therapy has presented an annual symposium, supported in part by grants from the US Department of Health and Human Services, Maternal and Child Health Bureau. Keynote speakers have included Stephen Hawking, world-renowned physicist; Jane Goodall, primatologist whose work with chimpanzees in the wild and in captivity has received international acclaim; and Mary Catherine Bateson,[33] noted anthropologist whose book *Composing a Life* emphasizes the complexity of the daily improvisations from which our life patterns emerge. Their work, along with other invited and peer-reviewed presentations, provided an interdisciplinary stimulus for the development of dialogue concerning the focus and range of occupational science. It is hoped that these papers, which are included in this volume, will engage others in this same dialogue.

The USC doctoral program in occupational science contributed to the process of developing the academic discipline. Seminars with outstanding faculty and students provided beginning synthesis as well as debate around topics at the core of occupational science such as temporal adaptation, information processing for occupation, development of adaptive skills, work, and play. In papers developed out of such seminar discussions, new and experienced scholars share their ideas, hypotheses, and preliminary research. Papers representing all of these influences form the content of this book.

Section I, "Importance of Occupation," addresses the general issue of the importance of occupation from a variety of interdisciplinary standpoints as eminent individuals from the disciplines of anthropology, art, and international relations celebrate the centrality of occupation. This section reminds us, as occupational therapists, not to minimize our work but rather to celebrate, in occupational therapy practice, the significance of occupation for individuals, for society, and for the planet.

In Section II, "Defining and Classifying," the process of defining terms in the construction of a new science is represented. Key concepts such as occupation, play, work, and adaptation must be defined so that those working in the discipline will have a shared sense of meaning and be able to communicate with clarity and precision. While all of the papers in the section are concerned with definition, they approach the task using different methodologies. Parham[34] has identified the theme that, as practitioners, we must name and frame the treatment concerns we will address. Definitions constructed in occupational science will give us a vocabulary with which we can become fluent. The discourse, then, can be used both for conceptualizing treatment and for communicating to others our goals and purposes.

In Section III, "Dimensions of Occupation," papers draw on interdisciplinary knowledge to shed light on aspects of occupation that therapists may never have considered. A perspective is provided on how time and space, habits, routines, emotions, and even prior engagement influences participation in occupation. The papers provide a rich array of concepts and perspectives that have potential for application to or incorporation in treatment.

Section IV, "Biology and Occupation," reminds us that a base of our occupational selves is in our physical and biological nature. Whether viewed from an evolutionary biological direction, from the biophysiological functioning of neurohormonal systems, or from sensory integrative approach, we can see the links between these underlying processes or mechanisms and our performance as occupational beings. Humans as complex living systems cannot be fully understood for their unique qualities without a thorough comprehension of the biological processes they share with other living things.

Section V, "Co-occupations of Mothers and Children," reflects the fact that most of occupation is not an isolated experience. Rather, social aspects of shared occupation are an inherent part of occupational experiences. The interaction of mothers and their children, in caregiving-receiving, in play, and in their daily routines, illustrates the temporal and spatial synchrony that develops. Further, there is the psychosocial impact of the co-occupations on both members of the pair. The papers in this section present these elements through empirical data, literature review, and phenomenological reflection.

Section VI, "Perspectives on Occupation," includes papers developed from seminal work examining the complexity of occupations. Historical perspectives, personal narrative, action theory, Edelman's theory of the biological basis of meaning, and the interaction of human subsystems in occupation provide a wide range of options for occupational scientists and therapists to consider. Additionally, the core assumption of hierarchy as a basic element of the General Systems perspective that has been used for model development and theorizing is questioned. Dynamic Systems theory is proposed as an alternative view for understanding the occupational nature of the human as an open system.

Section VII, "Occupational Science: Mapping New Directions for Occupational Therapy," offers a number of papers exploring the links between occupational science and occupational therapy. Papers presenting the concept of the transmission, through generations of a family, of values enacted in occupation and concepts about the meaning of occupations in old age reflecting themes of a lifetime of meaning. These concepts provide ideas for strategies to apply in the practice of occupational therapy. The concrete example of lack of attention in an intensive care unit to the temporality as a locating factor for optimum cognitive function reminds us that such concepts have potentially strong health implications. Techniques developed using a grounded theory approach provide clear-cut clinical direction arising out of a highly conceptual occupational science approach to patient treatment.

Section VIII, "Wilma West Lectures," includes an invited series of papers presented at the Occupational Science Symposia. Honoring a leader who has had a definite influence upon the development of knowledge in occupational therapy and occupational science, this series begins with a tribute to Wilma West. It includes reminders of aspects of occupation important to the practice of occupational therapy with children. It also includes papers of a broader nature, discussing the scope of occupational science and the question of balance in occupation. The papers in this section make a contribution to the developing field of occupational science and its application in occupational therapy, as do the other papers in this book.

This book does not provide a definitive and carefully controlled developmental style, which some readers might wish for from occupational scientists. Instead, it provides an exciting, in-process source of stimulating ideas about occupation and its implications for health and the practice of occupational therapists. Discussion questions at the end of each paper provide a basis for the reader to join in the process of professional growth possible through exploring these ideas.

Ruth Zemke
Florence Clark

References

1. Clark, FA, Parham, D, Carlson, ME, Frank, G, Jackson, J, Pierce, D, Wolfe, R, and Zemke, R: Occupational science: Academic innovation in the service of occupational therapy's future. Am J Occup Ther 45:300, 1991.
2. Yerxa, EJ, Clark, F, Frank, G, Jackson, J, Parham, D, Pierce, D, Stein, C, and Zemke, R: An introduction to occupational science, a foundation for occupational therapy in the 21st century. Occup Ther in Health Care 6:1, 1989.
3. Csikszentmihalyi, M: Paper presented at Occupational Science Symposium V. Loyola University, Chicago, IL, September 25, 1992.
4. University of Southern California, Department of Occupational Therapy: Proposal for a Ph.D. degree in occupational science, 1989. Unpublished manuscript.
5. Hoshmand, LT, and Polkinghorne, DE: Redefining the science—Practice relationship and professional training. Am Psychol 47:55, 1992.
6. Yerxa, EJ: Nationally speaking: Seeking a relevant, ethical, and realistic way of knowing for occupational therapy. Am J Occup Ther 45:199, 1991.
7. Gallimore, R, Weisner, TS, Kaufman, SZ, and Bernheimer, LP: The social construction of ecocultural niches: Family accommodation of developmentally delayed children. Am J Ment Retard 94:216, 1989.
8. Ruddick, S: Maternal thinking. In Thorne, B, with Yalom, M: Rethinking the Family: Some Feminist Questions. Longman, New York, 1982, pp. 76–94.
9. Langness, LL: The Life History in Anthropological Science. Holt, Rinehart & Winston, New York, 1989.
10. Langness, LL, and Frank, G: Lives: An Anthropological Approach to Biography. Chandler & Sharp, Novato, CA, 1981.
11. Chalmers, AF: Science and Its Fabrication. University of Minneapolis Press, Minneapolis, MN, 1990.
12. Carlson, ME, and Clark, FA: The search for useful methodologies in occupational science. Am J Occup Ther 45:235, 1991.
13. Clark et al., p. 304.
14. Yerxa et al., 1989, p. 4.
15. Yerxa, EJ (ed): Occupational Science: The Foundation of New Models of Practice. Haworth Press, New York, 1990.
16. Mosey, AC: Partition of occupational science and occupational therapy. Am J Occup Ther 46:851, 1992.
17. Hoshmand and Polkinghorne, p. 58.
18. Clark, F, Zemke, R, Frank, G, Parham, D, Neville-Jan, A, Hedricks, C, Carlson, M, Fazio, L, and Abreu, B: The issue is: Dangers inherent in the partition of occupational therapy and occupational science. Am J Occup Ther 47:184, 1993.
19. Ayres, AJ: Sensorimotor foundations of academic ability. In Cruikshank, WM, and Hallahan, DP (eds): Perceptual and Learning Disabilities in Children: Research and Theory, vol 2. Syracuse University Press, Syracuse, NY, 1972.
20. Schor, JP: The Overworked American: The Unexpected Decline of Leisure. Basic Books, New York, 1991.
21. Giddens, A: Modernity and Self-identity: Self and Society in the Late Modern Age. Stanford University Press, Stanford, CA, 1991.
22. Giddens, p. 81.
23. Heidegger, M: Being and Time. Macquarrie, J, and Robinson, E. Trans. Harper & Row, New York, 1962. Original work published 1927.
24. Calhoun, C, and Solomon, RC: What Is an Emotion: Classic Readings in Philosophical Psychology. Oxford University Press, New York, 1984, p. 232.
25. Reilly, M: Eleanor Clarke Slagle Lecture—Occupational therapy can be one of the great ideas of 20th century medicine. Am J Occup Ther 16:1, 1962.
26. Murphy, RF: The Body Silent. WW Norton, New York, 1990.
27. Murphy, p. 108.
28. Sarbin, TR: Emotions as narrative emplotments. In Packer, MJ, and Addison, RB (eds): Entering the Circle: Hermeneutic Investigation in Psychology. State University of New York Press, New York, 1989, p. 185.

29. Stegner, W: The Spectator Bird. Penguin Books, New York, 1976.
30. Stegner, p. 89.
31. Stegner, p. 26.
32. Sarbin, p. 193.
33. Bateson, MC: Composing a Life. Atlantic Monthly Press, New York, 1989.
34. Parham, D: Theory and therapy: An essential partnership. Keynote address, annual meeting of the Occupational Therapy Association of California, Los Angeles, CA, November 1992.

Acknowledgments

The authors wish the thank the following reviewers:

Diana M. Bailey, EdD, OTR
Associate Professor
Boston School of Occupational
  Therapy
Tufts University
Medford, Massachusetts

**Janice P. Burke, MA, OTR/L,
  FAOTA**
Assistant Professor
Department of Occupational Therapy
Thomas Jefferson University
Philadelphia, Pennsylvania

**Jerry A. Johnson, MBA, EdD,
  OTR/L**
Professor and Coordinator of Graduate
  Education
Department of Occupational Therapy
Thomas Jefferson University
Philadelphia, Pennsylvania

**Ellen Berger Rainville, MS, OTR,
  FAOTA**
Assistant Professor and Academic
  Fieldwork Coordinator
Department of Occupational Therapy
Springfield College
Springfield, Massachusetts

**Elizabeth J. Yerxa, EdD, LHD(Hon),
  OTR, FAOTA**
Professor Emerita
Department of Occupational Therapy
University of Southern California
Los Angeles, California

We wish to recognize the Department of Health and Human Services, Maternal and Child Health Bureau, Grant MCH 009048, for its support of the occupational science doctoral program through which occupational science was established as an academic discipline and the annual occupational science symposia for which many of the papers included in this book were prepared. In particular, the support of James J. Papai, Chief of the MCH Research and Training Services Branch, and Elizabeth Brannon, Director of the MCH Training Program, has been constant and encouraging. We also wish to acknowledge the support of *ADVANCE for Occupational Therapists*, especially E. J. Brown, Editor, for support for the 1991 Occupational Science Symposium IV in Philadelphia and of Loyola University Chicago, especially Sarah Skinner, MEd, OTR/L, Director of Occupational Therapy, for support of the 1992 Occupational Science Symposium V in Chicago.

Our thanks go to Wendy Wood, Loree Primeau, Elizabeth Larson, Deborah Mandel, Brian Young, and many other occupational science and occupational therapy students who assisted in the preparation of this book. We found it a collegial learning experience and hope that they did too.

Without the assistance of Marion and Jim Karsjens, this book, as well as many of our other publications, would not have been possible. To suggest that their help, along with that of Janice Wise and Robin Turner, was clerical in nature would grossly underestimate the many forms of their support, which we deeply appreciate.

We wish to thank Professor C. S. Whitaker, Dean of Social Sciences, in the University of Southern California College of Letters, Arts and Sciences at the time of the early Occupational Science Symposia and University of Southern California Vice President of Health Affairs, Joseph P. Van Der Meulen, who is also the Director of the Division of Independent Health Professions, for their administrative support of the occupational science program launched at USC.

Our husbands, Wayne Zemke and John Wolcott, deserve our constant thanks for their patience and understanding throughout this and all of our other occupational science and occupational therapy projects.

Contributors

Mary Catherine Bateson, PhD
Clarence J. Robinson Professor in
   Anthropology and English
George Mason University
Fairfax, Virginia

**Janice Posatery Burke, MA,
   OTR/L, FAOTA**
Assistant Professor
Department of Occupational Therapy
Thomas Jefferson University
Philadelphia, Pennsylvania

Mike Carlson, PhD
Research Assistant Professor
Department of Occupational Therapy
University of Southern California
Los Angeles, California

**Arnold S. Chamove, MA, MPhil,
   PhD, CPsychol, FIBiol**
Lecturer
Psychology Department
Massey University
Palmerston North, New Zealand

**Charles H. Christiansen, EdD,
   OTR, OT(C), FAOTA**
Professor and Dean
School of Allied Health Sciences
University of Texas, Medical Branch
Galveston, Texas

**Florence Clark, PhD, OTR,
   FAOTA**
Professor and Department
   Chairperson
Department of Occupational
   Therapy
University of Southern California
Los Angeles, California

Michael Dear, PhD
Professor of Geography
University of Southern California
Los Angeles, California

Anne Dunlea, PhD
Research Assistant Professor
Departments of Occupational
   Therapy, Linguistics, and
   Psychology
University of Southern California
Los Angeles, California

**Bridget Larson Ennevor, MA,
   OTR/L**
Occupational Therapist
Avon, Connecticut

**Linda L. Florey, MA, OTR,
   FAOTA**
Chief
Rehabilitation Services
UCLA Neuropsychiatric Institute
Los Angeles, California

Doreen Fraits-Hunt, MA, OTR
Occupational Therapist
Northern Nevada Easter Seals
Lake Tahoe, Nevada

Gelya Frank, PhD
Associate Professor
Departments of Occupational
   Therapy and Anthropology
University of Southern California
Los Angeles, California

Nedra P. Gillette, MEd, OTR, FAOTA
Director of Research Services
American Occupational Therapy
    Foundation
Bethesda, Maryland

Joshua S. Goldstein, PhD
Professor of International Politics
School of International Service
The American University
Washington, DC

Jane Goodall, PhD, CBE
Distinguished Adjunct Professor
Departments of Occupational
    Therapy and Anthropology
University of Southern California
Los Angeles, California

Julie McLaughlin Gray, MA, OTR
Adjunct Instructor
University of Southern California
Los Angeles, California

Stephen William Hawking, CH, CBE, FRS
Lucasian Professor of Mathematics
Department of Applied Mathematics
    and Theoretical Physics
University of Cambridge
Cambridge, United Kingdom

Cynthia A. Hedricks, PhD
Assistant Professor
Department of Occupational
    Therapy
Second Vice-President
Society for Menstrual Cycle Research
University of Southern California
Los Angeles, California

Anne Henderson, PhD, OTR, FAOTA
Professor Emeritus
School of Allied Health Professions
Boston University—Sargent College
Boston, Massachusetts

Jeanne Jackson, PhD, OTR
Assistant Professor
Department of Occupational
    Therapy
University of Southern California
Los Angeles, California

Jerry A. Johnson, EdD, OTR/L, FAOTA
Professor and Graduate Coordinator
Department of Occupational Therapy
Thomas Jefferson University
Philadelphia, Pennsylvania

J. Seward Johnson
Sculptor
Princeton, New Jersey

Bonnie L. Kennedy, MEPD, OTR
Doctoral Candidate, Occupational
    Science
Assistant Professor
Occupational Therapy Program
University of Wisconsin—
    Milwaukee
Milwaukee, Wisconsin

Susan H. Knox, MA, OTR, FAOTA
Doctoral Candidate, Occupational
    Science
Clinic Coordinator
Hyland Clinic
Van Nuys, California

Martin H. Krieger, PhD
Professor of Planning
School of Planning
University of Southern California
Los Angeles, California

Sheama Krishnagiri, PhD, OTR/L
Occupational Therapist
Lucille Murray Child Development
    Center
Bronx, New York
Adjunct Instructor
Department of Occupational
    Therapy
New York University
New York, New York

Zoe Mailloux, MA, OTR, FAOTA
Director of Administration and
  Practice
The Ayres Clinic
Torrance, California
Adjunct Instructor of Occupational
  Therapy
University of Southern California
Los Angeles, California

Alexander Moore, PhD
Professor and Chairperson
Department of Anthropology
University of Southern California
Los Angeles, California

Valerie J. O'Brien, MS, OTR
Program Director
Occupational Therapy Assistant
  Program
Army Medical Department Center
  and School
Fort Sam Houston, Texas

**Kenneth Ottenbacher, PhD,
  OTR/L, FAOTA**
Professor and Associate Director
Departments of Rehabilitation
  Medicine and Occupational
  Therapy
SUNY at Buffalo
Associate Director
Center for Functional Assessment
  Research
Buffalo, New York

**L. Diane Parham, PhD, OTR,
  FAOTA**
Associate Professor
Department of Occupational Therapy
University of Southern California
Los Angeles, California

**Heidi McHugh Pendleton, MA,
  OTR**
Doctoral Candidate, Occupational
  Science
Assistant Professor
Department of Occupational Therapy
San Jose State University
San Jose, California

Doris Pierce, MA, OTR
Doctoral Candidate, Occupational
  Therapy
Department of Occupational Science
University of Southern California
Los Angeles, California

Loree A. Primeau, PhD, OTR
Assistant Professor
School of Occupational Therapy
Dalhousie University
Halifax, Nova Scotia
Canada

Penelope L. Richardson, PhD
(Posthumously)

John A. White, Jr., MA, OTR
Assistant Professor
School of Occupational Therapy
Pacific University
Forest Grove, Oregon

Wendy Wood, PhD, OTR
Assistant Professor
Department of Medical Allied Health
  Professions
Division of Occupational Therapy
University of North Carolina at Chapel
  Hill
Chapel Hill, North Carolina

Ruth Zemke, PhD, OTR, FAOTA
Professor and Graduate Program
  Coordinator
Department of Occupational
  Therapy
University of Southern California
Los Angeles, California

Contents

Importance
of
Occupation

In the preface, the justification for establishing a science of occupation is presented. The following selections provide widely differing perspectives on what can be attained by developing a full-orbed understanding of human occupation.

In the first paper, Mary Catherine Bateson calls occupation the "web and woof" of the tapestries we weave, which are our lives. In this statement and others, she accords occupation a position of centrality in understanding the framework of human experience. Human life is seen as a complex tapestry in which work, pleasure, and the sense of identity are woven together in a kind of art form. An implication of her work is that if occupational therapists want to help their patients reconstruct a meaningful life following traumatic injury or disease, it may help them to think of the lives of their patients as progressive compositional art forms, in which in the next movement or phase, old strands or themes can be recycled and new ones simultaneously introduced.

For example, following open heart surgery, an 82-year-old woman felt smothered by her protective spouse who was watching over her, doing everything for her, and insisting that she restrict her activity. Having enjoyed a career as a high-powered executive, this woman felt humiliated by her dependence. Although she had always dismissed women's clubs as frivolous, she realized they provided a viable escape from her husband's watchful, though loving, eye and a context in which she might be able to reassert her independence. In this new "movement" in her life composition, for the first time, she joined a women's club (a new theme) but shortly thereafter convinced the members to start a recycling program, which, of course, she directed (recycling her role as executive).

Mary Reilly[1] once suggested that, unlike the king's men who were unable to put Humpty Dumpty together again, occupational therapists seem able to put their patient together, as a whole, through occupation. Bateson assists us in ap-

1

proaching therapy with a perspective implying that therapists must understand occupation within the framework of human lives. She also tells us that, although occupations in the lives of men may occur in "chunks," women's occupations are often enfolded one on another, so women typically perform multiple occupations in a given time frame. Discontinuities and disruptions punctuate human lives, but these can be bridged by reshaping dreams, retooling old skills, and developing new approaches. Finally, Bateson speaks of the potency of occupation as a therapeutic medium. In occupational contexts, multiple positive effects can accrue from a single occupation. Occupation, from Bateson's perspective, is worthy of study because it represents the core of human experience.

Goldstein addresses the importance of occupation in an international context rather than focusing on occupation within the framework of individual lives. He argues that the world of international relations produces scripts for daily life experience and vice versa; everyday choices of occupation affect the course of international politics. However, he echoes Bateson when he states that "the dance we do here on earth before we move off stage is a statement, or artistic expression of who we are." In keeping with his view that daily occupations shape international relations, Goldstein asks what practical activities can help to develop a human or global identity. What is needed, he argues, are rituals, symbols, and everyday occupations that link humans all over the planet.

Although Goldstein speaks most obviously and explicitly about issues of great interest to political scientists, the points he makes also can form a view of how therapists might help patients reconstruct meaningful lives. Goldstein accords powerful, even potentially international, significance to the choices that individuals make in their daily experience. Therapists using an occupational science perspective will be interested in analyzing the impact of international and global issues on their patients' valuing of activity. For example, an interest in macrobiotic gardening or zoo enrichment might be engendered in a patient through reference to global environmental concerns. A patient may choose to join a political movement as a way of dealing constructively with tensions between society's expectations and what he or she perceives is a biologically determined sexual orientation. Goldstein's work alerts us to think about our own patients' occupations in a global and political context.

The selection by Seward Johnson, in contrast with Goldstein's, directs our attention from the planet back to the individual but is no less powerful in its claims of the importance of simple occupations. Johnson has chosen to celebrate in bronze sculptures familiar acts (or occupations) of rest, play, or breaks from work.

When describing the message he communicates through his sculptures, Johnson states his belief that the quality of our lives can be changed through "minute vacations" and acceptance of the small joys of the mundane. The sculptor sees simple acts like resting in a park, getting out of a building, or fishing as opportunities to free oneself from the "ordered jail of . . . life." For Johnson, the more primal the act, the more therapeutic it is as an antidote to a technologically saturated world. He celebrates simple acts as opportunities to reclaim our animal nature. Johnson's work reminds us that humans may have a primordial need to connect with nature. Occupations like stretching out on the grass and gazing at the sky, engaging in outdoor sports, strolling with family, or embracing or talking with a loved one remind us of how basic human needs are met in simple activities.

Johnson's view is particularly useful for therapists using an occupational science perspective for several reasons. Can therapists begin to help their patients enhance their lives by encouraging them to take "minute vacations" from stressful routines? Exposure to the sculptures provides an aesthetic reminder of the multiple dimensions of occupation. In each sculpture, the emotional rewards and bonds that are associated with particular occupations are captured in bronze as is the form of the occupation itself. Each sculpture reminds us of the infinite rewards of ordinary experience.

The next selection, by the eminent physicist Stephen Hawking, provides a perspective on how technology can enhance, even make possible, the sense of being fully human after a traumatic degenerative disease. Just as enthusiastically as Johnson celebrates ordinary experience as a way of escaping the technological world, Hawking praises technology for enabling him to continue to be a part of the world of activity and accomplishment. Hawking was diagnosed as having amyotrophic lateral sclerosis (ALS) in 1963 when he was 21 years old. Two forms of ALS have been identified. In the first, patients typically die of pneumonia or asphyxiation following rapid voluntary muscle degeneration within 4 years of onset. Although initially Hawking was given this diagnosis, it now appears that he has the second form, in which survival is expected to extend beyond 15 years. Defying all expectations, Hawking has remained enormously productive for more than 20 years while his body has become progressively weaker.

Hawking expresses his view that the role of the occupational therapist is to help individuals with disabilities participate fully in society, a role for occupational therapy that he did not experience. Maybe, he says, he "just didn't encounter the right therapists." He believes the availability of technology has rendered the need for muscle power obsolete; therefore, the point of focus for therapists should be to encourage the "right mental approach" and to help patients achieve their potential and enter the world of normal activity. Hawking's ideas are compatible with other authors in this section because he also endorses the key role of activity (or occupation) in the construction of a meaningful life.

The last selection by the eminent ethologist Jane Goodall turns our attention from human to chimpanzee occupations. Once again, however, the power and potency of ordinary activity are depicted. Goodall describes the co-occupations of mother and infant chimpanzees. She describes feeding, grooming, travel, climbing, tool using, child play, and weaning. Goodall believes that these day-to-day ordinary activities are the contexts within which the adaptation of the young is fostered. For example, daughters seem to mimic the maternal style of their mothers when they have infants of their own.

Jane Goodall, it appears, has done the most thorough study of the customary round of activities of any species. We expect that occupational scientists will conduct similar observations of humans, documenting not only what they do daily, but also uncovering how social relationships are negotiated, development fostered, and a sense of meaning attained within these contexts.

Reference

1. Reilly, M: The educational process. Am J Occup Ther 23:299, 1969.

by Mary Catherine Bateson, PhD

1

Enfolded Activity and the Concept of Occupation

In a marvelous poem by Robert Frost called "Two Tramps in Mud Time,"[1] Frost describes himself outdoors on an early New England morning splitting wood. There is the feeling of spring about to come—mud time, of course, is spring time. The air is brisk, and buds are on the trees; he's working, using his muscles, and it feels wonderful. Two tramps come along to ask for the job of splitting wood, and Frost feels that he has no right to go on doing this task, which he is enjoying immensely, when somebody else needs money for food or shelter. He talks about feeling that he has no right to do for pleasure "the work another man does for pay." He ends with a line about uniting vocation and avocation:

> Only where love and need are one,
> And the work is play for mortal stakes,
> ₁ Is the deed ever really done
> For Heaven and the future's sakes.[2]

If you know the work of Robert Frost, you know that his poetry is built on the experiences of the outdoors in New England. He isn't chopping wood for pay, for the pleasure of the moment, or to burn it, he's chopping wood because this is essential to the business of being himself, of being Robert Frost. Being Robert Frost does, among other things, result in the activities for which he is paid. Of course, poets don't get paid much for writing poetry, but eventually they get paid for giving readings and teaching college courses, so this is all an indirect process in which one kind of activity is folded into others. The experience that he is having out there, of feeling his juices flow as he is engaged in physical labor, does have as one strand the issue of earning a living. Keeping those juices flowing is, however, something to live for, synonymous with living. The complex weave of work, pleasure, and personal identity is unraveled by the challenge of the two tramps who come along and impose, implicitly of course, a different system based on mutually exclusive categories, one that is powerful because it ties in tightly with how society is organized.

5

It seems to me that members of the occupational therapy profession are subject to issues of categorization: how your profession is categorized, how your activities are categorized, how your clients understand what they are doing with you, and what they believe it's all for. We live in a society that divides these things rather sharply. It makes a vast difference whether something is primarily labeled work, play, learning, therapy, exercise, or stress reduction, even though it is intuitively clear that many activities belong experientially to more than one category.

These labels are of immense importance in terms of insurance and tax and legal structures. If I enter psychotherapy, for instance, I may be forced to make the case that I am there because I am sick and not because I am learning something, because education and training for a profession are not deductible (although they may become deductible once I begin earning a living in that profession because only pretraining is not deductible). This is nonsense in terms of any sensible view of how a human life fits together, yet in the workplace these are important categories. It is also terribly important how the members of other professions with whom you work are categorized, because they carry invisible union cards defining what they do. First, there are the physicians, the ones who think they really help people, and who largely control the category systems that have to do with health. All the others who play supportive roles, including nurses, social workers, chaplains, and of course occupational, physical, and art therapists, may be treated as peripheral in the medical paradigm, as providing a frill, or as keeping the patients occupied. The categorization system, by dissecting and analyzing the texture of human life and putting things in boxes, creates the possibility of devaluing them. A component, when you separate it, may seem rather unimportant, yet whatever is essential cannot be seen as *merely* a part, because life can take place only in wholes. You have to struggle day in and day out to affirm that occupation is the "web and woof" of being for humans and not an instrumental component that is inserted here or there.

There is an interesting complementarity between what you have been doing and what I have been trying to do. As an anthropologist, I reject all the subdivisions of the human sciences and claim the right to be a scientist and a humanist simultaneously. An anthropologist needs to attend to human biology, to the work of all the social sciences, and to such issues as narrative and aesthetic tradition and self-expression. I have an appointment now, which is jointly in anthropology and english, that liberates me from the category system of departmental boundaries, so if anybody says that some piece of my work is not anthropology, I can smile sweetly and say that it is intended as literature. However, I have to do that less and less because increasingly in anthropology, we recognize that the study of human behavior has been hurt by the insistence that politics can be separated from economics and that psychology can be separated from social structure. As an anthropologist, even though clearly I have to narrow in for specific pieces of research, I can insist that the study of human behavior is not divisible into separate sciences.

Now you are in the process of proclaiming yet another new science. To redefine the focus of your discipline to gain a theoretical grounding for what you do and establish a distinctive framework for drawing on all the other disciplines, it is critical that you identify your work as scientific rather than as a collection of techniques. Even though the transition you are making in self-definition is critical, I would beg of you not to let the establishment of occupational science become a reason not to talk to people who define their disciplines under a different name. Keep the interdisciplinarity; do not erect new boundaries. Use the definition of your work as grounded in science as a point of entry to the dialogue, the multilogue, of all the human sciences. You want to be a full guest at the feast, with full courtesy and privilege, not to go off and eat alone in a corner.

Recently, in balancing my position between the social sciences and the humanities, I have been talking about the composition of a life as an art form. After viewing information about occupational science, it is clear to me that when I talk about composing a life, about how individuals weave together and combine many different kinds of activities, I am talking about occupation, particularly about how occupations fit together in the framework of a life. I, too, am engaged in this activity of category creation. My book, *Composing a Life*,[2] is based on the experiences of five women, but that does not mean that it is applicable only to women. I believe that just as we have all often had to understand human beings on the basis of research focused on men, much can be understood about human beings starting from research focused on women. Women are not a special case of humankind, but in some cases they may be the pioneers. I am convinced that many of the key points in *Composing a Life* are applicable and transferable to the experience of larger numbers of men.

Men have traditionally had two privileges that interest me here: The first has been the privilege of having a single, clear career line, in which you get educated and then become established in a career. Your career advances and improves, and when you die, your career can be summed up in the *New York Times* with one phrase—corporate lawyer, judge, author. The *New York Times* is going to have trouble with my obituary because you cannot put a laundry list, which is what my career feels like, into a headline. Many men, especially in the professions and skilled trades, have had the comfort of a single career trajectory, but fewer do today, because more have to start again, reshaping their careers, learning new skills, dealing with various kinds of uprooting and disruption. Even now, however, women's lives provide more immediate available material for studying how people adapt to discontinuities and disruptions than men's lives. Continuity has been a privilege that many men have had, never all men and now fewer, but enough so that we have tended to think of it as the norm.

Another privilege that men have had is being able to delegate many aspects of life to a wife. Therefore, they have had the extraordinary privilege of thinking about one thing at a time. The definition of women's work, cross-culturally, is that it consists of all that can be done while caring for a child. Men's work has been focused on activities that cannot be done while caring for a child, often because they involve danger and require mobility. Therefore, if you are a man, you make war, you hunt animals, and while you are doing those things, you are concentrating on one thing at a time. You think of killing the animal, winning the war, getting the Iraqis out of Kuwait—these are single-purpose activities.

During Operation Desert Storm, the generals were clear that one should not make war without clearly defined goals, because only then can one know when the job is done. They were both right and wrong, of course. They were right because clear goal definition allowed extraordinarily effective mobilization and tactics, the application of technology, and an extremely successful campaign; they were wrong because the definition of a narrow purpose allowed them to proceed without attending to a whole range of related issues with which those of us who are prepared to maintain attention will have to deal for years to come. Men have had, on the whole, the privilege of walking out the door and assuming that they could concentrate during some period, whether it was a workday or a military campaign, and someone else would take care of the children, the laundry, the elderly, tonight's dinner, calling the plumber, and getting on with the neighbors. We may be getting away from that. It is especially interesting in the criticism of the Bush administration that followed the war that people increasingly feel it is not legitimate to ignore domestic issues during wartime.

Among the San people of the Kalahari (who used to be called Bushmen), the men hunt, which requires great skill and a narrow purposive concentration. They come back having killed a large animal that will provide a lot of meat, and there is a great celebration about this achievement. People like the San use to be called "hunting" people until it was discovered that more than half of their subsistence came from the work of the women gathering, which was more or less taken for granted, and much less of their nutrition came from the much celebrated and admired activity of hunting.[3] It isn't just that when the men go off on the hunt, they are freed for that concentration by the women caring for the children, the old people, and the sick, and bringing water and firewood, it is also that the women are doing all of that while providing more than half of the food needs of the community. The women are simultaneously gathering a variety of food and caring for children, and when they are in the camp, they are preparing food and looking after the children and keeping track of things—doing a variety of tasks in an enfolded manner.

I am concerned about the centrality of the notion of "chunks of activity" in occupational science, because it is so much easier to delimit the chunks of activity in the men's day than in the women's day. The possibility of delineating clearly defined "chunks of activity" may be exceptional or in other cases, illusory, just as it is illusory to think of Robert Frost as chopping wood, which should perhaps be delegated, instead of seeing all the other things he is doing at the same time. Women do not stop caring for children when they start cooking dinner. Generally, the reason women have traditionally gotten so much done and that this has been so undervalued is this characteristic of doing many things at the same time. Doing a task like shelling peas or raking the lawn alongside a child often makes for a deeper companionship than the current ideal of "quality time" (Fig. 1–1). Many men left in charge of children convert that into a full-time activity and reject the suggestion that they could have cleaned the house or prepared dinner at the same time.

An example is a village woman in Iran in a household with several children, at least one other woman, and one or two elderly people. In the course of a day's work, she prepares food, keeps track of the children, cares for the elderly people, and if she has an hour here or there, she sits down at the carpet loom. She can be interrupted at any moment, yet after a few months, she has a valuable carpet, which is a unified work of art. At the end of a day, an onlooker might say that she did not get much done, because everything she did was enfolded in these interlocking patterns. Even more easily, the onlooker might dismiss the human and social value of the constant flow of conversation and gossip through the day that keeps the system functioning smoothly, but this, too, is essential to her occupation.

I meet and talk to many women who now do not say "I don't work; I'm just

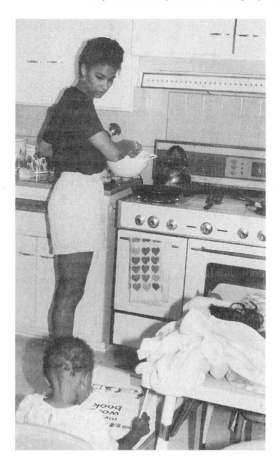

Figure 1–1. Mothers typically enfold one occupation within another. Here a mother cooks while she simultaneously keeps a mindful eye on her daughter. (Photo by John Wolcott.)

a housewife"; however, that is still the reaction they get if they try to get a job, as if they have been doing nothing for the last 20 years. Even when these women acknowledge that they have been working hard, they still talk as if they have been doing the *same thing* for 20 years, just being "a wife and mother." In fact, the shifts in skills needed to be a wife, a mother of a newborn, mother of a 2-year-old child, mother of a teenager, mother-in-law, no children, one child, two children, three children, and children grown up and moved out are major job shifts, each one requiring new skills. If you went through that kind of shift of responsibilities in the corporate world, you would get a new "title on the door and a Bigelow on the floor," and you certainly would not say, "I've been doing the same thing for 20 years."

From my point of view, it has been important to provide a vocabulary that values the achievements of women in particular, but also men whose lives do not follow the model of a successful career that our society has developed. Holistically, the composing of a life, the combining of the elements, and the balancing and harmonizing of them is in itself an art form. The concept of composition refers to pattern across time, such as that which a composer creates, with ongoing themes and variations and different movements, but all are part of the whole. It also refers to patterns such as a visual artist creates, putting together elements that seem disparate. I really wanted the cover of my book to be a classic still life, maybe a mandolin and some apples and drafting tools, arranged apparently casually but actually artfully on a table. That is the kind of combining and arranging that I think we do. We have to get beyond thinking that the mandolin and the fruit belong to different aspects of life and think of the composition that brings them together.

The explanatory category that I have tried to make available for people thinking about what they are doing when they bridge discontinuities and deal with conflicting priorities is the metaphor of artistic creation, of composition. Although you can do the statistics and show that a high percentage of homemakers also are wage earners, the way women actually put these things together in their lives is still individual, idiosyncratic, and often intricately enfolded. The way in which the Iranian village woman puts together her different activities and occupations is not idiosyncratic—she watched her mother doing it. In contrast, we are inventing it as we go along, which involves an extra level of creativity.

I do not see any reason to believe that a new pattern will be crystallized and everyone will be able to follow. Some things will settle down, but the task of composing a life is going to remain an individual task that can reasonably be thought of as the creation of an art work. This is true of a life that is publicly regarded as highly successful and high achieving or of lives that are not under any kind of spotlight, whether life is approached with a full range of physical possibilities or reinvented in the face of a physical challenge or handicap. There is always some element of composing when putting together the human rhythms of rest and effort, with an element of learning and some of the kinds of satisfaction that Frost was getting each time he split a log of wood or that the Iranian woman gets from serving a meal or completing a carpet.

Idiosyncratic composition does not mean that there is not great scope for studying lives scientifically, but it does suggest the value of retaining a humanistic point of view and resisting some of the temptations that can be called "scientism," the inappropriate application of scientific techniques. I felt that unless I started by looking closely at a small number of lives, I would be imposing analytic categories that might be inappropriate, derived perhaps from obsolete or gender-specific social arrangements. It is a mistake to start counting and measuring before you have understood what you are going to count. I hope that within 5 years, a whole cohort of people in psychology, sociology, economics, and occupational science will write dissertations in which they say that some hypothesis they are carefully testing came out of *Composing a Life* and out of the new way of focusing their attention and sensitivity that I was trying to achieve in that book. I do not, in that sense, think that the aesthetic emphasis and the scientific emphasis are at odds, but I do think that much in the traditional model of science does not fit.

A simple way of saying this is to think about the difference between adding and subtracting on the one hand and multiplying and dividing on the other. When you make it possible for clients operating under some extreme disability to perform some simple function or to engage in some craft activity for a portion of the day, you are not simply *adding* something to their life, which would imply that the balance of life remains unchanged. What you are doing is *multiplying* making a change in the whole. You may have the experience of doubling or tripling what someone is able to do—their competence, their ability to function as a person. Sometimes you are only multiplying by 1.2 or even 1.02, but you should still think of it as multiplying, because the whole is changed, whether by an hour a day of participating in a craft activity and talking to other people at the same time or by the sense of having finished something as simple as a pot holder or as complex as a doctoral dissertation.

This thinking in terms of multiplication is critical for our society. We hurt ourselves immensely by the way things are separated and considered in terms of addition and subtraction. One of the things I found most deeply shocking in some of the earlier newspaper discussions of the AIDS epidemic was the statement that the transfer of federal funds to AIDS programs was causing an increase in other sexually transmitted diseases (STDs). This is a giveaway that the people working on AIDS were ignoring syphilis and gonorrhea and the people in the existing venereal disease programs were ignoring AIDS (except of course for competing for the same funds). Any rational analysis of AIDS or STDs says that these are closely related societal problems that have to be addressed in combination. Dollars were being subtracted from one program and added to another, and no one was trying for synergy. Working that way also means losing sight of many other potential benefits that might come out of STD programs, through giving people control over their own bodies, their health, and sexual choices.

It seems to me that as occupational scientists, you have to move on two fronts. First, in terms of the development of the discipline, you must use the concept of occupation for a broad understanding of human completeness and health. The capacity to do something useful for yourself or others is key to personhood, whether it involves the ability to earn a living, cook a meal, put on shoes in the morning, or whatever other skill needs to be mastered at the moment. I think it is critical to argue for the holistic concept of health that is implied by the range of activities that you recognize as occupation so that those activities can be strengthened, empowered, freed up, by a variety of techniques. This is not peripheral to health and wholeness but absolutely central; doing surgery to fix a person's legs, hands, or eyes is only valuable if that person's legs, hands, or eyes can then be used in the total range of activities that goes with being human. That is half of your task: finding the concepts and the language to insist on that point.

Second, you must at the same time find a place to stand in terms of the full range of tools of scientific investigation and artistic perception that will allow you a full voice in the dialogue about human growth and healing and protect you from being denigrated or ignored. Sometimes there is a loss from focusing narrowly on solutions to particular problems. When I speak about the effect on women and men of being forced to pay attention to many things at the same time, as women traditionally have been, I use the phrase "peripheral visionaries."[4] This is what you are all called to be. Many of the organizations and institutions in which you work regard your activities as peripheral. However, in a fundamental sense, that peripheral position allows you a breadth of vision that those who think they do the only important thing do not have. It allows you to think of complex wholes and to do what you do, in Frost's words, "for Heaven and the future's sakes."

There are two kinds of visionaries: those who go after the holy grail without caring who they stomp on in the process, because their eye is on some specific future goal and those I call peripheral visionaries who work on the tasks of today and tomorrow with their eyes open, with a breadth of attention and vision that is inclusive and holistic. Occupational scientists and occupational therapists are called to be the second kind of visionaries, to bring the breadth of their attention and an inclusive holistic vision to bear on occupation in human life and in health.

Discussion Questions

1. What are ways in which engagement in therapeutic occupations may be said to multiply, rather than merely add to, patients' abilities to function as whole human beings?
2. What are ways in which the current health system allows or does not allow occupational therapists to concern ourselves with generating patients' abilities for engaging in enfolded occupations?
3. How might we optimally incorporate knowledge of enfolded occupations into daily occupational therapy practice?
4. What research strategies can be used to document the effectiveness of occupational therapy that are additionally sensitive to the pervasiveness of enfolded occupation in daily life?

References

1. Frost, R: Two Tramps in Mud Time: A Further Range. Holt, Rinehart, & Winston, New York, 1936, pp 16–18.
2. Bateson, MS: Composing a Life. Atlantic Monthly Press, New York, 1989.
3. Lee, RB: The Dobe !Kung. Harcourt Brace Jovanovich, New York, 1984, p 540.
4. Bateson, MC: Peripheral Visions: Learning Along the Way. HarperCollins, New York, 1994.

by Joshua S. Goldstein, PhD

International Relations and Everyday Life

Scripts as Structure for Daily Life
International Effects of Daily Choices
Developing a Global Identity

It is a truism that the world is getting smaller, that there are greater international influences in our lives, and that trade is increasing. Products cross borders, information crosses borders, people cross borders, and we all feel greater international influences in our lives in a variety of ways. We travel more, we have products on our tables from different parts of the world, and so forth. However, these aspects of the internationalization of our lives do not seem, on a more superficial level of analysis, to relate to occupation. These are external, objective things. Occupation deals with more subjective realities: the chunks of activities to which we give names, the actions we take on our environment, the responses to its challenges, and the ways we orchestrate our daily lives in this environment. Occupational science concerns more active things than just having a product from another country on our table. Occupations are goal directed, self-initiated, and involve rules, habits, and skills we develop to facilitate our actions in the social and physical environment in which we live.

How, then, might we enrich our understanding of occupation by considering the specifically international aspects and nature of the environment in which our occupations occur? Three aspects of this question will be considered to address the deeper relationships of our occupations to the internationalization of our lives: first, how the world of international relations provides *scripts* for our daily lives; second, how the everyday *choices* we make affect the nature of international relations; and third, how individual *identity* is beginning to change for many people as a result of the interaction of their daily lives with the international context.

Scripts as Structure for Daily Life

What meaning do people attach in their normal lives to international affairs? Why do international affairs matter to people? How do people use international relations in orchestrating their everyday activities? How do international relations impinge on and help shape people's rules, habits, and skills that they develop for coping with their everyday lives? In other words, how do international relations reverberate down and help to shape the flow of our daily lives?

Most fundamentally, international relations provide us with scripts that we use in our everyday lives to attach meaning to the activities in which we take part and to the environment in which we find ourselves. Even when the international things themselves are beyond the sphere of our daily lives, they provide scripts and themes that give deeper meaning to the things that are close at hand. Why do Americans watch the news when so much of the news now is international? What do they get from watching? A colleague who studies media and politics, including what meanings people attach to things they see on television, said that people watch the news so they can talk about it the next day without looking like they do not know what is going on in the world. We have two international occupations in which many of us engage: First, we sit down and watch the news; second, we talk about it the next day. When we talk about these things in our small circle with our friends, coworkers, and partners, we agree on meanings that we can attach to the international things that we saw on the news, such as great leaders or the unfolding of great historical events.

We also use these meanings to help structure our local social and political environments. For instance, recently a United States–Soviet summit meeting dominated our news and was a big international event. Few or none of us have any contact with the tangible aspects of a summit meeting, yet if the summit goes well, it uplifts us, gives us hope, and influences our mood the next day. Our thinking that there will be peace and not war changes how we relate to the people around us and what sort of future hope we have for the activities in which we are engaged. If the summit goes badly and we think that the superpowers are confronting each other, creating a danger of war, then we will be afraid the next day; we will be down, and we will reflect that in our mood.

Alternatively, the summit may go well, but we may decide, as many in the Soviet Union have done recently, that big international politics do not affect us. A Moscow engineer whose comments were reported in the newspaper and on television said "I don't give a damn about the summit. It's okay, but there are so many problems in this country." Someone else suggested, "This summit will not change our lives here." These people thus used the summit as a different kind of tool to generate a script of, "the big leaders carry on a summit, but it doesn't help our miserable lives" and then acted on that script by being depressed, queuing up for food, grumbling about those with political power, and so forth.

Scripts and themes are generated from international affairs in other ways as well. A few of these are especially potent in childhood. As children, we develop our view of the environment in which we live and attach social meaning to things in our lives. International scripts and themes help to shape our view of the world as it is formed in our childhood years.

First is the theme of good guys and bad guys. We externalize the bad guys beyond international borders. We have countries out there that are bad, are evil empires, or are run by crazy dictators, and we consequently construct domestic society in that context, believing that it is safe within our borders. We develop a feeling of belonging, safety, and domesticity within the borders of our nation-state and feelings of anarchy, chaos, war, and terrorism beyond our nation-state. Defining our daily lives in terms of this dichotomy of the safe world at home versus the dangerous world outside helps to shape our views of family, home, and neighborhood. Feminist theorists offer some interesting thoughts on domestic versus external environments, private versus public spaces, and ways in which scripts pertaining to these environments interact with gender roles in our daily lives. International relations are central in this "in and out" dichotomy. We have our nation, which defines "us," and beyond us is some other "them," which becomes a shadowy presence in our lives. This phenomenon also plays a role in something that occupational therapists deal with frequently: stigmatized groups.

A second theme is multicultural understanding and tolerance of diversity; this theme runs counter to the theme of good guys versus bad guys. From international relations, we learn that we live in a big world full of different people, cultures, and customs. We learn not only to tolerate that diversity, but also to celebrate it. Finding out about the lives of Mongolians, Russians, or Italians changes how we interact with diversity in our local environment. In effect, we become more accepting of local diversity because of our international script of a big, diverse, and interesting world. Contrary to the theme of good guys and bad guys, the theme of multicultural understanding and tolerance of diversity thus demonstrates that international influences cut both ways. In fact, bad guys become good guys. My book, *Three Way Street*,[1] shows how United States–Soviet–Chinese relations evolved from hostile confrontations to eventual cooperation. The themes and scripts for evolving international cooperation and conflict resolution can be applied at the local level as well, between street gangs, partners, and parents and children. If international cooperation can take place in that nastiest of worlds in the international environment, then surely parent and child can learn to get along.

Third, and perhaps most importantly, war and the threat of war provide a potent script that shapes the way we view our world. The scene in Figure 2–1 could occur in any toy store or playground, especially with little boys or even bigger boys in it. When one considers the extent to which the military mindset has come to dominate our lives in ways we do not even think about, it is clear that the militarization of our society is profound. This is a result of international relations and the fact that other nations may wish to destroy us. We need to be militarily strong to protect ourselves. This is reflected in sports, especially in the great emphasis on winning and the terrible dejection that people sometimes feel if their team loses. However, in international relations, these emphases are quite justified. If you lose a war, you could be dead, and your society could be overrun and conquered by terrible people. Indeed, your nation could lose its existence. Even though none of this is true in sports, business, or other competitive arenas, we have internalized the belief that we must win from that dangerous world of international relations. We thereby experience desperation in our daily lives because of the threat of war.

The military system also has a profound impact on gender roles in our society due to its heavily gendered nature and masculine character. Men fight wars;

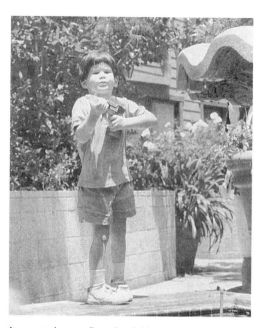

Figure 2–1. The military mindset is reflected in children's play. Here a young boy enacts a military "script" as he positions a toy gun. (Photo by John Wolcott.)

women stay home. Boys must be outwardly strong and must learn to fight; girls must learn how to take care and how to hold the home life together. While there is some truth to the idea that gender roles are actually what create international wars and militarism, indeed the whole war system, there also is some truth to the idea that because wars and militaries have been around for so long, they have profoundly influenced the development of gender roles in human society. In other words, because causation runs in both directions, the effect of international relations on gender roles in society has to be considered.

Particular wars also provide scripts that affect daily lives, moods, and decisions. World War II cast a long shadow over my generation, even though we did not live through that war. People born long after that war still speak with a German accent to convey evil nature because doing so is portrayed in films, television, and other cultural forms that reproduce scripts of World War II, replete with its evil Germans and good Americans. Because these television shows are rerun, there is a kind of stickiness in the culture. This stickiness, of course, also reinforces sexism and racism. For example, many television shows made in the 1950s and 1960s, such as "The Flintstones," "Get Smart," or "Mr. Ed," are rerun endlessly and explicitly translate cold war themes from that era into everyday experiences. The effect is that when Mr. Ed helps catch a Russian spy, we are reminded to be alert in our own lives to the dangers of our nation's enemies within our midst.

After World War II, the Vietnam war provided a different set of scripts about power, imperialism, and the meaning of patriotism that impacted my generation when we were in college. The uncertainty of national purpose and the tragedy (or crime) of war reached right into all of our lives and shook us up, especially draft-age men. Families and generations split, people's world views changed, the counter-culture flowered, and returning soldiers faced hard adjustments and isolation. Battle lines seemed to be drawn over all our lives, not just in a distant war.

Perhaps most interestingly, the threat of nuclear war affects our daily lives in pervasive ways. The film "The Atomic Cafe,"[2] made in the early 1980s, has a segment from a 1950s civil defense film. This civil defense film has a cartoon turtle character that teaches children how to duck and cover in the event of nuclear attack. My generation learned to put our heads under the desks in the event of a nuclear attack. We learned that at any moment, a certain whistle could blow, meaning you had 30 seconds before civilization was destroyed, so to be in the proper posture for this activity, you would put your head under the desk. Is it an occupation? As various children are shown jumping into duck-and-cover positions while blasts go off, the narrator says, "Paul and Patty [the little children] know this: No matter where they go or what they do, they always try to remember what to do if the atom bomb explodes right then. It's a bomb! Duck and cover! Here's Tony going to his Cub Scouts meeting. Tony knows that the bomb could explode at any time of the year, day, or night. Duck and cover!"[2] Then as a flash is shown, Tony jumps off his bike as the narrator says, "Atta boy, Tony! That flash means, act fast! Sundays, holidays, vacation time: We must be ready everyday, all the time, to do the right things if the atomic bomb explodes."[2]

That credo "we must be ready everyday, all the time, to do the right thing if the atomic bomb explodes" pervades our everyday lives in ways of which we are quite unaware, especially after decades of living this way. We share an occupation as potential victims of nuclear war, even though the event has never occurred and likely never will.

International Effects of Daily Choices

Now let me talk briefly about the *choices* people make in their everyday lives and how those choices reverberate into international relations. How do people in their everyday lives, through the choices that they make about their occupations, help to constitute or change the international scene and its meanings? I am not talking about diplomats, soldiers, and anchor people on the news who deal professionally with international relations but about "ordinary" people. How do occupational changes in the lives of ordinary people reverberate up and change the nature of international relations?

A colleague of mine in international relations at University of Southern California, James Rosenau, has written that most legitimacy in politics, most compliance with authority, is a matter of habit. When coming to terms with recent technological and political changes in the world, Rosenau argues that individual habits are breaking down worldwide because of changes in daily life, technology, communications, and the growing skills of individual citizens. Individuals are becoming empowered and undermining the old state system of international relations. They have changed traditional habits and have developed new skills to perceive and interact with the world. As a result, a new order is growing up that is more transnational, subnational, and multinational.[3] By emphasizing the skills and habits for interacting with the environment, this phrase sounds like the concept of occupation. For Rosenau, these skills and habits are the fundamental forces leading to the profound changes taking place in the world today.

We have seen enormous changes in the international environment in recent years. Some of these changes were brought about as a result of the Tiananmen square incident. Chinese students created an effective and powerful political demonstration simply by seizing control of a central location, Tiananmen square, which was considered a kind of center of the universe. The students' "occupation" of the square was itself an occupation. The meanings of such political demonstrations or of similar political occupations run much deeper than the sundry superficial activities that accompany them. These occupations are most effective, moreover, when demonstrations transform demonstrators' everyday lives. When people go to a different place and start living there through sit-ins, hunger strikes, or encampments, it captures people's imaginations. The Chinese students captured the world's imagination and changed the terms of how ordinary people relate to political authority in many countries. In many ways, the Tiananmen protest fueled the nonviolent revolutions in Eastern Europe that followed. The simple fact of some students in Beijing changing their everyday lives with respect to where they slept and what they ate exerted a force on international relations around the world.

Also on June 4th, but in 1968 in Los Angeles, Robert Kennedy was assassinated. I worked on his campaign, and as with the Chinese students (though less dramatically), we campaign workers hoped that our personal activities would aggregate up to the macro level and change the world. One of my important occupations while growing up was "licking stamps," which was shorthand for all the petty little tasks that had to be done to make a campaign work. Undeniably, the sum of all these little political acts, from voting to writing checks to knocking on doors, profoundly influences the course of history.

Occasionally these big social outcomes can be seen in the microcosm of small actions. When Robert Kennedy ran for President, I was assigned to walk a precinct in East Palo Alto. I would knock on a door, and a person would come to the door and look at me suspiciously. When I said, "I'm with the Kennedy campaign," the door would magically open, and I would find myself in the living room, sitting with a cold drink and talking about Bobby. That is the glimpse I got when walking through the door, of how my mundane political work could alter the big social forces. Just by knocking on a door or inviting a person in for a drink, we would together change the world; we would elect Robert Kennedy as President, we would end the war in Vietnam, and we would redefine America's place in the world. Like the Chinese students, we failed that time, but I am convinced that ultimately the stamp lickers will inherit the earth.

Beyond the political choices we all make in a democracy, our superficially nonpolitical choices also shape, in the aggregate, the international environment in which we live. A striking example is the way we think about and deal with poverty in the third world in relation to the choices we make in our everyday lives. In our world today, a child dies every 3 seconds from malnourishment.[4] In a sense, then, every 3 seconds of our lives, we deal in some way with how we are going to come to terms with that or choose to ignore it. People in the southern hemisphere and the poorer parts of the world occupy themselves with coping, or starving, that is, with trying to get by. People in the northern hemisphere occupy themselves with ignoring or rationalizing this problem, as we have learned to numb out nuclear war, or perhaps with grappling with it or even changing our lives to deal with it.

Few people join the Peace Corps, but many people choose what kind of new car to buy. So many expensive cars are being driven, and each one represents a choice to spend precious resources on a luxury car rather than to address world poverty. This choice requires special habits and skills, including the art of denying that one even makes such a choice. Nobody sits down in the showroom and decides that by purchasing a $20,000 car instead of a $40,000 car, they could donate the balance to Oxfam and save more than 100 children's lives. The salesperson does not point this out! Rather, the skills and habits we develop for interacting with our environment enable us to isolate our lives from the larger international context. However, the choices we deny making are the building blocks out of which, in the aggregate, the North–South division is constructed.

To take a happier example, we have begun to accept that our daily actions with respect to the environment can ultimately affect the global environmental problem. By conserving energy, we can reduce the number of oil spills and maybe even the number of Middle East wars. By recycling and planting trees and by using the right hair spray, we can slow global warming. Just a few years ago, these concepts had not taken hold, but today a large part of the public sees the global environment as their responsibility and sees their daily choices as influencing that global problem.

With time, this concept of responsibility for the environment can develop along parallel lines as responsibility for third world poverty, war, and other international problems. People can increasingly take responsibility for international relations through their everyday choices. We always have choices in any of these issues about how we live our lives and about how we occupy our time. These choices not only create the world in which we live, but they percolate up to change international relations.

Developing a Global Identity

As our choices increasingly have international ramifications and the international scene increasingly provides context and meanings for our lives, our identities are changing. The meaning of how we see ourselves and who we think we are takes on an international character. Ultimately, the actions we take and the choices we make matter because of what they say about our identity. What matters is not so much what our actions accomplish, but how we live our lives. The dance we do on earth before we move off stage is a statement or artistic expression of who we are. Today, not only is our stage an international one, but the identity we express also is internationalized.

It is not simple to define who we are. We actually have multiple identities, much like a mosaic, with interpenetrating meanings. International forces play a greater role in shaping those meanings today. And nowhere is this truer than in Los Angeles, where the North meets the South, the third world meets the industrialized world, and the Atlantic meets the Pacific: truly a "world capital." In Los Angeles, about 100 major language groups coexist, and new linguistic phenomena are popping up for the first time in human history. It is not uncommon to listen to someone speak to someone else and switch languages once or twice, sometimes several times, in one sentence. Where else in the world does an over-the-air international television channel play a Korean film about something in Africa with Japanese subtitles? It is wonderful.

The multilingual phenomenon reflects multiple international identities. A friend who works at a bank in downtown Los Angeles tells me about the little dance that her supervisor, who is a Filipino, does with a Filipino person who comes in to deliver a package. They eye each other, looking each other over, and think, "Well, I am . . . but are you?" So they talk about the package, then one slips in a word or two from their native tongue to test the ground, and the other slips in a word, and then, boom, they switch over into the other language, bonded into that other identity. Equally quickly they will jump back out of that identity again.

As the world becomes smaller, our identities become larger and more complex. This process is just getting started, and the ethnic and language communities do not freely intermingle most of the time. As technology and communications develop, the world trend will increasingly reflect what is starting to emerge here. Intercultural marriages give us a taste of the environment in which human beings will increasingly form their identity. Imagine a Salvadoran Catholic and a Russian Jew who marry and raise a child in a largely Korean neighborhood. Who is that child? That child is "a human being" and a Hispanic Jew who loves Russian food and speaks Korean. In other words, from this crazy quilt of mixed-up identities, what may emerge is a global identity that is truly human yet celebrates all the diversity of the different cultures that make up our world. We can have both a celebration of individual and cultural identity on the one hand and a truly human or global identity on the other hand.

To make global identity into an occupation and not just an idea, what we need are symbols, rituals, and everyday activities that affirm our nature as human beings. We have those things in our religious identities, our ethnic identities, and our national identities: liturgy, slang, and the flag. However, we lack those symbols and rituals for global identity. We do not yet fly the United Nations flag above our national flag or pledge allegiance to the human race. Politicians do not declare that "human beings are the greatest species in the universe." Discovering what practical activities can help people to develop a global human identity is, perhaps, a contribution that occupational scientists can make toward furthering our most important occupation, being human.

Discussion Questions

1. In what ways are most people's daily occupations influenced by international relations?
2. Can you identify ways in which you use scripts provided by international relations to attach meaning to your daily activities and the sociocultural environment in which you undertake those activities?
3. What scripts provided by international relations are particularly germane to the experiences of people with disabilities?

References

1. Goldstein, J: Three Way Street: Strategic Reciprocity in World Politics. University of Chicago Press, Chicago, IL, 1990.
2. *The Atomic Cafe* [Film]
3. Rosenau, JN: Turbulence in World Politics: A Theory of Change and Continuity. Princeton University Press, Princeton, NJ, 1990.
4. UNICEF: The State of the World's Children, 1993. Oxford University Press, New York, 1993.

by J. Seward Johnson

3

Realistic Expressions
Statements of Being

Imperceptibly, and not so imperceptibly, our life patterns are evolving further away from our animal state. We gratefully accept the changes of the past into which we were born—changes that made us have to worry less about shelter and food procurement. We gratefully accept heat in the winter and air conditioning in the summer, knowing somewhere in our collective subconscious that even these measures of civilization are encroachments on the most basic sense of ourselves.

We were born into accepting ourselves as only part animal, which is a denial of our true selves. On top of that, we exist in abstractly controlled environments, with air conditioning adjusted with the attitude that more is better. We watch the news on television defensively, preparing for society's next trend or demand on us. We are continuously aware, sometimes unconsciously, how we are not ready to adjust. We wake up each morning under subconscious challenge, fundamentally alienated from our roots.

How do we reclaim ourselves and fight back? *I recommend minute acts of "regression"*: counting one's toes, sitting out in the air and in the sun (Fig. 3–1), swimming in the ocean or a pond or a brook, and walking barefoot in the sand. These are touchstones of fundamental *re*-recognition. However, because we were born into a relatively high state of evolution, reclamation can happen through reaching less far back to less primal experiences: sitting on a park bench and watching passersby, listening uninterrupted to music, or feeding pigeons in the park. Even these "time outs" are sometimes difficult to achieve without embarrassment if you are at all spiritually timid. Another approach might be to take your "responsibility" into nature and claim your own nature sideways through your senses, as you keep up with the world in your newspaper, write your correspondence, read your magazine, or possibly just fake busyness to ward off interruption.

When the spirit grabs you, a more obdurate, or purposeful, statement can be made: taking time lighting a pipe (especially when someone is waiting for an answer), lying on one's back in the park and studying the clouds, sleeping in a pub-

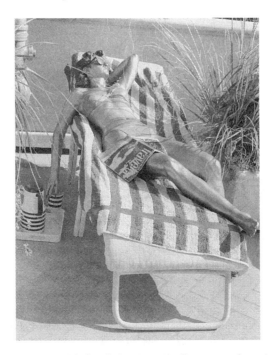

Figure 3–1. Johnson recommends so called minute acts of regression for reclaiming oneself. In this sculpture, a woman is captured in bronze, soaking in the sun. (Photo by John Wolcott.)

lic space, painting a picture on a sidewalk, formally setting a table in a public environment to eat out of doors, or holding a class in a park. These are not only expressions of being, these are *declarations of being*. Microexpressions of being can be in the choice of clothes you wear and the rakish angle of a hat (correction—the wearing of a hat is a declaration these days).

As a sculptor, I celebrate these acts in bronze. I do it in a two-step communication: First, I fool you into thinking there is a real person breaking loose from the ordered jail of his or her life; then, while you are still feeling foolish, I let you know that this act is more. This act is noble enough to be consecrated in art, permanent, expensive art.

Mine is the art genre of social statement. Its antecedents date back to the Greek heroic sculpture that celebrated the best in early human aspirations, but existence, and how we might artistically celebrate it, has different requirements today. The biceps have gone down in value, while a strong central nervous system has gone up. The model for the hero and the heroic act has changed with the challenge. It is a matter now of digging in our heels as we are dragged to extinction through the deanimalization of our species.

How does our work, yours and mine, our message, relate? We each are here to remind each other, and all the rest, of our human animal essence and the acts of reclamation of that essence that will be so psychologically therapeutic.

In occupational science and its therapeutic application, we know that what we do describes, in great part, who we are. It is one of the blunt social questions asked when getting to know one another: "What do you do?" This is a shorthand for "Who are you? Are you an actor or a neurosurgeon?" Depending on your answers, I will expect different things of you and be better able to characterize your responses either negatively, to package and dismiss you, or positively, to credit you with whatever individuality breaks out of your professional mold.

Nevertheless, identity first issues from our human animal heritage and then is *primarily conditioned* by what we do. This not only includes our specialty, which actually is the most superficial part, but more importantly, the simple, everyday things we do that describe our existence as we as individuals have developed. The more primal the act, the more therapeutic the reclamation of that act.

I will continue to produce my gentle, but persistent, bronze reminders. You in occupational science categorize and organize them and other acts of self-recognition and continue to discover the hidden, not yet acknowledged, acts of self-acknowledgment. They can be retaught by therapists where they have atrophied by alienation or have been severed by trauma.

We've got work to do!

Discussion Questions

1. Why, in your opinion, does Seward Johnson believe that it is important for human beings to accept our basic animal state? Do you agree with him?
2. In what "minute acts of regression" might occupational therapists engage hospitalized patients (or people living within institutions) so that they might experience declarations of being and of life?
3. In what ways do or do not Seward Johnson's "statements of being" interface with the concept of occupation proposed by Clark et al.[1]?

Reference

1. Clark, F. et al: Occupational science: Academic innovation in the service of occupational therapy's future. Am J Occup Ther 4S:300, 1991.

by Stephen William Hawking, CH, CBE, FRS

4

Striving for Excellence in the Presence of Disabilities

I suppose the idea of asking me to do this paper was to get the viewpoint of a recipient of the services of occupational therapy. However, I feel like what I imagine Margaret Thatcher would feel if asked to address a conference on women's rights: What have they ever done for me? She has gotten where she is without any help from the feminist movement. Similarly, I have not received much help from people calling themselves occupational therapists.

Still, both Margaret Thatcher and I have benefited from a general movement in favor of groups, like women and people with disabilities, that were disadvantaged. A hundred years ago, it would have been against the law in Britain for a woman to be a member of Parliament, let alone Prime Minister. Even 50 years ago, it would have been unthinkable, although it was technically possible. Similarly, there was a prejudice against disabled people. Disability was an embarrassment to be kept out of sight. Franklin Delano Roosevelt felt he had to conceal his disability, even though it did not affect his capacity to perform his duties as President of the United States. Now, however, people with disabilities and other previously disadvantaged groups, such as women and blacks, are demanding that they should be able to play a full part in society. As I see it, your job as occupational therapists is to make sure that they can. I cannot say that professional occupational therapists have been much help in my case, but maybe I just did not encounter the right therapists.

I shall concentrate on physical disability because that is what I know most about. Some people might say that I am mentally disabled as well, but if so, I am too far gone to know about it. There are two aspects to physical disability: the mechanical difficulties from limbs and muscles not working properly and the psychological problems from being different and not being able to take part in many activities.

In the days when people had to lead troops into battle, it was reasonable to discriminate against women and people with disabilities, because they could not do that, but times have changed. The development of machines has made muscle power obsolete and having an able body unnecessary. With modern technology, it ought to be possible for many people with disabilities to lead a life in the community and to contribute to society. It is the task of occupational therapists to enable them to do this. The important jobs involve mental and organizational abilities rather than physical strength or dexterity. This is the direction in which people with disabilities should be encouraged rather than being put onto carpet making and basket weaving, which are inappropriate for those who are mentally alive.

The two aids that are most important to me are my wheelchair and my communication system. The advent of electric wheelchairs in the last 20 years has greatly increased the mobility and independence of people with disabilities. Wheelchair design is a compromise between speed and range on one hand and compactness and the ease of transport on the other. The chair I use is one of the most compact available. It can be collapsed quite easily to go in a car or airplane. I use gel batteries because the airlines do not like liquid acid burning a hole in their airplanes.

Even more important to me than my wheelchair is my communication system. I have amyotrophic lateral sclerosis, or motor neuron disease. This is a progressive disease that affects all the motor functions, including the voice. My voice was getting more and more difficult to understand. Then, in 1985, I had a tracheostomy operation, which removed my voice completely. However, I still have enough movement in my hands to operate a switch. With this, I control a computer. My system also could be operated by head or eye movement.

On the computer, I run a program called Equalizer, written by Walt Woltosz, of Words Plus, in Lancaster, California. I have a menu on the upper part of the computer screen. When I press the switch, a cursor scans down the screen. When it gets to the row I want, I press it again, and it scans across the row. When it gets to the position I want, I press again, and it selects the option at that position. In this way, I can choose words, which are printed out on the lower part of the screen. When I have built up what I want to say, I can send it to a speech synthesizer.

It takes six to 10 presses of the switch to select most words, but there are 36 common words that can be selected with only three presses. There also are six words that the computer thinks are likely to follow the most recent word I have used. These can be selected with only three presses. You can select up to 2750 words. The program comes with a basic dictionary of about 1500, but you can spell words you do not have and add them to the dictionary. I can also use this system to write things, including mathematical papers. To handle equations, I use a formatting program called Tex. I write the equation in words, like alpha over 2 equals gamma. The program translates this into the appropriate symbols and prints it out. In addition, I can write speeches in advance and save them on disk. I can then recall them, and speak them as a connected unit, like a lecture. This is an example of such a previously prepared speech. I can get up to half an hour in a single file, but I can use more than one file. I can then answer questions at the end, but that takes longer because I have to select each word.

The quality of the speech synthesizer is important. Speech synthesizers convert text to sound, using a number of rules, although English is not a phonetic language. The synthesizer therefore has to have a table of exceptions (the bigger, the better). However, pronouncing individual words correctly is only half the story.

That would give a very machine-like sound, which would be difficult to understand. To sound human and be understandable, the synthesizer has to break each sentence into phrases, and put the stress in the right place. The synthesizer I'm using is by far the best I have heard. It is made by Speech Plus of Sunnyvale, California. When I hear how other synthesizers or even recordings of my own voice (before I had a tracheostomy), I realize what a difference it must make to what people think of me. A slurred voice really turns people off. It makes one an object of pity or revulsion.

The great thing about this communication system, which distinguishes it from most other computer-based systems, is that it is mounted on my wheelchair. I have a small lap top computer in a box on the back of my chair. The screen has been taken off and mounted on the arm of the chair. It runs from a battery under the chair. The system is pretty rugged. It has survived many trips abroad and has even gone to Disneyland. I just wish it would speak English with an English accent.

Aids like wheelchairs and computers can play an important role in overcoming physical deficiencies, but the right mental approach is even more important. It is not useful to complain about the public's attitude toward people with disabilities. It is up to disabled people to change awareness in the same way that blacks and women have changed public perceptions. To do this, it is essential to present a positive image of people with disabilities as normal people who have certain mechanical difficulties.

I have been fortunate in several respects. First of all, I did not become disabled until I was in my 20s. This meant I had a normal childhood. Although I was never very athletic, I took part in the usual games and had a circle of friends. I was not isolated and set apart as often happens with those who have disabilities from an early age. It is important that children with disabilities are helped to join in with others of the same age. It determines their self-image. How can a person feel like a proper member of the human race if he or she is set apart from an early age? It is a form of apartheid.

As I said, I was fortunate in not being disabled until after childhood. I was also fortunate to have chosen to work in theoretical physics and that I was good at it. My scientific reputation increased as my physical abilities decreased. This meant that I always had a job, which is vital to keeping self-respect. Of course, I was lucky: There's not room for too many cosmologists in the world. However, most people, disabled or not, have something they are good at. It is up to occupational therapists to identify this and to help people achieve their potential. In my opinion, people with disabilities should concentrate on what they can do well and should not try to compete in areas in which they will necessarily do less well than able-bodied people. They should aim to be the best, not the best of those with disabilities. That is why I think the para-Olympics are a mistake. The ordinary Olympics are ridiculous enough with people competing to run fastest when any fool on a motor bike can go four or five times as fast. Sport is about the only area in which the doctrine of "separate, but equal" for men and women still prevails. However, sports for the disabled are third and fourth class, coming below sports for able-bodied women. I know this will upset those who have put a lot of effort into sports for those with disabilities, but I think this is the wrong direction. Of course, I'm prejudiced, because I was never any good at sports, but I think people should aim for the real top, not just the top of a second-class field. I would like to be thought of as a scientist who just happens to be disabled, rather than as a disabled scientist. I think I have succeeded in that. It is your job, as occupational therapists, to help other people do the same.

Discussion Questions

1. Should occupational therapists abandon the use of activities in lieu of reliance on technological solutions to problems posed by severe disability, especially for those people with strong cognitive abilities?
2. What fundamental lessons might be derived from this paper with respect to practice and to our understanding of occupation as a central phenomenon of adaptation and personal development?

by Jane Goodall, PhD, CBE

5

Occupations of Chimpanzee Infants and Mothers

Chimpanzees are our closest living relatives. We share with them 97.6% of our genetic material. In other words, their DNA and ours differ by as little as 2.4%. The anatomy of the chimpanzee brain is more like that of the human brain than that of any other living creature. We now know from nonhuman primate research designed to study language acquisition that chimpanzees show many cognitive abilities that we used to think were unique to humans. As these abilities have been described in the last 15 or so years, they have initially been greeted with scientific hostility. The hostility occurs because the discovery of similar behavioral or biological characteristics in a nonhuman animal seems to be an affront to people who are trying to preserve the unique place of humans in nature. In fact, one of the things that a long-term study of chimpanzees has done for me is to provide a humbling influence. Clearly, humans are unique, but we are not as unique as we once thought. We are no longer standing on an isolated pinnacle separated from the rest of the animal kingdom by an unbreachable chasm. We now know from many sources that chimpanzees are like us in their cognitive abilities. For example, chimpanzees can reason and solve simple problems; can plan, to some extent, for the immediate future because of their excellent long-term memory; and can understand and use abstract symbols. This cognitive ability has been demonstrated in their communication with language trainers and in their communication with each other. Chimpanzees even have a sense of humor. In fact, they show many social behaviors much like our own.

Chimpanzees also progress through life stages much like those of humans. When I started my research at Gombe in 1960, I quickly became fascinated by the development of infants, the relationships between infants and their mothers, the different types of mothering, the development of relationships between family members with time, and perhaps most interesting of all now that I have been there for nearly 29 years, the effects of various early life experiences on adult behavior. In particular, I am interested in the different types of mothering techniques and how these affect behavior in adult chimpanzees.

I think one of the big surprises in the early data that came from observations of Gombe chimpanzees was that of the infant's long-term dependency on the mother. We also discovered rare cases in which the mother actually became dependent on her child. I am intrigued by this state of reverse dependency and by how the relationship between mother and child changes as the child grows older and is weaned, by how the emotional dependency of the offspring on the mother continues up to early adolescence, and by how the affectionate bond between mother and offspring actually persists throughout life. Before I begin to discuss child development and the occupation of chimpanzee infants and their mothers, I want to construct a framework in which to view mother–infant relationships of chimpanzees. This framework consists of the ecology and the social structure of chimpanzees living in large social groups. It is extremely important to understand the ecological environment in which chimpanzees live and their social structure because it is unique even among nonhuman primate species.

Social Behavior

Chimpanzees, not only at Gombe but everywhere they are being studied in their natural environment, live in large social groups we call communities. At Gombe, the size of the social group has, over the years, averaged about 50 individuals. Of those 50 individuals, between 6 and 10 have usually been fully adult male chimpanzees, about twice as many have been fully adult female chimpanzees, and the remaining group members have been juveniles, adolescents, and infants. A small chimpanzee social group may be composed of two mothers and their offspring and may remain together for a few hours or even a few days. During this time, the composition of small groups is continually changing as individuals or groups of individuals move away to travel on their own or to join up with other individuals. We also have observed changes in group composition when there is a particularly favorite food or when food is available in large amounts but is located only in one portion of their territory. Chimpanzees will congregate there in large numbers in a highly excitable noisy state and then separate again into smaller groups.

The only chimps that remain together for months and years are mothers and their dependent young, that is, youngsters up to 7 or 8 years old. We have observed that while some female chimps are far more solitary than others, all female chimps at Gombe spend a great deal of time traveling, away from other members of their community, with just their own infant or infants and older dependent young. I want to emphasize that an infant may spend hours or days away from other infants, with just the company of its mother, particularly if it is a first-born child.

One of the fascinating things about the study of chimpanzees is that every individual has his or her own personality. They are as different one from the other as humans. Individuals of a community, even though they may be scattered about feeding in different parts of the home range, keep contact with one another using a long-distance vocalization called a pant-hoot. Because pant-hoots can be heard from long distances, chimpanzees out of visual range can identify each other by their individually distinctive calls. As we examine the stages of chimpanzee growth and social development, keep in mind that chimpanzees are individuals, and the degree to which they differ is reflected in social behaviors, such as mothering.

Nursing and Grooming

The chimpanzee infant nurses for about 3 minutes every hour for the first 3 years of life. After age 3, the infant continues to nurse but less often and with less regularity for another 2 or 3 years. This is obviously a very long period of nursing and infant dependency which equals that of the cultures of San people (previously called Bushmen) or pygmies in Africa.

During the period of nursing, mothers are almost always with their young infants. When the infant is fussy or restless, mothers start to groom their young child, which calms and relaxes the infant. In fact, often when a child becomes restless, for example, if the youngster wants to run off and join a group of other older infants, or if the mother gets nervous with her child's activity, she will nurse the youngster and begin to calm him or her by grooming. Under the gentle caress of the mothers' fingers, the child will usually relax and become more tractable.

Cradling and Traveling

The efficacy of maternal behavior to the extent to which they cradle their child differs tremendously from one chimpanzee mother to another. Some female chimps seem very inept at providing good secure laps. Very often an infant traveling around with its mother begins to slip until finally it is dangling by one or both hands before the mother reaches down and gathers it up again. However, many mothers demonstrate secure cradling behaviors. During the first few weeks of life, an infant chimpanzee often loses his or her grip while the mother travels, but the mother quickly reaches up to support the child. In fact, during the first few weeks, the mother typically places her hand under the infant's back to support it for at least a few steps. Then she will let go of her infant and continue to travel about normally (Fig. 5–1).

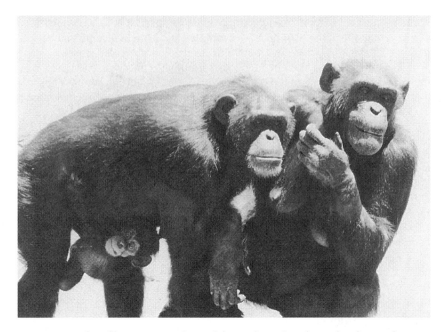

Figure 5–1. Infant chimpanzee traveling with his mother. (Photo by Paula Schoenwether.)

Often after nursing, an infant falls asleep, and the mother places her hand in a position to provide support for the infant's head and back. As the infant grows older, the location of the infant's body on the mother's lap is left increasingly to the infant to establish. Likewise, when the baby is tiny, the mother almost always supports the infant's head and neck, yet as the infant grows older, it assumes the support of its own head and neck and gets into a comfortable and secure position supported by the mother's thigh. There is a great deal of variability between mothers in the length of time that they are attentive to the slightest movements or cries of distress in their infants. Some infants are pushed toward earlier independence than others.

When the infant starts to ride on the mother's back, which is between 4 and 5 months of age normally, he or she often slips down and hangs on precariously in all kinds of unusual positions. Often the mother pauses and pushes the infant back up onto her back or presses it firmly back into the natural riding position. Small infants are gathered up when the mother moves on. As the infant gets older, he or she learns to follow the mother and climb onto her back while she is traveling. By the time the child is 6 to 9 months old, the infant is usually able to ride securely on the mother's back.

Climbing

Chimpanzee infants start to climb when they are around 6 months old, just about the same time they start to ride on the mother's back and take their first tottering steps. Young infant chimps, like children and kittens, sometimes find it easier to climb up than they do to climb down. In fact, we find exactly the same behavior among chimpanzees housed in cages. They climb to the top of the cage, then turn and whimper in fear and become distressed. In the wild, most chimpanzee mothers are extremely attentive to the needs of their small infants. Many mothers keep a watchful eye on their children when they practice climbing and often reach up and pull down an infant who is climbing too high, long before the infant shows any signs of distress.

As a mother travels through the branches of a tree or between trees with her infant following her, the mother must often make large jumps or cross fairly large gaps. For the first 3 years of the child's life, chimpanzee mothers almost always make these long jumps, keeping a grip on the branch of the tree that she just left, while making a bridge for her infant to follow along behind. As the child gets older, about 3 years of age, mothers no longer provide this assistance. Infants still desiring this kind of attention often become frustrated and distressed; their frustration may result in temper tantrums.

We have seen some wonderful examples of infant tantrums at Gombe. Tantrums are attempts of infants to manipulate their mothers in various situations. Obviously, it is easier for the child to sit on the branch and scream for the mother to extend a helping hand than it is for the infant to retrace its steps along the tree branch, back to the trunk of the tree, and climb down to cross at a more suitable place.

As the infant gets older, he or she spends more time away from the mother and more time with other individuals. I think it is because of the long years of infant dependency on the mother that later on in life, when he or she is frightened and the mother is not there to offer embraces, reassurance is sought from other familiar individuals. This is why friendly physical contact is immensely important to maintain close and friendly relationships between the adult chimpanzees of the community.

Feeding Traditions

Chimpanzees eat different foods in different areas, even though the same foods are present in both places. Chimps are omnivorous but they feed mostly on fruits, leaves, grasses, stems, vines, and pith. They eat several species of insects and often hunt and kill young mammals and then feed on their flesh.

Initially, the child learns which foods to eat by tasting food from its mother's mouth, watching the eating behavior of other members of the social community, and then imitating what it has seen. Infants repeatedly beg from their mothers by reaching up with little hands and extracting food from their mother's lips. Usually, the mother then discards half of the food she is eating for her child. Sometimes a mother will actually take food from the baby's mouth that is not a part of the traditional diet of that particular community.

Chimpanzees love to eat some hard-shelled fruits. However, the outside cover of these fruits are so hard that the chimpanzee cannot bite them open to extract the fruit inside. Being highly intelligent creatures, chimpanzees solve this problem by using a rock as a tool to crack open the hard shells and gain access to the fruit. Learning by imitation, or observational learning, thus provides a mechanism for passing along food preferences from one generation to another among members of a chimpanzee community. It is not surprising that in the different geographic areas of Africa where chimps are being studied, we have observed different feeding traditions. In addition to learning by imitation, chimpanzees also learn from trial and error, just like humans.

Tool Using

Chimpanzees in the wild use more objects for a greater variety of purposes as tools than any other creature except humans. The most commonly seen tool-using behavior in Gombe is termite fishing. Some termites live in large nests or mounds, which make it difficult for chimpanzees to catch and eat them. With time, chimpanzees have developed a technique of altering natural objects to produce a tool to enable them to reach the insects inside the mound, while preventing painful bites from the insects.

To obtain mound-dwelling termites, the chimpanzee must first select a stick or blade of grass and break it off to the approximate size needed. The next step is to remove leaves from the stick and, if necessary, further reduce its size to the proper length for the particular situation. With the tool completed, the chimpanzee may use a fist or the knuckles to tap several times along the surface of the termite mound to arouse the termites inside. Using one or two fingers, the chimpanzee then bores a hole into the mound to insert the newly constructed termiting tool. At this point, highly excitable termites swarm up from the nest onto the stick or fishing wand. The chimpanzee removes the fishing wand from the hole in the termite mound and places the stick laden with stinging termites carefully between the teeth and lips. The termites are extracted from the wand and the process begins all over again.

Chimpanzees learn termite fishing techniques by watching their mothers, siblings, and peers. They begin to imitate fishing behavior when they are about 2 years old. Gradually over the next 2 years they become increasingly proficient so that by the time they are 4 years old, they have usually developed successful termite fishing techniques. Like food preference traditions, there are different tool-using cultures in different parts of Africa. These are traditions passed on from one individual to another through observational learning and practice, and they originated in the distant past as a result of an original performance by a chimp of genius.

To summarize thus far, young chimps, like human children, have a great deal to learn, which is undoubtedly why the longer span of childhood is extremely adaptive for primates. They not only have to learn the feeding and tool-using traditions of their society, they also have to learn social behaviors that will help later with adult social interactions. Several years ago, experiments were conducted raising infant chimpanzees in complete isolation for the first 2 years of their lives. After several years, the chimpanzees in this experiment exhibited many of the social behaviors that we observe among chimpanzees raised under normal conditions, but these same social behaviors were used out of context and often not in the proper sequence. These deprivation experiments have demonstrated that chimpanzees may be born already having some social gestures; however, they also demonstrated that chimpanzees must learn, during their long childhood, to use these behaviors in the appropriate situation and in the appropriate behavioral sequence.

Child Play When Mothers Are Occupied

Chimpanzee mothers show great variability in their mothering behavior. Some chimpanzee mothers are playful and some are not. There are times when chimpanzee mothers are not in the mood to play. In fact, some mothers are seldom in the mood to play. The infant chimpanzee must therefore be able to occupy many hours by itself when his or her mother is not prepared to play, groom, or pay any attention to it. This is particularly true of the child of a rather asocial and aloof mother. Of course, in the wild, in a lush forest vegetation, there is plenty for infants to do. For young infant chimpanzees, sticks, stones, and fruits are toys, just as these kinds of objects are playthings for children who, in African society, cannot easily go to stores and have expensive toys bought for them. Of course, there are trees, branches, vines, and an unlimited opportunity for developing acrobatic skills during play. First-born infants truly are inventive when their mothers are otherwise occupied. For example, sometimes a child chimpanzee will spend 30 minutes playing and investigating a trail of ants. The chimpanzee will get a little stick and poke it into the ant trail and watch the ants scurry in all directions. Sometimes, if the ants head toward the chimp and start biting its toes, the youngster will start leaping about in the branches, slapping at the offensive ants. When the ant trail settles back into its old pattern, the chimp youngster will go back and poke the stick in it again, to start the game all over. Young chimpanzees also play games with members of other species. Often young chimps and young baboons play with one another, despite the fact that adult chimpanzees sometimes hunt, kill, and eat infant baboons.

On occasion, two adult female chimps meet when traveling through the forest with their dependent young. The youngsters take advantage of the chance meeting to run and chase each other in play. This is probably the most preferred type of play activity for young chimps between the ages of 2 and 5 years. After a while, the play becomes increasingly wild and acrobatic, with the excited youngsters running, climbing, and jumping among the tree branches. When one youngster finally catches the other, the game of chase quickly turns into a high-spirited bout of wrestle, tickle, and poke with intermittent bouts of running around tree trunks, chasing each other up into high tree branches, dropping out of branches to the ground, and then beginning the whole series of events again. Like human children, the play of chimpanzee youngsters is frequently punctuated with the sound of laughter.

Weaning and Movement Toward Independence

For about the first 3 or 4 years of life, the chimpanzee child has a wonderful life because the mother is always there to meet its needs. In addition, other individuals of his or her society are very tolerant and protective of him or her too. They can even approach an adult male chimp without the danger of being threatened. Thus, the infant chimpanzee's world is a very warm and secure place. Then comes the first traumatic experience, at least for most infants, of being weaned. At about 3 years of age, the infant may occasionally be rejected when it tries to suckle or ride on the mother's back. During the fourth year of life, weaning intensifies, and the mother rejects the child more frequently and more vigorously. For some youngsters, this is an extremely disturbing period, which peaks when the child is about 4 years of age.

Weaning also is disturbing for the mother because at all other times, the mother–infant relationship is very pleasant. Some youngsters throw violent temper tantrums, hitting and stamping on the ground, grabbing onto tree trunks, slapping their heads, screaming loudly, and occasionally hitting and biting their mothers. The mother's discomfort with her child's violent behavior shows on her face; she often wears a fear grin. If the child runs off screaming in frustration, the mother almost always follows and reaches out and embraces the child, holding it close to her until the screaming subsides and the child is calm again. It is as though she is telling the child, "You may no longer ride on my back or suckle, but I do love you anyway." Whatever the exact message may be, it helps to smooth over the rough edges of a difficult time and restore the typically peaceful and harmonious relationship between chimpanzee mother and child.

It is also during the weaning period that the mother begins to spend more time grooming her child. As I mentioned previously, grooming is a reassuring and relaxing behavior. Therefore, it is used by the mother to lessen her child's fear and frustration. Play also is another way chimpanzee mothers distract infants, at least temporarily, who are persistently seeking to nurse.

Family and Supportive Bonds

Chimpanzee youngsters often attempt to touch and later hold newborn chimpanzee siblings. Sometimes they can be very persistent and vigorous in their demands to play, woo, and try to pull the infant away from its mother. In these instances, chimpanzee mothers attempt to distract their attention away from the newborn by gentle grooming or play. Mothers deal with this situation more frequently with persuasion techniques rather than with punishment techniques. When mothers do punish their infants, it is usually by seizing a hand and giving a quick and relatively gentle bite. The bite elicits a little shriek from the infant but does not harm the child.

After the birth of the new infant, the older child continues to be emotionally dependent on the mother. The mother increases the time she spends caring for her older child in the form of grooming, playing, and sharing food. She may actually spend more time attending to the needs of the older child than she does to her infant. Of course, the baby is always attached to her body, and she must nurse it frequently, but she is still able to give attention to the older child.

To compare infant behavior related to birth order, I will describe the family life of Fifi. When her first son, Freud, was little, he constantly pestered her for attention. The birth of a second son changed things for Fifi. Frodo, her new son, pestered Freud for play, and Fifi was left alone for hours, during which time she could just sit and relax peacefully while the youngsters played nearby. Later infants are blessed with a sort of "built-in" playmate, whereas the first born has only its mother for companionship. Thus, infants with older siblings are not confined to pestering their mothers for play. Older siblings also serve as role models. The infant learns a great deal from watching and imitating the behavior of its mother and from watching and imitating older brothers and sisters.

When Frodo was only 5 years old he began to leave Fifi sometimes for 2 or 3 days at a time to travel around the border of the home range with groups of adult male chimps. Young male chimps do not normally leave their mother's company for long periods of time until they are at least 8 years old. Some remain close to their mothers until they are 10 or 11 years old. Frodo was unusually precocious in this respect because he had an older brother, Freud, to keep him company as he traveled around patrolling the home range with the older male chimpanzees. If the big male chimps became socially excited and Frodo grew fearful, he had his big brother nearby to offer him reassuring gestures.

We will move ahead a few years. Fifi has now given birth to her third infant, a little daughter named Fanny. Frodo is still spending most of his time with Fifi, and he is fascinated by Fanny, just the way Freud was by him. Frodo spends time grooming the little infant and playing with her. When Fanny was 5 months old, Fifi allowed Frodo to carry Fanny, just as she allowed Freud to carry Frodo when he was an infant.

Once again several years have passed. Fanny is old enough to be weaned and Fifi is pregnant again. Frodo continues spending time with his mother. Freud is still spending a good deal of time with his family. Family bonds are formed during the many years when older children continue to spend time with their mother and her dependent young. This is exemplified in the close bond that has formed between Frodo and Fanny, who is nearly 10 years younger than he. Hence, Fifi's family, like other chimpanzee families, spends a great deal of time together and supports each other in social altercations. Fifi, like her mother, continues to play with her young children and spend a great deal of time with her daughters. She spends less time with her sons, who patrol the territory boundaries with the other adult male chimps.

Fifi gives birth to another daughter, Flossy. When Flossy is 5 years old, Fifi becomes pregnant again. Flossy has been trying to suckle but has given up. While it appears that Fifi can no longer produce milk, there is still a close affectionate bond between Fifi and Flossy even though she has been weaned.

Unusual Mothering Behavior

We have observed some unusual mothering behavior among Gombe chimpanzees. The first example is Melissa, the only female chimpanzee at Gombe who has given birth to twins. We named the twins Gyre and Gimble. From birth, Gyre was the weaker twin. Melissa could not produce a sufficient amount of milk for two infants. One or the other of the twins was constantly suckling and often both of them were nursing at the same time. We think that Gimble, the more active twin, obtained more than his fair share of the milk from the start.

Transportation of the twins also was a problem for Melissa. She had great difficulty trying to carry both twins at the same time. This problem was exacerbated by the fact that the twins could not grip well enough to hold on to her securely. Often we would see Melissa traveling with one infant hanging precariously from her body. The twins would start to whimper, cry, or scream. Melissa would be forced to stop and readjust their positions before she could move on. Often they would grip on to each other, and then, of course, both would start to fall; they would then commence whimpering, crying, or screaming again. However, in this instance, Melissa, despite the problems she had carrying the two babies, seemed determined to keep up with the adult male chimps. I think this was because at this time, there was another adult female chimp, Passion, and her adolescent daughter, Pom, who were attacking other female chimps in their own community. Passion and Pom would seize, kill, and eat newborn babies. The infant to whom Melissa had given birth before the twins had been a victim of the murderous mother and daughter pair, and Melissa was clearly frightened of Passion.

At 10 months, Gimble was just beginning to climb tiny saplings. He had not been out of his mother's contact and had just taken one or two tottering steps beside her, but little Gyre remained constantly on his mother's lap. Although the twins were 10 months old, developmentally, they appeared to be only 4 or 5 months old, with Gyre appearing to be even younger than his heavier twin, Gimble. It was just about this time that Gyre fell sick. He showed signs of a cold, which quickly turned to something like pneumonia, and then he died. Gyre's death was quite clearly to Melissa's advantage, because she could concentrate her energy on feeding and caring for just one infant. After Gyre died, Gimble began to grow and quickly began to make up for lost time. Gyre's skull, which is being studied by anthropologists, is apparently about the same size as a 1-month-old infant, although he was actually 10 months old. Today, Gimble, from lack of proper early nourishment, remains tiny.

Old Flo is the second example of a female chimpanzee who had an unusual and difficult mothering experience. When Flo was already at an advanced age, probably around 40 or 45, she gave birth to her last infant, a little female named Flame. Because she was so old at the time, she lacked the energy and determination to wean her juvenile son, Flint, properly. He would throw violent temper tantrums, the worst of any we have seen at Gombe. Flint would repeatedly hit, bite, and shove his mother. With her reserve worn down, Flo would give in one more time and let him suckle and ride on her back. Unfortunately for Flo, he continued behaving this way when Flame was born.

Flint became increasingly depressed after the birth of the new baby. Unlike most older siblings, who by this time had started sleeping on their own at night and traveling on their own when their mothers moved through the forest, Flint pushed his way into Flo's night nest and pestered Flo until she let him ride on her back. Flame was only 6 months old when she died, and Flint, who had been so depressed, became cheerful again but remained abnormally dependent on Flo. He continued to ride on her back and sleep with her at night. Flint was 8.5 years old when Flo died. It seemed that Flint was unable to cope with the psychological blow caused by the death of his mother. He showed signs of clinical depression; he huddled, rocked, shunned social interaction, began eating less and less, and in this state of grieving and with his immune system depressed, he fell sick and died about 1 month after his mother.

Another infant who lost his mother is Pax, Passion's last son. Passion died when Pax was 4 years old, and it seemed that he might be unable to survive. He traveled around for a while with his older sister, Pom, and adolescent brother, Prof. After a few months, his depression lifted and he became quite active and cheerful again. This story ended delightfully when Pom immigrated to another community, which female chimps sometimes do, after her mother's death. At the time she moved to a neighboring community, little Pax had already bonded firmly with his brother, Prof. Today, Prof, 19 years old, and Pax, 15 years old, are virtually inseparable. For many years, Prof has assumed the maternal role and has protected and nurtured little Pax. It is interesting to see the male chimp, who usually plays no special role in the rearing of a child, show protective and maternal behaviors. Perhaps I should say Prof is showing paternal chimpanzee behavior.

Still another example of unusual mothering behavior occurred when an old female died and left a 3.25-year-old infant, Wolfie. This is a young age for a chimpanzee to be orphaned. Luckily, Wolfie was always close to his 8-year-old sister, Wanda, who frequently carried him with her. Normally, a female chimp does not enter menarche until she is about 10.5 years old. This means that Wanda was behaving as a mother 2 to 3 years before she could possibly give birth. This situation was more interesting because Wanda appeared to have started to lactate. We couldn't be certain that she did lactate, but we observed the infant approach and suckle for 3 to 4 minutes at a time, every 2 hours or so. If Wanda tried to prevent him from suckling, he became quite hysterical, cried, and threw tantrums.

The last example of unusual mothering behavior is an infant male chimp, Mel, who also lost his mother when he was 3.25 years old. Mel was left alone in the world. He had brothers and sisters, but the oldest sister in the family had transferred to a neighboring group, and the next born son and daughter had died of various diseases. Thus, when his mother died, Mel was alone. Moreover, he was a sickly infant and heavily infested with a number of internal parasites. We all thought that Mel would die.

Mel spent 3 weeks wandering alone after his mother's death. Sometimes he would follow one adult, sometimes another. The adults showed concern for him and would wait for him to catch up with them, especially if he whimpered. Occasionally, he would jump on one of their backs hoping for a ride. He would beg for food and sometimes receive some, but there was no special chimp that he followed more than another.

Then one day, when he was looking very sickly, he met a young adolescent male chimp who was 12 years old, named Spindle. Spindle began to nurture Mel. We do not know why this happened. There had been no close relationship of any sort between Spindle's mother and Mel's mother; nevertheless, Spindle took charge of caring for little Mel. He carried him from place to place. Spindle not only allowed Mel to ride on his back but sometimes actually gathered him up. When Mel found it somewhat difficult to climb up some of the taller trees, he would whimper, and Spindle would come and reach out a helping hand. There was absolutely no question that Spindle saved Mel's life. He shared food with him, he shared his nest at night with him, he waited for him during travel, and if Mel got in the way of an adult male chimp performing one of his vigorous charging displays, he would risk being attacked by rushing up and seizing Mel out of the way and carrying him to safety.

After 1 year, when Mel was quite clearly going to survive, Mel formed another relationship. At this time, the relationship between Mel and Spindle was quite strong, but when Mel was not with Spindle, he could be found with a sterile adult female chimp named Gigi. Gigi has, in fact, taken over two little orphans to raise. She has no children of her own, although she's been having estrus cycles since 1965. Now she is traveling around with another infant who lost its mother in the pneumonia-like epidemic that killed Mel's mother. If Gigi comes into estrus and goes off with the adult male chimps, then these two little orphans are on their own. They are so small and helpless that they are really like two little babes in the woods.

I might add that, although we don't know why Spindle adopted Mel in the first place, he did lose his mother during the same epidemic that killed Mel's mother. Although male chimpanzees at 12 years old do not spend much time with their mothers, adolescent male chimps do seek out their mothers when things get tense and difficult in adult male society, so perhaps the relationship with young Mel developed to fill an empty space in his life.

I must end the stories of maternal behavior with a comment. It has been extremely pleasing to watch the continued development of these young orphans whose lives we feared were lost. The many years I have spent at Gombe observing wild chimpanzees have brought many surprises and taught me that there is still much more to learn about chimpanzee behavior. If I had not remained there for a prolonged study, we would not have learned how chimpanzee communities split up, about civil war, about enduring family bonds, and about the plasticity of chimpanzee behavior, which allows them to adapt to meet such crises as those presented by orphaned infants.

Discussion Questions

1. Do you agree with Goodall that the occupations of chimpanzee infants and mothers show evidence of rudimentary culture?
2. What implications for humans can be derived from the occupations of chimpanzees?
3. What do Goodall's accounts suggest concerning the adaptive value of play?

Defining and Classifying

In the development of a science, a starting point is the defining of major concepts. One of the primary challenges in occupational science is defining the elusive term "occupation." Kielhofner has written that occupation "refers to human activity" but not to all human activity.[1] He excludes from his definition survival, spiritual, sexual, and social activities, leaving only activities "occupational in nature" as fully within the category of occupation, although he acknowledges that certain nonoccupational activities may have an occupational nature. Activities that have an occupational nature are those that are serious and productive or playful, creative, and festive.

Clark et al.[2] define occupation more inclusively as the "chunks of culturally and personally meaningful activity in which humans engage that can be named in the lexicon of the culture." Here, the emphasis is on occupation's meaning, rather than on its nature as in the Kielhofner definition. Sexual activity, social activity, and spiritual activity are included in the general category of occupation, and the focus is placed on such issues as how individuals choose and orchestrate occupations in the stream of time and how, over a lifetime, occupations define the essence of the person, are emplotted by issues of moral identity, and give rise to certain modes of thinking.[3]

The selections in this section are unified by their concern with definition. First, in Frank's paper, a definition of adaptation is provided for occupational science. In the paper "The Concept of Adaptation as a Foundation for Occupational Science Research," Frank eloquently defines the term "adaptation" from an occupational science perspective using the situation of Paul Longmore, a historian with a disability, who burned papers as a protest against a social security administration policy that required cutbacks of his disability benefits because he was receiving modest royalties on a book he had written. Longmore's action, Frank argues, reveals the nested nature of adaptation. She points out that adaptation, from the perspective of occupational science, should be defined in relation "to what occupations and outcomes" are best. Second, she argues, it should include discovery of "what is adaptive about occupations as they occur." She then proposes the following definition:

> Adaptation is a process of selecting and organizing activities (or occupations) to improve life opportunities and enhance quality of life according to the experience of individuals or groups in an ever-changing environment.

The emphasis here, as Frank points out, is on "orchestrated" activity, and therapists who begin to adopt this perspective will see themselves as concerned with helping patients put their daily activities together in a way that improves their life circumstances. Frank states that the definition puts "the emphasis on adapting while doing things, in the way we turn the pieces of a jigsaw puzzle around, fiddling with them until we get them to fit."

Frank's thinking does not stop here. She then defines the terms "adaptive strategies" ("chunks of action to improve life opportunities") and "person-oriented adaptive systems" (a person's "full range of activities and resources needs to be considered an orchestrated whole"). She has studied the adaptive strategies and the more complex adaptive systems of women with disability in her ethnographic research. She found that the adaptive systems, which subsume strategies, involve complex arrangements of activity in a variety of domains, including material culture or technology, the division of labor in subsistence activities, kinship, and aesthetics, including activities of play, leisure, religion, and politics. These may constitute useful domains around which occupational therapists can organize their work as they attempt to help their patients maximize life opportunities.

Primeau's paper deals with clarifying the term "work" and its conceptual distinction from leisure. The focus of the paper is on household work and illustrates another approach to defining concepts in the furthering of occupational science. Here, theory (in this case, feminist theory) is used to show the problematic nature of defining household work using terms that emanate from the traditional androcentric perspective represented in the social sciences. Androcentric social science constructs concepts that are based on male activities and the male social world. The classification of human activity as work, leisure, or self-care, which fits the experience of men who typically work for pay and then do other things, does not capture the inherent nature of household work. When examining housework carefully, elements of leisure seem to be embedded in household work and work can be part and parcel of what women call leisure. For example, a woman might experience cooking the family meal as a playful episode or work hard at embroidering a bath towel.

Primeau argues that it may be more accurate to examine household work in a fresh way, without relying on the traditional classification system that partitions activity into work or leisure. Instead, one could study the activities called housework from the standpoint of their meaningfulness, their value, and how they fit into the framework of a life. Therapists influenced by the thinking presented in this paper might view the lives of the women they treat in a different light. For example, they might take more time to discover what their patients do all day long and the extent to which these activities are experienced as having playful or worklike qualities.

Like Primeau, Parham challenges our conventional ways of classifying occupation. Here, the focus is on play, rather than work, and rather than relying on one theoretical framework for her analysis, Parham draws on several to tackle the problems inherent in defining play, explaining play, and assessing its value.

Initially, Parham points out the difficulties in identifying play when we rely solely on the generally accepted definition "that it involves intrinsically motivated activity which is experienced as pleasurable." After viewing a videotaped sequence of a cat interacting in a yard with the carcass of a dead squirrel, more than 50% of Parham's students judged the observed behavior to be predatory, although Parham was convinced the cat was playing. As Parham points out, consensus was difficult to achieve because the "ultimate motive of the cat (to eat or not to eat)" was unclear. The videotaped sequence illustrated the difficulties inherent in deciding whether an observed behavior constitutes play.

Next Parham tackles the problems inherent in defining play as one end of a continuum with work on the opposite side. In this model, a behavior is more playful if it is voluntary, pleasurable, relaxing, and improvisational. It is more worklike if it is obligatory, productive, effortful, and rulebound. However, using logical arguments, Parham uncovers the problem with dichotomous thinking and ultimately defines play as "intrinsically motivated and pleasurable" but also potentially "productive, embedded in obligatory roles or tasks," requiring effort and involving rulebound behavior. Finally, Parham urges us to be wary of play theories that relegate play to a secondary focus; rather, she urges occupational scientists to search for theories in which the nature of play is the focal concern. Parham concludes that play must be valued for its own sake as an occupation that is central to experiencing a healthy and satisfying life and not simply because it subserves other functions. This paper not only provides an innovative definition of play but also justifies the need for further research on the phenomenon and the importance of it as a crucial component in the attainment of quality of life for patients.

Also concerned in a sense with play, Knox's paper illustrates how qualitative research using a grounded theory approach[5] can be used to flesh out a definition of playfulness. In the study, Knox asked two research questions: 1) How is playfulness manifested? and 2) How do adult involvement and environment influence a child's play? The first question is concerned with the nature of playfulness. What Knox proposes, after having observed and interviewed children and caregivers and analyzing her data, is that playfulness is characterized by exhibiting verbal and social flexibility, taking command of and elaborating on play sequences, experiencing joy in physical activity, and using imagination. Her paper illustrates how qualitative research can be used to build definitions.

Further, the study in a sense demonstrates how qualitative research methods can be used to begin to detect the influences of the environment and caregivers on playfulness. The respondents identified the following caretaking behaviors as those that evoke play: "being loving, nurturing and relaxed" and joining the child in play. Also, the availability of toys and objects, novelty, and options in the environment was considered by the respondents to have an impact on playfulness. Respondents also believed that the home environment was key in encouraging playfulness. These insights may provide hints to therapists about strategies for encouraging playfulness in their practice.

Thus, through this qualitative approach, not only does a definition of playfulness emerge, but factors that evoke it are identified. We believe that therapists reading the paper can gain insights into how to recognize playfulness in their patients and what they can do to maximize its presence in their lives.

In summary, the papers included in this section represent attempts by occupational scientists to define key terms. The definitions are developed through a variety of approaches, but in each case, what results is "meat" into which therapists can begin to sink their conceptual teeth. What kinds of definition of occupation is best, one that is exclusive or broad? What kinds of classification systems should be used when grouping occupations? How can the process of definition building influence practice? Words may be considered the foundation for conceptualization, and conceptualization, in turn, is essential for guiding approaches to treatment.

References

1. Kielhofner, G: Occupation as the Major Activity of Humans. In Hopkins, HL, and Smith, HD (eds): Willard and Spackman's Occupational Therapy (8th ed). JB Lippincott, Philadelphia, 1993, pp 137–144.
2. Clark, F, Parham, D, Carlson, M, Frank, G, Jackson, J, Pierce, D, Wolfe, RJ, and Zemke, R. Occupational science: Academic innovation in the service of occupational therapy's future. Am J Occup Ther 45:300, 1991.
3. Sarbin, TR: Emotions as narrative emplotments. In Packer, MJ, and Addison, RB (eds): Entering the Circle: Hermeneutic Investigation in Psychology. State University of New York Press, New York, 1989.
5. Strauss, A, and Corbin, J: Basics of Qualitative Research: Grounded Theory Procedures and Techniques. Sage Publications, Newbury Park, CA, 1990.

by Gelya Frank, PhD

6

The Concept of Adaptation as a Foundation for Occupational Science Research

Defining Adaptation
Adaptive Strategies and Adaptive Systems
Conclusion

For roughly 2 decades, the field of occupational therapy has undergone a period of intense self-reflection. Dialogues in the literature among theorists have focused on identifying concepts and themes of professional unity against considerable pressure toward technical specialization and fragmentation.[1-3] One theme of professional unity to emerge during this period is that of adaptation.[4-9] Many occupational therapists see as their goal to elicit or foster adaptive responses of individuals with disabilities to environmental challenges through purposeful, meaningful activities. Occupational science is intended to embrace the spectrum of human activity, but the lives of people with disabilities offer a particularly clear window for defining adaptation from an occupational science perspective.

Defining Adaptation

Lorna Jean King defined adaptation from an occupational therapy perspective in her Eleanor Clarke Slagle Lecture in 1977.[5] Adaptation, she suggested, is an active response to a challenge in the environment that is self-reinforcing and that becomes most effective when it is organized subcortically as an unreflected habit. The example she cited is given by Elizabeth J. Yerxa in her Slagle lecture 1 decade earlier: that of a brain-injured patient unable to open her fingers on command who nevertheless extends her hand to grasp a cup of water that she is offered.[10] With this example, King emphasized the purposeful yet unconscious organization of an adaptive response compared with decontextualized muscular movement. This example captures the clinical moment in which an individual with a disability performs a meaningful action that, when repeated, will become one among many graded skills, eventually organized as habits, to support maximal function and independence for the individual. Anne Henderson (in Section VIII of this book), in her Wilma West Address at Occupational Science Symposium III, further developed the analysis of this level of adaptation; she used Bronfenbrenner's[11] ecologic approach to describe the proximate environments in which occupational therapists closely focus with patients to perform fundamental activities of daily living in an adapted manner.

Although it is a new discipline, occupational science emerges from occupational therapy in the endeavor to define the field and give a central place to the concept of adaptation.[12,13] Occupations are defined as "chunks" of activity within the stream of human behavior that are named in the lexicon of the culture, for example, "fishing" or "cooking" or at a more abstract level, "playing" or "working."[13] Just as occupational science has developed around a definition of occupation as "chunks of activity,"[14] adaptive responses have begun to look "chunkier" from our newly adopted perspective. Identifying the occupations in "chunks of activity" can be like taking apart the famous Russian lacquer dolls that nest one inside the other. From the standpoint of occupational science research, adaptive responses are nested within "adaptive systems." Such nestings make it possible to address the complexity of adaptation as meaningful action in the range of actual life situations beyond discrete functional activities in proximate environments.[15–20]

The following is an example of how these nested concepts of occupation and adaptation may be used. In the *Los Angeles Times* on October 19, 1988, there was a news photo in which a man with a beard, dressed in a suit and tie, was burning a stack of paper on the grill of a kettle barbecue (Fig. 6–1). As identified in the accompanying article, the man was Paul Longmore, "a 42-year-old historian whose upper body is twisted and partially paralyzed from polio." The object going up in flames was a copy of Longmore's book, *The Invention of George Washington*, which had taken the historian 10 years to write. Longmore was joined by 40 people, many of them disabled, to protest a Social Security Administration policy under which royalties earned on his book could end his disability benefits.[21]

The occupations performed by Paul Longmore are nested. He set a fire and managed it very effectively for someone who cannot use his arms. The proximate occupation in which Longmore was engaged was burning his book, but the purpose was far from functional in a proximate sense. The book was burned not for food, light, or heat, but to make a protest: Is it adaptive for a scholar with a severe disability to bother writing books when faced with work disincentives by which eligibility for Medicaid and personal assistance services might be forfeited for a modest gain in income earned through royalties? That is the question with which Longmore was occupied, and his action was strategically designed to provoke others to reflect and act.

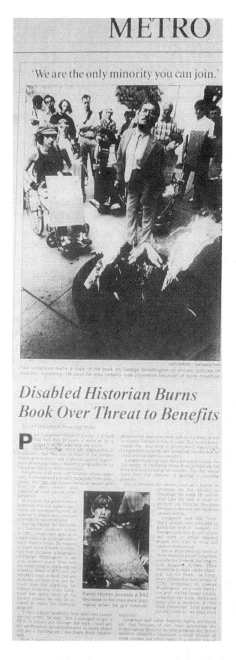

Figure 6–1. Clipping from the *Los Angeles Times,* October 19, 1988, in which Paul Longmore is burning a book he has written in protest of Social Security Administration benefit policies, which constitute a disincentive to his productivity. (Reprinted with permission from the Los Angeles Times Syndicate, Los Angeles, CA. Photo by John Wolcott.)

Paul Longmore did not know on October 19, 1988, whether his actions would actually contribute to eliminating work disincentives. For that reason, his actions help highlight some interesting points about adaptation for occupational science research:1) Actions are symbolic as well as functional; 2) actions can and perhaps must be interpreted within more embracing adaptive strategies and adaptive systems; and 3) the success of our actions is sometimes indeterminate if we consider only empirically verifiable, proximate, functional outcomes.

As a matter of record, the book burning incident was used by Los Angeles-based disability rights activist Douglas Martin to lobby successfully in Washington, D.C., for legislation to remove work disincentives for recipients of Supplemental Security Income (SSI). Among the technical changes introduced was the "Longmore Amendment," which redefined royalties and honoraria for speaking engagements as wages rather than gifts, allowing a beneficiary who earned royalties of $600 a month to retain needed Medicaid and personal assistance services, with SSI cash benefits reduced on a sliding scale rather than eliminated.

Occupational science will need to go beyond the definitions of adaptations that occupational therapists have insightfully developed through clinical practice. This expansion will be welcomed because occupational therapists work with a background view of the patient's world or environment as a constellation of challenges and resources toward which the single adaptive response or act is ultimately directed. Before defining adaptation, we need to discuss what kind of discipline occupational science is. Occupational science has been launched as a social science, but it also may be viewed, in common with its occupational therapy roots, as an applied form of moral philosophy. Its central tenet is the idea that human adaptation through occupation, that is, adaptation through mindfully organized action, is necessary for the good life. In this view, purposeful engagement in occupations is preferred over more randomly organized or disorganized activity, behaviorist manipulations, and wholesale use of technological controls over the human organism, such as drugs and surgery. The concept of adaptation in occupational science involves moral agency: Someone's action and experience must be taken into account, even when it is a matter of the occupational therapist acting as a surrogate or proxy for an incapacitated patient until he or she can gain more control in his or her environment. (For example, see White's paper "Temporal Adaptation of the Intensive Care Unit" in this book.)

A definition of adaptation in occupational science will need to balance a teleological impulse from moral philosophy to define what occupations and outcomes are best with an empiric impulse from the social sciences to discover what is adaptive about occupations as they actually occur. A definition of adaptation for occupational science may be as follows:

> Adaptation is a process of selecting and organizing activities (or occupations) to improve life opportunities and enhance quality of life according to the experience of individuals or groups in an ever-changing environment.

What is distinctive about this definition of adaptation, compared with definitions of adaptation in other disciplines, is its emphasis on orchestrated activity. Such a definition overlaps and diverges from concepts of "coping" and "adjusting" that stress cognitive skills and resolution of emotional states.[22–24] Occupational scientists put the emphasis on adapting while doing things, in the way that someone might turn pieces of a jigsaw puzzle around, fiddling with them until they fit.

Adaptive Strategies and Adaptive Systems

Adaptive strategies are sequences or chunks of action to improve life opportunities or enhance quality of life, often becoming part of a repertoire or style. The idea of adaptive strategies was central to Edgerton's study of adults with mild to moderate mental retardation living in the community.[25] Some individuals in the cohort studied by Edgerton could not tell time but wore wrist watches anyway. When they wanted to know the time, they approached someone and said, "My watch stopped. Could you tell me what time it is?" This was one of many adaptive strategies to enhance function yet avoid the negative consequences of being identified and stigmatized as retarded. Interestingly, when Edgerton and his research assistants ranked the nearly 50 members of the cohort, they found adaptability to be independent of IQ.

With time, when working well, adaptive strategies can acquire a coherence and elegance of style that is every bit like a personality or a piece of music. I learned this in my research on the life of Diane DeVries, a woman now in her 40s who was born with quadrilateral limb deficiencies. One aspect of my research with Diane concerns the way she presents herself through her choice of clothing.[26] Diane has always preferred wearing shorts and tops that fit her body to emphasize her assets rather than wearing shapeless skirts where her legs should be or covering her upper extremity stumps with bolero jackets (a strategy vigorously endorsed in childhood by her rehabilitation team). I was touched when Diane sent a musical toy for my daughter Rebecca's third birthday and was delighted that the green dinosaur with the goofy eyes did not require a key to make the music come out. You bat the creature's leg, and it plays a song. Diane selected a toy that she could play with. She was pleased that I noticed this detail, and we agreed that the dinosaur was something like the commercially available brass table lamp she owned that you can turn on and off with only a tap. The ready-made clothes Diane buys and wears, the dinosaur, and the lamp reflect a characteristic kind of adaptive strategy to reconfigure her environment to be maximally functional and essentially normal. On Diane's birthday, I asked for her wish list. She wanted either a compact disc (CD) of the Phantom of the Opera or a hanging silk plant. These are gifts in the key of "D"—that is, attuned to Diane's abilities—the selections on a CD player can be easily accessed by Diane, in contrast with a record turntable or even a cassette player, and silk plants never need to be watered.

The idea of an adaptive system—or "person-centered adaptive system"—embraces and goes beyond the idea of an adaptive strategy. To think in terms of adaptive systems means to consider activities in all the domains of life in a kind of ecologic niche.[27,28] A person's full range of activities and resources needs to be considered as an orchestrated whole that promotes, to the extent possible, the individual's life goals. Perhaps an overly single-stranded and conscious choice is suggested by the term "goal." It might be just as helpful to think of the configuration of activities and resources as promoting the individual's quality of life.

"Quality of life" is where our definition becomes fuzzy or relativistic and open to interpretation. Mainstream American society places a high value on success or prosperity, often wishing or striving for productive growth of some kind, relative to that with which one began. "Quality of life" may be experienced materially and spiritually, however, with the outcome being anything from building a more valuable portfolio of investments to establishing strong ties with friends and family to polishing one's capacity to find meaning and value in a constricting universe of resources and function. The latter may be particularly true for persons with severe disabilities and chronic illnesses. As anthropologist Gregory Bateson[29] has pointed out, however, an orientation toward unchecked growth and productivity in any dimension of life is neither culturally universal nor desirable. If a system is to survive, balance is needed.

Person-centered adaptive systems became a working concept in a study of long-term polio survivors with respiratory quadriplegia.[30] This was a population with residual functional capacities that were relatively stable postrehabilitation, although some were reporting a sudden loss of muscle strength with aging, known as postpolio syndrome. Three individuals studied in depth were members of a self-help group, nominated by other polio survivors as exemplars of adaptation. They were mature women, divorced or widowed, heading single-person households with live-in or rotating part-time help. The core constellation of resources necessary to their adaptation in Los Angeles was finite and could be identified fairly simply.

For each, the federal and state governments provided a stable and predictable substructure of support through SSI, Medicare, Medi-Cal, and In-Home Supportive Services, the state personal assistance services program. Essential technology involved little more than power wheelchairs with head rests, foot rests, and modified controls; intermittent positive pressure ventilators; power beds; phones, sometimes with modified switch and headset; televisions with remote control; and, if affordable and a driver was available, vans with lifts or ramps. Most of this technology was available through the state, but sometimes only after ferreting out information about how to acquire it.

Beyond this, each of the three women had worked out, depending on socioeconomic class related to resources acquired during the prior marriage, how to gain sufficient personal assistance services with attendant care for her around-the-clock needs, despite inadequate funding. One had established what anthropologists call a "fictive kin" relationship with her attendant, providing her with a sense of home and mothering in return for a greater amount and quality of services than could be purchased strictly on an hourly basis. Another had relied on her daughter for evening care to supplement paid day attendants until her daughter left for college; at that point, she took in friends of her daughter, providing room and board in return for services. The third woman was wealthier than the others and possessed a biting wit; she was able to pay for as many attendant hours as needed but seemed to wear out her helpers and had to find replacements more frequently. All three women had well-developed strategies for advertising, interviewing, and hiring help.

The temporal factor in these polio survivors' adaptive systems is striking. Not all disabilities and chronic illnesses follow a stable trajectory.[31,32] These polio survivors had the benefit of slowly developing and refining their adaptive systems within a relatively stable pattern for 30 years or more. The wealthier woman had an electric door opener. The less wealthy women left the door open during the day or had their attendant answer it. All had a primary command position in their homes, either an armchair or bed, fully facing the television and the front door. Each woman organized the activities of her day and week according to personal preference, taking into consideration her energy level and the availability of help; this included making grocery lists, supervising cooking, getting a bath, having a shampoo, and going out to attend meetings or visit friends. What stood out most was that each woman could recite precisely on which day, at what time, and for how long each of these activities or occupations would occur. Although the personal routines of these polio survivors were varied, the women were alike in having developed one.

Conclusion

Adaptive systems are more complex arrangements than adaptive strategies. They involve, from the individual's point of view, complex balanced arrangements of activities within the array of domains that characterize society. These domains include, for example, material culture or technology; the division of labor in subsistence activities; kinship; aesthetics, including activities of play and leisure; sexuality and reproduction; religion; and politics. Adaptive systems undergo periods of stability and instability. In the life of Diane DeVries, sudden changes in a key element of her adaptation could send reverberations through her system in a domino effect. Diane's separation and divorce from her husband, for example, destabilized her psychologically, landed her in a mental health unit for depression, interrupted her studies, left her without personal transportation, and made her almost entirely dependent on part-time paid attendants. However, within 2 years, Diane had reestablished a stable system by which she had returned to graduate school, relocated to an apartment at the nexus of several transportation lines, established a workable routine with a reliable attendant, and was not only in charge of her functioning again, but was in a growth mode toward fulfilling her professional career aspirations.

If the idea of person-centered adaptive systems proves foundational for occupational science research, it will invite us to think more in terms of the vocabulary of play and creativity.[33,34] Implications for occupational therapy will be to support patients' capacities for organizing human and material resources and establishing reliable but flexible routines that are open enough to allow for innovation and growth. When occupational therapists propose that the patient be viewed as a consumer and manager of services, a redefinition advocated by the Independent Living Movement, they are taking a person-centered adaptive systems approach.[35]

As a final note, I must add a warning that the concept of person-centered adaptive systems alone strikes me as dangerously solipsistic. Even the most creative adaptors innovate by recombining the inherited adaptive strategies and adaptive systems of their families, communities, ethnic traditions, and national cultures. This is not the place to debate the Hobbesian doctrine of methodologic individuals, the idea that society is nothing but the sum of its individual constituents.[36] Occupational scientists today may appear to focus on individuals, but interdependence is the essence of human society. How individuals select and orchestrate their occupations is important, but adaptation depends crucially on relations with one another.

Discussion Questions

1. Given Frank's definition of adaptation as a process that is concerned with improving life opportunities and quality of life, what do you imagine is the relationship of adaptation to

health? In other words, in what ways are adaptation and a state of health the same or
different kinds of phenomena?
2. How might occupational therapists primarily concerned with eliciting adaptive responses in the
here and now of the treatment session be enhanced by a rich understanding of adaptive
strategies and systems as defined by Frank?

References

1. Christiansen, C: Toward resolution of crisis: Research requisites in occupational therapy. Occup
   Ther J Res 1:115, 1981.
2. Kielhofner, G, and Burke, JP: Occupational therapy after 60 years: An account of changing
   identity and knowledge. Am J Occup Ther 31:675, 1977.
3. Mosey, AC: Occupational Therapy: Configuration of a Profession. Raven Press, New York,
   1981.
4. Fine, S: Resilience and human adaptability: Who rises above adversity? 1990 Eleanor Clarke
   Slagle Lecture. Am J Occup Ther 45:493, 1991.
5. King, LJ: Toward a science of adaptive responses. Am J Occup Ther 32:429, 1978.
6. Larson, E: The story of Maricela and Miguel: A narrative analysis of adaptation and temporality.
   Am J Occup Ther 50, April 1996.
7. Montgomery, MA: Resources of adaptation for daily living: A classification with therapeutic
   implications for occupational therapy. Occup Ther Health Care 1:9, 1984.
8. Schkade, JK, and Schultz, S: Occupational adaptation: Toward a holistic approach for
   contemporary practice, Part 1. Am J Occup Ther 46:829, 1992.
9. Schultz, S, and Schkade, JK: Occupational adaptation: Toward a holistic approach for
   contemporary practice, Part 2. Am J Occup Ther 46:917, 1992.
10. Yerxa, EJ: Authentic occupational therapy. Am J Occup Ther 21:1, 1967.
11. Bronfenbrenner, U: The Ecology of Human Development: Experiments by Nature and Human
    Design. Harvard University Press, Cambridge, MA, 1979.
12. Yerxa, EJ, Clark, F, Frank, G, Jackson, J, Parham, D, Pierce, D, Stein, C, and Zemke, R: An
    introduction to occupational science, A foundation for occupational therapy in the 21st century.
    Occup Ther Health Care 6:3, 1990.
13. Clark, FA, Parham, D, Carlson, ME, Frank, G, Jackson, J, Pierce, D, Wolfe, RJ, and Zemke, R:
    Occupational science: Academic innovation in the service of occupational therapy's future. Am J
    Occup Ther 45:300, 1991.
14. Yerxa et al., p 5.
15. Frank, G: The personal meaning of self-care occupations. In Christiansen, C (ed): Ways of
    Living: Self-care Strategies for Special Needs. American Occupational Therapy Association,
    Rockville, MD, 1994.
16. Jackson, J: Lesbian Identities, Daily Occupations, and Health Care Experiences. Doctoral
    dissertation, Department of Occupational Therapy, University of Southern California, Los
    Angeles, 1995.
17. Primeau, LA: The Orchestration of Work and Play Within Families. Doctoral dissertation,
    Department of Occupational Therapy, University of Southern California, Los Angeles, 1995.
18. Segal, R: Family Adaptation to a Child With Attention Deficit Hyperactivity Disorder. Doctoral
    dissertation, Department of Occupational Therapy, University of Southern California, Los
    Angeles, 1995.
19. Wood, W: Environmental Influences Upon the Relationship of Engagement in Occupation to
    Adaptation Among Captive Chimpanzees. Doctoral dissertation, Department of Occupational
    Therapy, University of Southern California, Los Angeles, 1995.
20. Wright, J: Occupational Restructuring by Older Adults After the Deaths of Their Spouses.
    Doctoral dissertation, Department of Occupational Therapy, University of Southern California,
    Los Angeles, 1995.
21. Goldman, J: Disabled historian burns book over threat to benefits. Los Angeles Times, October
    19, 1988, Part II, p 1.

22. Cohen, F, and Lazarus, RS: Coping and adaptation in health and illness. In Mechanic, D (ed): Handbooks of Health, Health Care, and the Health Professions. The Free Press, New York, 1983, pp 608–635.

23. White, RW: Strategies of adaptation: An attempt at systematic description. In Coelho, GV, Hamburg, DA, and Adams, JE (eds): Coping and Adaptation. Basic Books, New York, 1974, pp 47–68.

24. Wright, BA: Value Changes in Acceptance of Disability. Physical Disability—A Psychological Approach, ed 2. Harper & Row, New York, 1983, pp 157–192.

25. Edgerton, RB: The Cloak of Competence: Stigma in the Lives of the Mentally Retarded. University of California Press, Berkeley, 1967.

26. Frank, G: On embodiment: A case study of congenital limb deficiency in American culture. In Fine, M, and Asch, A (eds): Women with Disabilities: Essays in Psychology, Culture, and Politics. Temple University Press, Philadelphia, 1986, pp 41–71.

27. Frank, G: Life history model of adaptation to disability: The case of a "congenital amputee." Social Science and Medicine 19:639, 1984. Reprinted in Nagler, M (ed): Perspectives on Disability: Text and Readings on Disability. Health Markets Research, 1990, pp 608–617.

28. Gallimore, R, Weisner, TS, Kaufman, SZ, and Bernheimer, LP: The social construction of ecocultural niches: Family accommodation of developmentally delayed children. Am J Mental Health 94:216, 1989.

29. Bateson, G: Bali: The Value System of a Steady State. Steps to an Ecology of Mind. Ballentine Books, New York, 1972, pp 107–127.

30. Frank, G: Independent Living Environments for the Disabled: Self-directed Strategies. Session on "Dealing with Disability at the Individual and Systems Level." Annual Meeting, Society for Applied Anthropology, American Anthropological Association, Toronto, Ontario, March 14–18, 1984.

31. Strauss, A, and Glaser, B: Chronic Illness and the Quality of Life. Mosby, St. Louis, 1975.

32. Corbin, J, and Strauss, A: Unending Work and Care: Managing Chronic Illness at Home. Jossey-Bass, San Francisco, 1988.

33. Bateson, MC: Composing a Life. Penguin, New York, 1990.

34. Nachmanovitch, S: Free Play: The Power of Improvisation in Life and Art. Jeremy P. Tarcher, Los Angeles, 1990.

35. Burke, JP, Miyake, S, Kielhofner, G, and Barris, R: The demystification of health care and demise of the sick role: Implications for occupational therapy. In Kielhofner, G (ed): Health Through Occupation: Theories and Practice of Occupational Therapy. F.A. Davis, Philadelphia, 1983, pp 197–210.

36. Lukes, S: Methodological individualism reconsidered. In Lukes, S (ed): Essays in Social Theory. Columbia University Press, New York, 1977, pp 177–186.

by Loree A. Primeau, PhD, OTR

7

Work Versus Nonwork
The Case of Household Work

"Men may work from sun to sun, but woman's work is never done." So goes the old saying, and as with many old sayings, there is some truth to it. When work is defined as any activity or energy expenditure to produce services or goods of value to others,[1,2] it is clear that most women work throughout a great part of their waking hours, whether they are paid or unpaid.[3] Even so, women's work, especially unpaid work, is generally taken less seriously than men's work. Oakley[4] states:

> In relation to male labor, female labor is characterized as unproductive, marginal, trivial, temporary, intermittent, dispensable, less valuable, less skilled, and less physically demanding. . . . Most fundamental of all, . . . housework is not real work at all: In its unreality it is either not-work or an intrinsically trivial work activity.[5]

Social science research in general and research in the area of work in particular have traditionally focused on the male social world and men's activities.[1,6,7] "The circle of men whose writing and talk was significant to one another extends backwards in time as far as our records reach. What men were doing was relevant to men, was written by men, about men for men."[8] Smith argues that this androcentric focus in social science has led to the development of conceptual categories of human activity that do not accurately reflect women's experience. The social science dichotomy of work and leisure has excluded the category of housework. As Smith explains:

> The work-leisure organization applies to employment. . . . If we started with housework as a basis, the categories of "work" and "leisure" would never emerge. And indeed, it is hard to [imagine] how, using housework as our basic framework, it would be possible to make "work" and "leisure" observable. The social organization of the roles of housewife, mother, and wife does not conform to the divisions between being at work and not being at work.[9]

Thus, the dichotomy of work and leisure is a more accurate description of men's lives than of women's lives. A similar classification system appears to be developing within occupational science. Occupations have been conceptualized as work, rest, play, leisure, and self-care[10] or as work, rest, and leisure.[11] Where does household work fit into these conceptualizations? Household work not only contains aspects of work, leisure, and self-care, but also includes the unpaid labor of care for others, that is spouses, children, and perhaps aging parents. An understanding of how the occupations within the category of household work fit into the conceptual categories of work, leisure, and self-care may elucidate the nature of the conceptual categories themselves.

The term "household work" is used to describe the occupations and activities related to the home and family.[12,13] Other terms have been found in the literature, including family work,[14,15] household labor,[16,17] domestic work or tasks,[18,19] housework,[20,21] child care,[19,21] and childbearing work.[12] Household work is used in this paper to encompass the activities conducted to maintain the home and care for children and thus consists of housework (i.e., cleaning, cooking, and clothing care) and child care. Although household work may be done for pay, that is, by domestic paid workers, only the case of unpaid household work is considered here.

This paper explores the nature and meanings of the conceptual categories of work, leisure, and self-care through an investigation of the nature and meaning of household work. Household work has been chosen as a special case to demonstrate the interactions of work, leisure, and self-care within specific occupations. This paper demonstrates how the essential nature of an occupation cannot be explicated without an understanding of the meaning of that occupation to the individual engaged in it. Thus, occupations may elude facile categorization.

Conventional definitions of work, leisure, and self-care as found in the literature are reviewed. Next, the nature of household work, as described in the literature, is presented. An exploration of the meaning of household work follows. The meanings of household work to the person who is doing the work and the social meanings of household work as conceptualized by two feminist standpoint theorists[7,22] are discussed. Implications for occupational science conclude the paper.

Conventional Definitions of Work and Leisure

A review of the literature reveals that the categories of work, leisure, and self-care have been defined in various ways. Work may be broadly defined as purposeful and sustained activity that is the opposite of rest, or it may be defined narrowly as a means of earning an income and a living.[23,24] The latter definition of work as a form of paid employment has led to the development of a dichotomy of work time versus nonwork time in modern western culture.[23] The notion of work versus nonwork is socially determined within a specific culture. "Classification of any given task as work, rather than as leisure or obligation, is arbitrary and tied to a particular culture's basic values, division of labor, and sources of identity."[25] Nonwork time in western culture consists of leisure and obligatory activities, including self-care.[23-25]

Leisure has been defined as discretionary activity that is chosen and carried out in time that is free from obligations.[24] Leisure activity is that which "we want to do because we enjoy it."[26] Obligatory activities include self-care activities, such as personal grooming, eating, and sleeping, and activities that provide for the care of others and of nonhuman objects, such as children, pets, clothing, gardens, and homes.[23-25]

There is a significant lack of consensus within the literature on whether household work is work, leisure, or an obligatory activity. Daniels argues that household work is work but that it disappears from the traditional conception of work because it is a private, unpaid activity.[23] She believes that:

> any activity we do for pay, wherever it is found, even if we enjoy it, must, by definition, be work. But any effort we make, even if it is arduous, skilled, and recognized as useful—perhaps essential—is still not recognized as work if it is not paid.[26]

In contrast, Parker places household work in the category of nonwork obligations or semileisure.[24] He does, however, acknowledge that "the line between obligation and leisure is not always clear and depends to a large extent on one's attitude to the activity."[26] Nock and Kingston include all three definitions of work, leisure, and obligatory activities in their discussion of household work.[27] They state that household work involves work even though it is not paid, that it is discretionary and allows for individual preference, and that it is subject to general social and personal obligatory standards. In an effort to clarify these conflicting views of household work, the nature of household work is now explored.

The Nature of Household Work

Time-use studies and other studies of women's and men's participation in household work consistently indicate that women are responsible for most of it.[17,21,28] Two major time diary studies were conducted in the 1960s and provide comprehensive information of women's and men's time use in the home. The most significant finding of these studies was that when paid work and household work hours were combined, employed husbands of employed wives actually had a shorter work day than employed husbands of unemployed wives.[29,30] This finding is explained by the shortened paid work day of husbands with employed wives. It appears as if husbands with employed wives could afford to cut back on their paid work day because of their wives' income contribution. The surprising conclusion that husbands of employed wives did not participate in household work to any greater extent than did husbands of unemployed wives created a controversy and precipitated further research on household work.[15]

The Survey Research Center at the University of Michigan conducted time-use studies on American national samples in 1965, 1975, and 1985.[31] Comparisons have been made across all three studies reflecting historical trends in women's and men's participation in household work during the last 3 decades.[31-33] Employed women's participation in household work, including housework and child care, decreased from 28.2 hours per week in 1965 to 26.2 hours per week in 1985. Employed men's time spent in household work increased from 13.7 to 17.2 hours per week in 1965 and 1985, respectively. Unemployed women decreased their total time spent in household work from 53.7 hours per week in 1965 to 39.3 hours per week in 1985. The changes in women's and men's time use in the home between 1965 and 1985 occurred in the time spent on housework, while the time spent in child care activities remained constant.

These historical trends indicate a significant decrease in women's time spent on housework and a significant increase in men's housework time. Both of these changes occurred in the activities of cooking and cleaning.[31] Thus, employed husbands appear to be making their primary contributions to household work in the areas of cooking and cleaning. During the 20-year period, employed women's and employed men's time spent in child care remained constant, although women's weekly contribution to child care was more than three times that of men's contribution. These figures indicate that employed women work a "second shift" that adds up to an extra month of 24-hour days of work during a year.[21]

Hartmann summarizes the findings of time-use studies in terms of the differences between women's and men's participation in household work.[34] First, on the average, 70% of the time spent on household work is spent by the wife. Second, child care is largely the wife's responsibility. The wife adjusts her household work responsibilities according to family size and the age of the youngest child. The husband's contribution to household work varies little across the family life cycle. Third, the husband of an employed wife does not, on the average, spend much more time on household work than does the husband of an unemployed wife. Fourth, "husband care," that is, household work created by the addition of another person in the household, creates up to as much as 8 extra hours of household work per week for the wife. Fifth, on average, an unemployed wife works a minimum of 40 hours a week within the home. An employed wife, in addition to her paid work hours, spends a minimum of 30 hours per week on household work.[34] Thus, men and women differ significantly in their participation in household work.

Household work has been labeled inherently menial, boring, degrading, isolating, fragmented, repetitive, unskilled, and unrewarding in nature.[35-39] The skill level needed to do household work is assumed to be such that it could be acquired by anyone.[40] The conditions of household work, especially when child care is involved, require the worker always to be on call. The task at hand is frequently picked up and put down as other demands on the worker's time and attention are made.[35] Household tasks, such as cooking, washing the dishes, and cleaning, are constant and recurrent throughout the day.[41] Because most household work is conducted in the home, it is said to produce a sense of social isolation.[42]

Perceptions of household work frequently cited in the literature are that it is devalued, low in prestige and status, and to be avoided if possible.[39,40,43,44] Men perceive household work as demeaning and unmasculine,[37] whereas women perceive it to be degrading, simple, and trivial.[35,45] Schleuning, however, argues that although "both men and women belittle housework as unproductive and inefficient, . . . it also [offers] women an outlet for self-expression, creativity, and meaningful work."[46]

Household Work: Leisure or Work?

Leisure and work are frequently compared and contrasted with household work in the literature. The obligatory nature of household work is rarely discussed. While specific examples of the self-care nature of household work were not found in the literature, there were references to the leisure and work aspects of household work. These references are presented to explore the personal meanings of household work.

The boundary between household work and leisure is difficult to establish.[27,35,47–50] Time spent in household work is thought to be discretionary.[27,50] Once minimum personal and social standards and expectations have been met, the demands, amount, and scheduling of household work are subject to individual preferences.[27,50] Women engaged in household work define their leisure time as "those moments they can squeeze in among other activities (often while monitoring children's activities)"[51] rather than discrete blocks of time separate from their daily work.

Some household work activities may cease to be chores and become hobbies, while some activities during leisure time may be put to use in the course of household work.[27,48,50] Often household work tasks appear to combine work and leisure, as in the case of reading to a child or preparing food for a picnic.[35] On one hand, Nock and Kingston ask:

> Cooking meals, for example, is a central task in household production, but what if the cook enjoys the activity and goes beyond the requirement of providing sustenance, perhaps even with some creative flourish? Preparing a good meal may be the most pleasurable part of the individual's day—in effect, may be that person's leisure.[52]

On the other hand, Firestone and Shelton ask, "If a woman is reading a magazine but also noting recipes for use in future meal preparation, should that be classified as leisure time?" (p 480).[53] Thus, there are aspects of leisure in household work and aspects of household work in leisure.

To explore the meaning of work and leisure as experienced in the context of household work, Berk and Berk asked women in their study to identify household activities as work, leisure, neither, or both.[17] The women defined work activities as washing dishes, making beds, dusting, and cleaning the bathroom and leisure activities as reading, watching television, and visiting with friends. Activities considered by women to be both work and leisure were child care and meal preparation. Given that child care and meal preparation make up a large part of household work, Berk and Berk conclude that "a simple dichotomy between work and leisure (at least in the minds of our respondents) is inappropriate for much of what goes on in the home."[54]

The same two activities, raising children and cooking, were rated most positively of all household work by men and women in the 1985 time study conducted by Robinson et al.[31] Of the total sample of men and women, 55% reported liking to cook, and 51% reported liking to raise children. Women seemed to enjoy these activities more than men did. Only 26% of the total sample reported "liking housework, on the whole" (21% of the men versus 32% of the women).[31] These two studies indicate that individual perceptions of household work as work or nonwork are essential to the understanding of the personal meanings of household work.

Feminist activists were the first to question the unpaid nature of household work.[55,56] They argued that the fact that household work is unpaid results in its devaluation and lack of social validation and recognition as work.[23,44] The isolating nature of household work also has consequences for its recognition as work. Ferree states that "because housework is done in individual family units, there is no job to 'go to' nor coworkers with whom to share it. Thus the work becomes coextensive with the self and the distinction between working and not working blurs."[57]

As Daniels explains, household work is frequently "invisible work" that "is private; there is no audience beyond the family and the work is personalized for the family members who rate it as they please. . . . It is not hard to see why women . . . do not understand some aspects of their activity as work."[58] Daniels[23] and other feminist scholars have argued that a wide range of women's responsibilities have gone unrecognized as work or as effort of any type.[55] Examples of women's invisible work that have been studied at length are interaction work done to facilitate communication with men;[59] emotion work, that is, the management of feelings;[21] and the work of meal planning, preparation, and management that organizes family life.[35,60]

DeVault, in her analysis of the invisible work that goes into feeding and creating family life, states that expectations of the family to be a respite from work provide "an interpretive frame that allows the work done to meet those expectations to remain hidden."[51] Although the women in her study were aware of the amount of time, effort, and skill that feeding a family requires, "they talked about feeding as something other than work in the conventional sense, trying to explain how their activities are embedded in family relations. . . . They describe their activity as something different from work."[61] Feeding was described as motivated by love, but the amount of work that went into it also was recognized. Thus, feeding was not labeled as "love" or "work" alone. DeVault concludes that:

> Vocabularies of work come from the model of paid employment; there are few words with which to express the kind of effort that so many women put into their family lives. Since they have no vocabulary for their own activity, the women talk of their work at home in terms of "love."[62]

The literature indicates that perceptions of household work as work, nonwork, or leisure vary with the individual. Feelings about household work are not neutral; women attach meaning to their work in the home. Knowledge of the personal meanings of household tasks is essential to understand the significance of household work to the individual. Exploration of the social meanings of household work, as conceptualized by two feminist standpoint theorists, may demonstrate the significance of household work to society.

Feminist Standpoint Theories

The feminist standpoint theories of Aptheker[22] and Smith[7] aim to establish women's work as a basis for understanding women's consciousness, experience, and ways of knowing. Aptheker and Smith describe their theories as grounded in women's gendered experience in the context of their subordination to men. As such, their theories are representative of feminist standpoint theories. Standpoint theories argue "that men's dominating position in social life results in partial and perverse understandings, whereas women's subjugated position provides the possibility of more complete and less perverse understandings."[63] Transformation of women's perspective into a standpoint provides a more preferable moral and scientific understanding of social life than the dominant male perspective. The feminist standpoint is "grounded in the universal features of women's experience as understood from the perspective of feminism."[63]

A problem inherent in a feminist standpoint is its universalizing nature. Critics question if there can be a feminist standpoint given the variety of women's social experiences according to class, race, and culture.[6] Aptheker and Smith try to resolve the issue of universalism in different ways.[7,22] Aptheker refers to a way of knowing, which arises from the meanings women create through their work, as a woman's standpoint. She suggests that "this standpoint pivots, of course, depending upon the class, cultural, or racial locations of its subjects, and upon their age, sexual preference, physical abilities, the nature of their work and personal relationships."[64] Women's gendered experience creates a common center of thinking that pivots according to women's individual differences.[22] Smith states that she is not fully satisfied with her attempts to deal with class and racial oppression within the gender organization of society.[7] She does, however, believe that research of the everyday world as problematic would "have the capability of continually opening up a different experience of the world, as women who have not yet spoken now speak. Each speaker from a new site discloses a new problematic for inquiry."[65]

The feminist standpoint theories developed by Aptheker and Smith suggest that women have common experiences in their daily lives that give rise to unique ways of perceiving and knowing the world.[7,22] Aptheker suggests that understanding the complexity of women's lives and putting that understanding to use in daily life lead to the act of knowing from women's experience.[22] Embedded in traditional research materials and in poetry, literature, oral histories, plays, dances, and visual art, Aptheker discovered the details of the "dailiness" of women's lives. The dailiness of women's lives consists of patterns and meanings that women create through the process of carrying out their daily work during their lifetime. Included in Aptheker's definition of women's work are child care and other forms of caregiving, domestic work, emotional work, maintenance of personal relationships, shopping, and daily travel work.

A lifetime of women's work provides a legacy of female artifacts in the form of art, crafts, stories, gardens, letters, and recipes to name a few. In these artifacts, Aptheker finds:

> The evidence that there is and always has been another point of view, another record of social reality, a women's standpoint. This standpoint has always existed, but for thousands of years it has not been seen, even by ourselves. It has certainly not been seen as anything "important." Friendship, family, children, ritual, community, connection to the earth, a belief in life, the need for beauty and art are some of the most evident of women's values. There is also a focus on the practical, a continual analysis and reworking of context, which comes out of the particularity of women's labors and consciousness. This is the meaning of daily life.[66]

Like Aptheker, Smith discovers a women's standpoint based on women's work within the everyday world.[7] To obtain a woman's standpoint from the matrix of experience in the everyday world, a feminist mode of inquiry, specifically a problematic of the everyday world, is required. Rather than using artifacts of social life to find meaning in women's work, Smith suggests that research should "begin with women's experience from women's standpoint and explore how it is shaped in the extended relations of larger social and political relations."[67]

Based on her experience in her local and particular world of everyday life, that of an academic sociologist and mother of two children, Smith identifies two modes of consciousness.[7] One mode of consciousness is organized by actual position in the physical world. It is a local and particular consciousness concerned with the body and physical space. The second mode of consciousness is the ruling mode dominant in current society that transforms local and particular aspects of life into generalized and abstract forms.[7] Transcending the local and particular mode to move into the abstract and generalized mode requires a bifurcation of consciousness.

Bifurcation of consciousness occurs for everyone who chooses to participate in the abstract and generalized (or conceptual) mode of action. Women, however, had been forced into a specific relation to the conceptual mode of action. They have traditionally been assigned to the local and particular (or concrete) mode of action in the home and vocational options by virtue of male appropriation of the conceptual mode of action.[7] "If men are to participate fully in the abstract mode of action, they must be liberated from having to attend to their needs in the concrete and particular. . . . The direct work of liberating men into abstraction . . . is the work of women."[68] The unpaid and paid work of women consists of the facilitation of men's transition to, and maintenance in, the conceptual mode of action. Examples of such work include taking care of men's bodily existence through the domestic duties of a wife and creating concrete forms of conceptual activities through the vocations of secretary, nurse, or other health professions, such as social worker or occupational therapist.

Implications for Occupational Science

The historical development of the profession of occupational therapy as a predominantly female profession demonstrates the relationship of women's paid work and Smith's theory of two modes of consciousness and action.[7] Professions composed primarily of women, such as nursing, teaching, and occupational therapy, share commonalities in their historical roots.[69] These professions developed into their modern forms in the patriarchal society of the 19th century. Gender ideology at the time "viewed women as especially sensitive, moral and self-sacrificing by nature—an ideology that, when a need for women's labor arose, could be adapted to support their work in the serving professions."[70] In addition, predominantly female professions emerged within organizations in which men generally directed the female workers.

The conditions under which these professions evolved led to low wages, long hours, poor working conditions, and discrimination for the largely female workers. Problems within such professions continue to be manifested today in the form of "short career ladders, and modest earnings potential, considerable intraoccupational sex segregation by which the minority of men tend to rise to the top of the field, and difficulties in achieving consensus"[71] about the future of their professions.

Stromberg cites occupational therapy one of the nine professional specialties composed mostly of women.[69] Indeed, anyone familiar with the historical development of occupational therapy and its contemporary form could not help but agree with Stromberg's assessment of female professions. A male psychiatrist is credited with the establishment of the philosophy on which occupational therapy as a profession was built,[72] but occupational therapy has a long history of women workers. Women were initially recruited to work as reconstruction aides during World War I, and today 98% of occupational therapists are women.[73] Occupational therapy's interest in the development of the patient's competence and independence in daily activities, including self-care, dovetailed with the then-current gender ideology that prescribed women's responsibility for activities within the home.[74] As the need for reconstruction aides arose during World War I, the training of women to provide much-needed rehabilitation services to returning war veterans was justified by the same gender ideology. Women's nature made them especially suited to care for and nurture wounded and disabled soldiers.

From the beginning of the profession, occupational therapists were directed by male physicians in the course of their work. Applying Smith's feminist standpoint theory (1987), it is clear how female occupational therapists acted as mediators between the conceptual and concrete modes of action for male doctors.[7] Using nurses as an example, a male psychiatrist explained the relationship between doctor and occupational therapist: "so must he rely upon the therapists to administer the practical part of occupational therapy. . . . The occupational therapist, therefore, has the same relation to the physician as has the nurse, that is, she is a technical assistant."[75]

The local and particular details of the everyday world have always been the focus of occupational therapy. The view of the human as an occupational being "that maintains and balances itself in the world of reality and actuality by being in active life and active use"[76] was first proposed in 1922. In the early days of the profession, "the key role of occupational therapists was to guide patients in a customary round of balanced daily activity."[77] This tradition has continued with the occupational therapist's attention to "enhancing the individual's skills, competence, and satisfaction in daily occupations."[78] Concern for the concrete mode of action is evident in the occupational therapists' interest in the patient's ability to dress, feed, bathe, and groom herself or himself; to obtain and maintain employment; to participate in leisure activities; and to travel within his or her own community. The profession of occupational therapy would not exist today without the benefit of women's ways of knowing based on lived experience in the everyday world; thus, a feminist perspective may be a useful frame of reference for theory development within occupational science.

Given that the practice of occupational therapy is based on women's experiences and ways of knowing arising from the daily occupations of life and the everyday world, Smith's feminist standpoint theory, with the everyday world as problematic, may be a particularly fruitful frame of reference of occupational science. Already parallels between the work of Smith[7] and workers in the field of occupational science may be found. Smith, when discussing the problems inherent in shifting between the concrete and conceptual modes of consciousness while balancing her unpaid and paid work, states that the two modes of thinking often existed in the same person, in the same place, and competed with each other for time. In the course of examining the literature on the occupation of human daily travel, Primeau[79] found that working mothers frequently combined trips to their jobs with trips for other purposes related to their household work.[80] Also of note was the finding that women made an abrupt shift in their thinking from the home domain to the work domain during their morning commute, while men made a gradual shift in consciousness that began before leaving home.[81] Similarly, DeVault's research[35,60] on women's work to feed the family and to create family life, using Smith's[7] feminist research strategies, resonates with Pierce's theoretical papers on the occupations of food gathering and food preparation.[82,83]

Such patterns indicate a rich source of research questions that originate within the everyday world of women's experience. For example, how do working mothers orchestrate their paid and unpaid work? How is household work shared by family members within different types of families, such as single-parent families or dual-career families without children? Does children's participation in household work facilitate learning of self-care skills?

Conclusion

This paper began by reviewing the categories of work, leisure, and self-care. Next, the nature of household work and its personal and social meanings were explored. Two feminist standpoint theories and their conceptualization of household work were examined. The everyday world as problematic, a feminist standpoint theory developed by Smith,[7] was suggested as being particularly useful as a frame of reference for the incorporation of feminist theory into occupational science research. In conclusion, using the case of household work, this paper has attempted to demonstrate some of the problems inherent in the indiscriminate use of the conceptual categories of work, leisure, and self-care within occupational science. Because occupational science seeks to understand the experience and meaning of one's occupations and how they relate to one's values and sense of purpose in life,[10,84] occupational scientists must look beyond the conceptual categories of work, leisure, and self-care to explore fully the nature of the human as an occupational being.

Discussion Questions

1. What clinical implications can be derived from Primeau's deconstruction of work, leisure, and self-care as mutually exclusive categories of occupations?
2. If occupational therapists abandon their usual discriminations between work, leisure, and self-care, what kinds of evaluation tools might be generated?
3. How might Primeau's deconstruction of these categories relate to Bateson's concept of "enfolded occupations?"

References

1. Fox, MF, and Hesse-Biber, S: Women at Work. Mayfield, Palo Alto, CA, 1984.
2. Hall, RH: Dimensions of Work. Sage, Beverly Hills, CA, 1986.

3. Chester, NL, and Grossman, HY: Introduction: Learning about women and their work through their own accounts. In Grossman, HY, and Chester, NL (eds): The Experience and Meaning of Work in Women's Lives. Lawrence Erlbaum, Hillsdale, NJ, 1990, pp 1–9.
4. Oakley, A: Reflections on the study of household labor. In Berk, SF, (ed): Women and Household Labor. Sage, Beverly Hills, CA, 1980, pp 7–14.
5. Oakley, p 8.
6. Harding, S: The Science Question in Feminism. Cornell University, Ithaca, NY, 1986.
7. Smith, DE: The Everyday World as Problematic: A Feminist Sociology. Northeastern University, Boston, 1987.
8. Smith, p 18.
9. Smith, p 68.
10. Yerxa, EJ, Clark, F, Frank, G, Jackson, J, Parham, D, Pierce, D, Stein, C, and Zemke, R: An introduction to occupational science: A foundation for occupational therapy in the 21st century. Occupational Therapy in Health Care 6:1, 1989.
11. Clark, FA, Parham, D, Carlson, ME, Frank, G, Jackson, J, Pierce, D, Wolfe, RJ, and Zemke, R: Occupational science: Academic innovation in the service of occupational therapy's future. Am J Occup Ther 45:300, 1991.
12. Berch, B: The Endless Day: The Political Economy of Women and Work. Harcourt Brace Jovanovich, New York, 1982.
13. Nieva, VF: Work and family linkages. In Larwood, L, Stromberg, AH, and Gutek, BA (eds): Women and Work: An Annual Review (Vol 1). Sage, Beverly Hills, 1985, pp 162–190.
14. Barnett, RC, and Baruch, GK: Correlates of fathers' participation in family work. In Bronstein, P, and Cowan, CP (eds): Fatherhood Today: Men's Changing Role in the Family. John Wiley & Sons, New York, 1988, pp 66–78.
15. Pleck, JH: Working Wives/Working Husbands. Sage, Beverly Hills, 1985.
16. Berk, SF: Women and Household Labor. Sage, Beverly Hills, 1980.
17. Berk, RA, and Berk, SF: Labor and Leisure at Home: Content and Organization of the Household Day. Sage, Beverly Hills, 1979.
18. Delphy, C: Close to Home: A Materialist Analysis of Women's Oppression. University of Massachusetts, Amherst, MA, 1984.
19. Smith, AD, and Reid, WJ: Role-sharing Marriage. Columbia University, New York, 1986.
20. Cowan, RS: Two washes in the morning and a bridge party at night: The American housewife between the wars. In Scharf, L, and Jensen, JM (eds): Decades of Discontent: The Women's Movement, 1920–1940. Greenwood, Westport, CT, 1983, pp 177–196.
21. Hochschild, A: The Second Shift: Working Parents and the Revolution at Home. Viking, New York, 1983.
22. Aptheker, B: Tapestries of Life: Women's Work, Women's Consciousness, and the Meaning of Daily Experience. University of Massachusetts, Amherst, MA, 1989.
23. Daniels, AK: Invisible work. Social Problems 34:403, 1987.
24. Parker, SR: Leisure and Work. George Allen & Unwin, London, 1983.
25. Masur, J: Women's work in rural Andalusia. Ethnology 23:25, 1984.
26. Daniels, p 403.
27. Nock, SL, and Kingston, PW: The division of leisure and work. Social Science Quarterly 70:24, 1989.
28. Cowan, RS: Women's work, housework, and history: The historical roots of inequality in work-force participation. In Gerstel, N, and Gross, HE (eds): Families and Work. Temple University, Philadelphia, 1987, pp 164–177.
29. Robinson, JP: How Americans Use Time: A Social-psychological Analysis of Everyday Behavior. Praeger, New York, 1977.
30. Walker, K, and Woods, M: Time Use: A Measure of Household Production of Family Goods and Services. American Home Economics Association, Washington, DC, 1976.
31. Robinson, JP, Andreyenkov, VG, and Patrushev, VD: The Rhythm of Everyday Life: How Soviet and American Citizens Use Time. Westview, Boulder, CO, 1988.
32. Robinson, JP: Housework technology and household work. In Berk, SF (ed): Women and Household Labor. Sage, Beverly Hills, 1980, pp 53–68.
33. Robinson, JP: The hard facts about hard work. Utne Reader, (March/April), 70, 1990.
34. Hartmann, HI: The family as the locus of gender, class, and political struggle: The example of housework. In Harding, S (ed): Feminism and Methodology. Indiana University, Bloomington, IN, 1987, pp 109–134.

35. DeVault, ML: Feeding the Family: The Social Organization of Caring as Gendered Work. University of Chicago, Chicago, 1991.

36. Ferree, MM: Class, housework, and happiness: Women's work and life satisfaction. Sex Roles 11:1057, 1984a.

37. Ferree, MM: The view from below: Women's employment and gender equality in working class families. Marriage and Family Review 7:57, 1984b.

38. Perry-Jenkins, M, and Crouter, AC: Men's provider-role attitudes: Implications for household work and marital satisfaction. Journal of Family Issues 11:136, 1990.

39. Shehan, CL: Wives' work and psychological well-being: An extension of Gove's social role theory of depression. Sex Roles 11:881, 1984.

40. Hiller, DV: Power dependence and division of family work. Sex Roles 10:1003, 1984.

41. Keith, PM, and Schafer, RB: Housework, disagreement, and depression among younger and older couples. American Behavioral Science 29:405, 1986.

42. Ferree, MM: Working-class jobs: Housework and paid work as sources of satisfaction. Social Problems 23:431, 1976.

43. Reisine, ST, and Fifield, J: Defining disability for women and the problem of unpaid work. Psychol Women Quar 12:401, 1988.

44. Ross, CE, Mirowsky, J, and Huber, J: Dividing work, sharing work, and in-between: Marriage patterns and depression. Amer Sociol Rev 48:809, 1983.

45. Schleuning, N: Idle Hands and Empty Hearts: Work and Freedom in the United States. Bergin & Garvey, New York, 1990.

46. Schleuning, p 87.

47. Ferber, MA: Women and work: Issues of the 1980s. Signs: Journal of Women in Culture and Society 8:273, 1982.

48. Firestone, J, and Shelton, BA: An estimation of the effects of women's work on available leisure time. Journal of Family Issues 9:478, 1988.

49. Gronau, R: Leisure, home production, and work: The theory of the allocation of time revisited. J Pol Econ 85:1099, 1977.

50. Schooler, C, Miller, J, Miller, KA, and Richtand, CN: Work for the household: Its nature and consequences for husbands and wives. Am J Sociol 90:97, 1984.

51. DeVault, p 5.

52. Nock and Kingston, p 26.

53. Firestone and Shelton, p 480.

54. Berk and Berk, p 230.

55. Gerstel, N, and Gross, HE: Introduction and overview. In Gerstel, N, and Gross, HE (eds): Families and Work. Temple University, Philadelphia, 1987, pp 1–12.

56. Tong, R: Feminist Thought: A Comprehensive Introduction. Westview, Boulder, CO, 1989.

57. Ferree, p 432.

58. Daniels, p 407.

59. Fishman, P: Interaction: The work that women do. Social Problems 25:397, 1978.

60. DeVault, ML: Doing housework: Feeding and family life. In Gerstel, N, and Gross, HE (eds): Families and Work. Temple University, Philadelphia, 1987, pp 178–191.

61. DeVault, p 179.

62. DeVault, p 180.

63. Harding, p 26.

64. Aptheker, p 39–40.

65. Smith, p 223.

66. Aptheker, p 74.

67. Smith, p 10.

68. Smith, p 83.

69. Stromberg, AH: Women in female-dominated professions. In Stromberg, AH, and Harkess, S (eds): Women Working: Theories and Facts in Perspectives, 2nd ed. Mayfield, Mountain View, CA, 1988, pp 206–224.

70. Stromberg, p 207.

71. Stromberg, p 208.

72. Hopkins, HL: Historical perspective on occupational therapy. In Hopkins, HL, and Smith, HD (eds): Willard and Spackman's Occupational Therapy. J.B. Lippincott, Philadelphia, 1988, pp 16–37.

73. American Occupational Therapy Association: Occupational Therapy Manpower: A Plan for Progress. American Occupational Therapy Association, Rockville, MD, 1985.
74. Welter, B: The cult of true womanhood: 1820–1860. American Quarterly 18:151, 1966.
75. Dunton, WR: Prescribing Occupational Therapy. Charles C. Thomas, Springfield, IL, 1928, p 10.
76. Meyer, A: The philosophy of occupational therapy. Archives of Occupational Therapy 1:5, 1922.
77. Primeau, LA, Clark, F, and Pierce, D: Occupational therapy alone has looked upon occupation: Future applications of occupational science to pediatric occupational therapy. Occup Ther Health Care 6:21, 1989.
78. Yerxa et al., p 6.
79. Primeau, LA: Human daily travel: Personal choices and external constraints. In Clark, FA, (Chair): Occupational Science Symposium III: Ecology and occupation. Symposium conducted at the University of Southern California, Los Angeles, June 1990.
80. Rosenbloom, S: The growth of non-traditional families: A challenge to traditional planning approaches. In Jansen, GRM, Nijkamp, P, and Ruijgrok CJ (eds): Transportation and Mobility in an Era of Transition. Elsevier Science, Amsterdam, 1985, pp 75–96.
81. Richter, J: Crossing boundaries between professional and private life. In Grossman, HY, and Chester, NL (eds): The Experience and Meaning of Work in Women's Lives. Lawrence Erlbaum, Hillsdale, NJ, 1990, pp 143–163.
82. Pierce, D: The occupation of food gathering. Unpublished manuscript, University of Southern California, Department of Occupational Therapy, Los Angeles, CA, 1989a.
83. Pierce, D: The occupation of food preparation. Unpublished manuscript, University of Southern California, Department of Occupational Therapy, Los Angeles, CA, 1989b.
84. Clark, FA, and Jackson, J: The application of the occupational science negative heuristic in the treatment of persons with human immunodeficiency infection. Occup Ther Health Care 6:69, 1989.

by L. Diane Parham, PhD, OTR, FAOTA

8

Perspectives on Play

How Do We Define Play?
How Do We Explain Play?
Why Is Play Important?
The Functionalist View
Play For Its Own Sake

From the beginning of our profession, occupational therapists have touted a concern for the role of play in our patients' lives; we have advocated the use of play to promote health. Most of our knowledge about the clinical uses of play has come from clinical "folk knowledge" passed on from clinician to clinician. Only in relatively recent years, launched by the scholarly work of Mary Reilly[1] and her students, have occupational therapists begun to contribute to the universe of knowledge on play, and we have a long way to go in articulating an occupational science perspective on play. As we strike out on a path of inquiry, fundamental questions arise that must be considered before we can proceed. How can we explain the existence of play? Why is it important to us? What is it? These are the questions I consider in this paper. They are fundamental because they frame the way we understand play and hence how we approach the study of play. Ultimately, the ways we answer these questions will shape the design of our assessment tools and intervention programs.

How Do We Define Play?

Although play is a notoriously difficult construct to define, there is general agreement that it involves intrinsically motivated activity that is experienced as pleasurable. As Takata[2] has noted, it is not a specific behavior but an attitude or process. In fact, a particular behavior may or may not be play, depending on the motives and experience of the organism (Fig. 8–1). A child engaged in "playing" softball may not actually be playing if he or she dislikes the activity and is doing it only because adults require him or her to participate in the game during physical education class. In such a case, he or she might participate in the game but would not experience it as play.

A significant problem in operationalizing play is that the motives and experiences of the organism are not always accessible to the observer. When the organism is not able or available to verbalize how the activity is being experienced, we must rely on observable surface behaviors to draw conclusions about whether or not play is present; unfortunately, these behaviors are often ambiguous. This problem became clear to me the first year I taught a graduate course on play in our new doctoral program in occupational science at the University of Southern California. In class, I showed a videotape recording of a cat interacting with an object and asked the class to decide whether or not the animal was playing.

The videotaped episode begins with the cat lying outdoors in a sphinx-like pose, facing the object, which appears to be about 1 ft in front of him. He serenely lies still for a little longer than half a minute, moving only his head occasionally to survey the yard. The next 23 seconds of the cat's actions are transcribed below.

- Suddenly pounces on object, briefly mouthing it, then leaps to its right with his right paw outstretched
- Sinks claws of right paw into object and leaps, twisting his body and lifting object off the ground
- Grasps object in mouth and aggressively tosses head back and forth while making three powerful forward leaps in rapid succession, pushing off with hind limbs, and dropping object once, only to resume flipping it with claws of fully extended forelimbs

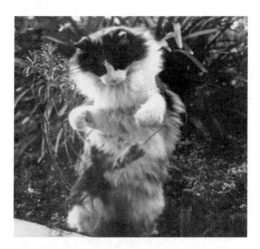

Figure 8–1. In this picture, it is unclear whether this cat is playing or hunting. (Photo by Susan Knox.)

- Makes a small leap while rotating body to roll to the ground, object in mouth
- Briefly seems to fight with object while sidelying, batting it with both forelimbs and hindlimbs
- Pauses and slowly lowers head to ground
- Rests in sidelying position for 5 seconds, as if going to sleep
- Suddenly, as if startled, raises head and outstretches right limbs
- Looks at object while quickly reaching forelimbs toward it
- Abruptly interrupts movement toward object before contact is made and arches away from object, pushing it away with hindlimbs
- Partially rolls while batting forelimbs toward object but does not move close enough to it to contact it; instead, seems to attack the air
- Abruptly gives a strong push of the hindlegs to leap away from the object
- Turns in midair with back arched dramatically and lands facing object defensively, as if threatened
- Looks away from object as if disinterested

The videotaped segment continues with the cat making a series of spectacular leaping attacks on the object, punctuated with periods of what appear to be bored disinterest. To my mind, this was a clear-cut case of play behavior.

The classic criteria for identifying play in animals, as outlined by ethologist Loizos,[3] seems to support my view that the cat in the videotape was playing. According to Loizos,[3] play in animals involves motor patterns usually used in "serious" context to achieve particular ends, for example, to obtain a meal, flee from a predator, or copulate. In play, however, these motor patterns are modified in peculiar ways, such as a reordered sequence of actions, exaggerated or uneconomical quality of movement, more repetition of certain movements (compared with movements in the "serious" context), fragmentation, and incomplete movements.

Before showing the videotape in class, I did not tell my graduate students how I interpreted it, nor did I review Loizos' criteria. Afterward, when asked whether or not the cat was playing, a little more than half of the students voted that this was not an example of play behavior. Some felt quite strongly that it was not play, just as I had felt strongly that it was.

Why the disagreement? In the discussion following the videotape, the students focused on the object with which the cat was playing. It was the carcass of a squirrel, and although we do not know whether the cat was responsible for its death or whether the cat later devoured the remains of the squirrel, the question was raised as to whether this was an example of real predatory behavior rather than play. Had the object been a toy squirrel, the behavior would have been more clearly classified as play by the students, they explained. The ultimate motive of the cat (to eat or not to eat) was of overriding concern to them in deciding whether or not play was taking place.

I bring up this incident to illustrate how difficult it can be to agree on whether or not observed behaviors constitute play. As we saw in the cat example, perceived motives affect our interpretations. A disadvantage in studying nonverbal animals like the cat is that they cannot tell us what they are experiencing or what their motives are. On the other hand, most human beings do have the potential to tell us. Human play is not necessarily easier to interpret, however. With humans, we may have to sift through thick layers of symbolism and elaborate sets of rules to detect the presence of play.

Perhaps rather than focusing on whether or not play is present in a situation, a more meaningful strategy might be to examine the extent to which the qualities of play permeate a situation. In common parlance and in the play literature, play is often treated as an antonym for work. For the sake of this discussion, let us conceptualize the two terms as poles on a continuum, rather than as discrete phenomena, and examine some well-worn descriptors for these polarities (Table 8–1).

One of the most commonly cited distinctions between play and work is that play is voluntary, that is, intrinsically motivated, whereas work is obligatory, or extrinsically motivated. I believe this might be the most important and essential distinction to make between play and work, yet this dichotomy is not always clear in real life. It breaks down, for example, when a person is asked to do a task as part of his or her employment and becomes so involved that he or she goes far beyond the requirements of the job. What started out as strictly extrinsically motivated has become intrinsically motivated. The opposite problem also can occur; that is, a person starts out doing an activity because he or she enjoys it (for example, playing baseball), makes it a job, and winds up doing it only for a handsome economic reward. The intrinsic motivation has been gradually replaced by extrinsic. Might there be a little of both types of motivation fueling such situations? Might an activity be both voluntary and obligatory at the same time?

Another dichotomy separating play from work is the characterization of their goals as pleasurable, in the case of the former, versus productive, for the latter. The presence of pleasure is another characteristic of play that I consider to be essential, yet we can easily see through the pleasure–productivity dichotomy as an illusory one. If a person loves work, won't he or she pursue it to experience pleasure and to be economically productive? Conversely, an occupation pursued as a hobby may generate pleasure while being quite productive: Consider pastimes such as ceramics, woodworking, cooking, and textile arts. Clearly then, play may be enfolded in work and vice versa.

The other dichotomies noted in Table 8-1 similarly have shortfalls. Play has classically been linked with relaxation and recreation, whereas work has been characterized as effortful. However, many play activities that require great effort easily come to mind, for example, chess, which requires deep concentration. Likewise, the conceptualization of play as improvisational[4] compared with work as rule bound falls apart when considering the multitude of games with complex rule systems. Indeed, Huizinga,[5] in his classic treatise, defined play as a phenomenon characterized by its own rules and proceeding within its own time and space boundaries.

Play is intrinsically motivated and pleasurable, yet also may be productive, embedded in obligatory roles or tasks, require effort, and involve rule-bound be-

Table 8–1   Play and Work as Poles of a Continuum

Play	Work
Voluntary	Obligatory
Pleasurable	Productive
Relaxing	Effortful
Improvisational	Rule bound

havior. The pleasure ingredient, by the way, is not trivial and should be taken seriously by occupational therapists, who use activities for their healing value. For example, considerable evidence points to the immune-enhancing power of favorite occupations, which Ornstein and Sobel[6] call "healthy pleasures." The pleasure ingredient may be an important key to the health-promoting properties of occupation.

How Do We Explain Play?

Let us move now from definitional issues to the question of how we explain play. Many theories are available to help us answer that question. Which ones are most relevant for occupational science?

To aid the process of selecting theories on which to build our knowledge and our practice, it may be helpful to sort out the scholars who focus directly on understanding play from those who address play as secondary to their main object of study. The latter group of authors is more plentiful. These writers deal with play as a byproduct or piece of something else. Typically they study play as a means to get at some other construct.

Groos,[7] for example, focused on explaining the instinctual basis of behavior, especially in relation to the evolution of human intelligence. His germinal work on the evolutionary significance of play presented it as pre-exercise or rehearsal of skills by juvenile animals (including humans) in preparation for adult behaviors. In this view, play assumes a critical role in the adaptation of species who do not depend on extensive wired-in behavioral routines for survival. Play, therefore, is related to phylogenetic status. Through play, the animal constructs skills for survival and adaptation. Animals who must adapt to complex social and physical environments will require more play ontogenetically than those who do not.

Nearly a century after Groos[7] published his classic treatise, the pre-exercise theory continues to be highly influential in play literature today. Contemporary refinements of his view are reflected in work by Vandenberg,[8] for example. Bruner[9] also has presented a modernized version of Groos' theory in his work on the development of problem-solving skills. Although Bruner's work is often cited by occupational therapists in relation to play, Bruner was centrally concerned with understanding the mind, not play.

Berlyne[10] is another prominent figure in the play literature whose interest in play was secondary to some other domain; in his case, it was the physiologic basis for attention and curiosity. His well-known studies of curiosity and arousal inspired other researchers to embark on a line of research and theory aimed at the physiologic dimension of play, particularly in relation to arousal. Hutt,[11] for instance, conducted laboratory studies with human children and theorized that play is a mechanism for modulating arousal level. Interestingly, Berlyne[12] originally suggested a relationship between arousal and play but concluded that play, because it is not easily operationalized, is not worthy of study.

A number of other authors are important contributors to the play literature yet were concerned with play only peripherally. Piaget[13] incorporated play into his elaborate theoretical framework of cognitive development. Play for him was narrowly defined as pure assimilation, distinct from imitation (which he viewed as accommodation). He considered play to be an infantile process that eventually merged with accommodation to produce game behavior. Erikson[14] used play to illustrate his concepts of ego development. For him, play in childhood was a vehicle for achieving mastery over traumatic events and developing a capacity for social adjustment. Bateson[15] is often cited for identifying the existence of the nonverbal message, "This is play" (evident, for example, in the "play face" used by primates to communicate that forthcoming interactions are playful rather than serious). His primary interest was in explaining metacommunication and mind, not play. Whiting[16] studied the relationship between sociocultural systems and personality; in the process, he constructed the view that desirability of social roles is mirrored within children's games.

Within the field of occupational therapy, Ayres[17] is sometimes cited as making contributions to the understanding of play.[18,19] Her interest was in the neurobiologic expressions of sensory integration, however. Although her work brought some new insights into the interpretation of children's play as a vehicle for sensorimotor competence, her theory was not about play. It was about sensory integration; therefore, like the work of most of the writers discussed thus far, it presented only a circumscribed understanding of play.

Now I will identify some of the scholars whose focus was on explaining play. Because their interest in play is primary rather than secondary to some other phenomenon, their approaches to play tend to be more integrative.

Dolhinow and Bishop[20] described the forms and functions of primate play. Their work is consistent with the early groundwork laid by Groos,[7] yet they provided a fuller understanding of play as occupation because of their focal interest in play itself. In their classic paper, they outlined the motor, manipulative, and social skills acquired in play and contextualized the acquisition of these skills within the particular characteristics of the environments of primates, both human and nonhuman.

Sutton-Smith[21] was one of the first scholars who sought to interweave folkloric and anthropologic studies with the biologic and psychological literature to produce a comprehensive view of play. He also called attention to the sociopolitical forces that influence patterns of play.

Another giant in the play literature is Huizinga,[5] a Dutch historian whose classic *Homo Ludens* presented the thesis that the impulse to play was the driving force in the emergence of civilization. Rather than consigning play to a supportive role in maintaining culture, Huizinga considered play to be the origin of cultural forms. His argument that civilization springs from play is bolstered by fascinating examples of the play element in such wide-ranging arenas of human experience as law, philosophy, poetry, myth, art, and war.

Although most writers in the field of psychology relegate play to a trivial, or at best secondary, position in relation to cognitive or sociobehavioral constructs, Csikszentmihalyi[22] is an exception. He began a distinguished career of scholarship with a focus on the dynamics of play in the creative arts. Over the years, his thinking about play was transformed into a sophisticated model of a process he calls "flow." A person who is in flow, according to Csikszentmihalyi, is completely absorbed in a satisfying autotelic activity. When this conceptual framework is adopted, the dichotomy between work and play dissipates, because flow can occur during activities conventionally classified as work just as easily as those considered play.

Another exceptional writer in the field of psychology is Cohen,[23] a filmmaker turned psychologist. In his qualitative study of his own children, he focused on the ecology of play in the home and pleaded that an individual's play be interpreted within the context of the everyday social environment.

Reilly,[1] of course, is the scholar within the field of occupational therapy who spearheaded an effort to develop a deep understanding of play as a cornerstone of occupational behavior. Her strategy for managing the "cobweb" of play was to use a systems approach to organize its biological, psychological, and social elements. Several of her students, such as Florey,[24] Knox,[25] Takata,[26] and Robinson[27] contributed influential papers on play that have shaped practice and theory development in the field.

My message in this cursory review is to take heed of where the primary focus of study lies when using the work of authors who have written about play. Those for whom play is a secondary concern make important contributions to our understanding of play, but they tend to present only a fragmented or incomplete picture. If we were to embrace wholly their perspectives on play, we may end up contributing more to knowledge of cognition, socialization, psychophysiology, or whatever the main interest is, rather than to play itself. A familiar example is the Piagetian approach to play assessment,[28] which all too easily slips us into evaluating cognitive stages. When such an approach is used in occupational therapy practice, we may end up looking like "minipsychologists," offering nothing unique to occupational therapy. Reliance on scholars for whom play is a focal concern is likely to be most valuable in our quest to understand play as occupation; that, naturally, is our goal in occupational science.

Why Is Play Important?

Now I will turn to the final question raised in this paper: Why is it important for people to play? Why is it so important for us, as occupational therapists, to understand it? Answers to these questions spring from the work of play theorists and become implicit assumptions underlying our clinical practices with play.

The Functionalist View

The most popular view of why play is important is that it serves other functions, such as motor or cognitive development. I call this the functionalist view of play. This view clearly dominates in our clinical applications of play. It may result in the fragmentation of play if functions are considered in isolation, for example, if play is used to assess or promote discrete gross motor, manipulative, self-care, social, or cognitive skills. Often, however, following in the footsteps of Reilly and her students, therapists using a functional approach consider play as a vehicle for integrating multiple developmental skills. The occupational behavior approach, for example, tells us that when the child is playing, she is learning rules—rules about how her body works, what she can do with objects, and how social interactions are systematically patterned.[1,27] An excellent example of a clinical play assessment that incorporates an integrative view of play is Knox's Preschool Play Scale,[25] which includes an ecologic component and developmental features that are intrinsic to the child.

Reilly's[29] dictum that play in childhood prepares the individual for the worker role epitomizes the functional view from an occupational perspective. This view, presaged by Freud and Piaget, tells us that play serves adaptation in the long run. It is tempting, and often appropriate, to use such a functionalist view to justify using play in our treatment programs. If this is our sole justification for using play, however, some important implications need reckoning. If preparation for an adult worker role is the only reason to use play, then we would not work as clinicians with terminally ill children (or at least we would not use play with them), because they are not the workers of the future.

What does a functionalist position tell us about adult play? Do adults play, and if so, is their play of any significance? The developmental continuum of occupational behavior from childhood play to adult work seems to exclude the notion of adult play.[29] It seems that in our literature, the term "leisure" replaces "play" in reference to adulthood, perhaps because "leisure" is considered to be more respectable than the frivolous term "play" in our culture. This is supported by the fact that many definitions of leisure are indistinguishable from definitions of play.[30] A closer look at the occupational behavior literature reveals that Reilly[31] did view leisure and recreation as important in adulthood insofar as they comprise pockets of time that are a separate framework and prepare the individual to return to work, having been refreshed and relaxed. Once again, we have a functionalist justification, with play (now called leisure or recreation) subserving work.

As compelling and essential as the functionalist view of play may be, I suspect that at the heart of occupational therapy values lies something that transcends it. Clinicians do encourage play in terminally ill children despite the fact that many developmental achievements, particularly those related to adult work skills and roles, will never be acquired.[32] Clinicians do value play in adult patients, albeit cloaked in the disguise of leisure and recreation, even when those patients are not workers and have little potential for becoming productive workers in the future. Why do occupational therapists think play is important in these cases, in which the functionalist justification falls apart?

Play For Its Own Sake

Play is important for its own sake, not only because it subserves other important functions. The experience of pleasure in the here and now, the expression of *joie de vivre*, is health promoting.[6] Furthermore, play is a vehicle for meaning. Watching a person at play reveals what is important to him or her, what provides satisfaction and makes life worth living. Occupational therapists would do well to identify the themes of meaning that occur during the play of adults and children with whom we work and to search for opportunities to incorporate or expand on these themes. From this perspective, play becomes a quality of life issue for the present and the future. It is an expression of our humanity throughout the lifespan, not simply a relaxing agent, but an active ingredient of a healthy, satisfying lifestyle.

Some may argue that reimbursement constraints mandate the functionalist view. My response is that we need to be more than pawns of the reimbursement system. If we believe that play is important in its own right, aren't we responsible as members of a profession to take an active stance in promoting this view? This responsibility will certainly involve generating knowledge regarding how play shapes quality of life and mediates health. Equipped with this kind of knowledge, we are empowered with the potential to influence public policy and private industry for the betterment of all.

One challenge to occupational science is to learn more about the process of play as it is experienced by individuals throughout the day. I am not referring to the traditional time log that neatly sequences occupations into discrete slots of time. Rather, we need to begin to examine how play is enfolded within many occupations, including what we typically call work. One avenue for this line of inquiry might be to study playfulness. Is it a quality that can be identified and nurtured? Should we be concerned with flow?[22] If so, we might strive to study how we can create flow experiences for our patients, whether they are children with learning disabilities or physically disabled men in rehabilitation programs.

Another path of inquiry for occupational science might be to identify play styles. Do children demonstrate clear preferences for play activities involving, for example, objects versus people or detailed precision versus broad gestalt configurations? If such play styles exist in childhood, is there continuity into adulthood? That is, do they predispose toward particular work habits and play preferences later in life?

Scholars in occupational science have their work set out before them: to gain clarity about the what, how, and why of play and to add knowledge of the when and where of play in relation to the everyday occupations of individuals. The knowledge that results will stimulate new avenues for occupational therapy practice—how to assess play, nurture it, and justify programs designed to promote health through play.

Acknowledgments

This work was supported in part by a grant from the Bureau of Maternal and Child Health (Grant #MCJ 009048).

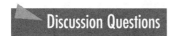

Discussion Questions

1. Parham discusses several advantages and limitations of the functionalist view of play with respect to its therapeutic applications. What are each of these, and what implications do they have for the practice of occupational therapy with children and adults?
2. What are critical dimensions of play? That is, what does and does not constitute play?
3. What does occupational therapy's historic use of play as a therapeutic medium convey about our understanding of play's importance?

References

1. Reilly, M: Play as Exploratory Learning. Sage, Beverly Hills, 1974.
2. Takata, N: The play milieu—A preliminary appraisal. Am J Occup Ther 25:281, 1971.
3. Loizos, C: Play in mammals. In Jewell PA, and Loizos C (eds): Play, Exploration, and Territory in Mammals. The Zoological Society of London, London, 1966, pp 6–8.
4. Nachmanovich, S: Free Play: Improvisation in Life and Art. Jeremey P. Tarcher, Los Angeles, 1990.

5. Huizinga, J: Homo Ludens: A Study of the Play Element in Culture. Beacon Press, Boston, 1950 (Original work published in 1938).
6. Ornstein, R, and Sobel, D: Health Pleasures. Addison-Wesley, Reading, MA, 1989.
7. Groos, K: The Play of Animals. Appleton, New York, 1898.
8. Vandenburg, B: Play and development from an ethological perspective. Amer Psychol 33:724, 1978.
9. Bruner, JS: Nature and uses of immaturity. Amer Psychol 27:687, 1972.
10. Berlyne, DE: Curiosity and exploration. Science 153:25, 1966.
11. Hutt, C: Exploration and play in children. In Jewell PA, and Loizos C (eds): Play, Exploration, and Territory in Mammals. The Zoological Society of London, London, 1966, pp 61–81.
12. Berlyne, DE: Laughter, humor, and play. In Lindzey G, and Aronson E (eds): The Handbook of Social Psychology (Vol 3). Addison-Wesley, Reading, MA, 1969.
13. Piaget, J: Play, Dreams, and Imitation in Childhood. (Gattegno C, and Hodgson FM, trans.). Norton, New York, 1962 (Originally published in 1951).
14. Erikson, EH: Childhood and Society, 2nd ed. Norton, New York, 1963.
15. Bateson, G: Steps to an Ecology of Mind. Ballantine Books, New York, 1972.
16. Whiting, JWM, and Child, IL: Child-training and Personality: A Cross-cultural Study. Yale University Press, New Haven, CT, 1953.
17. Ayres, AJ: Sensory Integration and the Child. Western Psychological Services, Los Angeles, 1979.
18. Lindquist, JE, Mack, W, and Parham, LD: A synthesis of occupational behavior and sensory integration concepts in theory and practice, Part 2: Clinical applications. Am J Occup Ther 36:433, 1982.
19. Sutton-Smith, B: The playful modes of knowing. In Curry, N, and Arnaud, S (eds): Play: The Child Strives Toward Self-Realization. Proceedings of the Conference Sponsored by the Arsenal Family and Children's Center, Western Psychiatric Institute and Clinic, School of Medicine, and Department of Child Development and Child Care, School of Health Related Professions, University of Pittsburgh, and the National Association for the Education of Young Children. National Association for the Education of Young Children, Washington, DC, 1971, pp 13–25.
20. Dolhinow, PJ, and Bishop, NH: The development of motor skills and social relationships among primates through play. In Hill, JP (ed): Minnesota Symposium on Child Psychology. University of Minnesota Press, 1970, pp 180–198.
21. Sutton-Smith, B: The Folkgames of Children. University of Texas Press, Austin, 1972.
22. Csikszentmihalyi, M: Beyond Boredom and Anxiety. Jossey-Bass, San Francisco, 1987.
23. Cohen, D: The Development of Play. New York University Press, New York, 1987.
24. Florey, LL: An approach to play and play development. Am J Occup Ther 25:275, 1971.
25. Knox, S: A play scale. In Reilly, M (ed): Play as Exploratory Learning. Sage, Beverly Hills, 1974, pp 247–271.
26. Takata, N: Play as a prescription. In Reilly, M (ed): Play as Exploratory Learning. Sage, Beverly Hills, 1974, pp 209–246.
27. Robinson, A: Play: The arena for acquisition of rules for competent behavior. Am J Occup Ther 31:248, 1977.
28. Parham, LD: Play Development and Sensorimotor Abilities in Autistic Children: A Piagetian Approach to Clinical Assessment. Unpublished master's thesis, University of Southern California, Los Angeles, 1980.
29. Reilly, M: Occupational behavior—A perspective on work and play. Am J Occup Ther 25:291, 1974.
30. Godbey, G: Leisure in Your Life, 3rd ed. Venture Publishing, State College, PA, 1990.
31. Reilly, M: A psychiatric occupational therapy program as a teaching model. Am J Occup Ther 20:61, 1966.
32. Pizzi, M: Pediatric AIDS: OT assessment and treatment. OT Week, pp 6–7, 10, November 23, 1989.

by Susan H. Knox, MA, OTR, FAOTA

Play and Playfulness in Preschool Children

Methodology

Findings and Data Analysis

Characteristics of the Playful Child and the Less Playful Child

Categories of Play and Their Effect on Playfulness

Environmental and Caregiver Influences

Issues of Credibility and Plans for the Future

Conclusions

- A group of boys is playing with tricycles. They are having a race on what they call "fast bikes." One boy says to his friend, "You get in back of me. We need more wheels."
- Two boys are playing in a child-sized kitchen, pretending to cook and set the table. All of a sudden one of them starts moving the furniture around and makes a climbing structure.
- Two girls are sitting on a suspended tire swing while a third girls spins them around. They are all squealing and laughing.

These three episodes illustrate some of the elements that make play fun for children: the imagination that turns tricycles into "fast bikes," the imitation of parents cooking, the fun of changing the rules in the middle of a game that turns it into a completely different game, or the joy of fast swinging and spinning.

Occupational science is concerned with the individual as an occupational being. The study of play behavior of children from a phenomenologic perspective is vital to understanding the occupations of children. Qualitative methods of inquiry are particularly appropriate for the study of play behavior and can capture the richness of this phenomenon. In this study, the phenomenon of play is explored in the preschool child using a qualitative approach. Playfulness is examined in terms of how it is manifested by the preschool child and in terms of adult and environmental influences.

Playfulness is present to some degree in all children. However, there is a continuum of playfulness, with children in certain situations showing greater or lesser degrees. Playfulness has been described in the literature from the perspective of personality characteristics or traits innate in the child. Lieberman defined five dimensions of playfulness: physical spontaneity, cognitive spontaneity, social spontaneity, manifest joy, and sense of humor.[1] Other studies by Truhon and Barnett[2-6] have used these categories and have elaborated on them. Barnett developed a rating scale on which teachers and caregivers can rate a child's playfulness.

However, playfulness cannot be viewed only in terms of inherent traits. A child's activity can never be isolated from the environment within which the child is playing nor from other familial, social, and cultural influences. The presence or absence of other people or animals, the physical setting, the availability of toys or other objects with which to interact, have a profound effect on children's play. Many studies have examined the effects of the quality of care and types of interactions between caregivers and children in play behavior. They found, among other things, that socioeconomic status, variations in home environment, and variations in the quality of day care programs have substantial effects on children's activities in terms of social interaction and levels of play, imaginary play, and creativity.

Methodology

This study uses a ground theory approach, as described by Glaser and Strauss[7] and Corbin and Strauss,[8] in which data collection and analysis are interrelated by allowing concepts to arise from the data, which are then analyzed and further developed. Concepts are considered provisional until they are proven through continued scrutiny. Because this was a preliminary work, the concepts developed from it are therefore still regarded as provisional.

The data were analyzed by open, axial, and selective coding. In open coding, the data are broken down analytically, compared, and given conceptual labels. Through open coding of field notes and interviews, play properties, actions, interactions, and characteristics of playful and nonplayful children were designated and grouped into categories. Two main research questions emerged: 1) How is playfulness manifested? and 2) How do adult involvement and environment influence a child's play? Axial coding relates categories and tests them against the data. Axial coding resulted in further delineation of categories relating concepts from personal experience, from experiences of people who were interviewed, and from the literature. When selecting coding, all the categories are unified around "core" categories. Three primary categories were selected, which are discussed later.

Two primary methods of data collection were used for this study: observations and interviews. The child care center for the children of hospital employees at Glendale Adventist Medical Center in Glendale, California, was chosen for the research setting. This setting is located on the hospital grounds in two old houses. This child care center is not typical of child care centers in many aspects and may represent more of an ideal setting due to the educational background of the staff, available resources, and amount of parent involvement. Another proprietary center was visited to note differences and similarities, while the perceptions of the director and the teachers, who also spoke of differences between this center and others from their experiences, were noted.

The Center was visited 15 times during 3 months for field observations and interviews. Interviews were conducted with the Director of the Center, one parent, three teachers, and one teaching assistant. Two older groups of children, ages 18 months to 3 years and 3 to 5.5 years, were observed.

Through the observations, certain children stood out as being very playful, and others always seemed to be on the fringe of activities. By attending to these polar types of children, elements of playfulness and influences that seemed to foster or inhibit play were identified. Through the interviews, the teachers' and parents' views of the same children were obtained. From observations and interviews, a number of environmental factors that affected playfulness, from parent and teacher encouragement to the way in which the physical environment was set up, were additionally gleaned.

Findings and Data Analysis

The data were analyzed from observations and interviews, and a number of conceptual categories were formulated. First, actions and behaviors that differentiated more playful children from less playful children were identified. Second, different categories of play that were observed in all the children were identified. Within these categories, certain activities seemed to provoke more playful behavior than others. Third, factors in the immediate environment and factors in the home environment that affected observed amounts of playfulness and observed types of activities were identified.

Characteristics of the Playful Child and the Less Playful Child

The playful child showed flexibility in play and often became the center of action (Fig. 9–1). Some of the characteristics observed in playful children included curiosity, imagination, joy, physical activity, and social and verbal flexibility. One teacher, when describing a playful child, said, "She takes such joy in things, in discovering things, in talking about things." The more playful children generally seemed to be in charge of the play situations. They were creative and often elaborated on games or episodes that others started, gradually making them their own. Playful children set up situations, and others often added to them, creating wonderful sequences. For example, some children constructed a "road" and pretended they were different kinds of vehicles going along it. A number of the playful children were described as leaders or "bosses."

Children who were less playful might start games, but as soon as someone else took the lead, they would retreat to following or onlooker status. These children often lacked spontaneity and flexibility to go with the flow of a play episode; as a result, their play was often more stereotyped and immature. Other character-

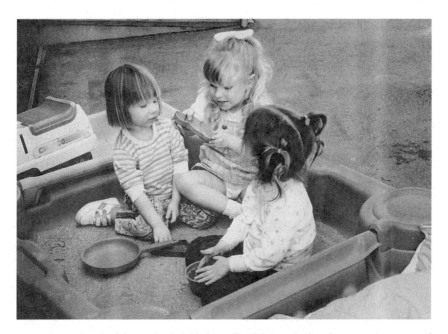

Figure 9–1. The playful preschool child shows flexibility and often becomes the center of attention. (Photo by Susan Knox.)

istics of the child with diminished playfulness included negative affect or verbalizations, physical or emotional withdrawal, lack of control over a situation, refusal to participate, preference for adults or younger children, and emotional immaturity. Less playful children were described as "solemn," "a solo artist," and "more into their own little world."

Although there were clear distinctions between playful and less playful children, most of the characteristics fell along continua with children being more or less playful at different times and under a variety of circumstances (Fig. 9–2). This led to investigation of how different types of activities, that is, categories of play, and different types of environment influence playfulness.

Categories of Play and Their Effect on Playfulness

Throughout the observations, the tremendous diversity exhibited in the children's play suggested why play is of such importance in a child's life. All of these children showed a rich repertoire of behavior and playfulness. I originally developed play categories in earlier studies, which were used to examine the kinds of play that seemed to evoke playful behavior.[9,10] These categories are space management, material management, imitation, and participation.

Space management refers to the way a child learns to manage his or her body and the space around him or her. The types of activities included in this category are gross motor actions, playground activities, activities that provide primarily sensory input, and exploratory activities. Examples might include climbing a structure

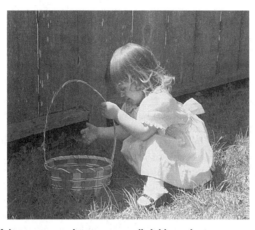

Figure 9–2. Playfulness seems to be present in all children, there is a continuum of playfulness with children in certain situations showing greater or lesser degrees. This preschooler engaged in solitary play shows a moderate degree of playfulness. (Photo by Shay McAfee.)

and sliding down, dancing, or spinning around to music. These types of activities elicited great playfulness, especially when more than one child was involved.

Material management refers to the manner in which a child handles material. This category includes sensorimotor manipulation of objects and construction activities, such as building sand castles. Certain materials that could be used in a variety of ways were part of the more playful activities. For example, depending on the imagination of the child, bristle blocks could be used as skates by attaching wheels, made into birthday cakes or guns, or used as lipsticks or baby bottles. Many activities in which the materials required more structured manipulation, such as puzzles or pegboards, did not evoke particularly playful responses. The children readily chose and participated in them, but their creativity, joy, and imagination were not as evident. Solitary activities, although they might be creative, did not evoke playful responses. On the other hand, many children entered into construction activities, particularly with large blocks, and often these became the setting for elaborate and playful imaginary sequences. Almost always at the end of these games, the children gleefully destroyed the structures they had built with great fanfare.

The category of imitation is important because through observation and imitation, children learn a great deal about their world. This category includes imitation of peers and adults, imaginative play, and dramatization. The children at this center spent a lot of time in activities that tapped their imaginations; even the younger children created long sequences with dolls and cars. Imagination also was evident when the children used play materials in unusual ways. One activity that almost always elicited joy and joyful movement was music. Books could evoke playful episodes when shared by two or three children, with the children dramatizing a story.

Participation refers to the amount and manner of interaction with people in the environment and includes the amount of independence and cooperation demonstrated in play. This category includes the social dimensions of play and language.

One important observation was that activities that evoked more playfulness were child initiated and directed. This has great relevance for the amount of and type of adult involvement in play and leads into the next area of discussion.

Environmental and Caregiver Influences

Environmental and caregiver characteristics that evoke or inhibit play are as important as the inherent characteristics of the child. In this setting, the repertoire of playful behavior was vast, partially due to the environment and partially to the director's and teachers' philosophy of learning and of play. All of the teachers and parents agreed that playfulness could be evoked or inhibited by the physical environment or people in the child's life. Environmental characteristics that affected playfulness were the presence of a variety of toys and objects, provision of novelty, and multiple opportunities. The teachers cited a number of caregiver behaviors that evoked play: being loving, nurturing, and relaxed; entering into play with the child, but on the child's terms; being an example for the child by being playful; enticing the child; picking up and responding to the child's cues and elaborating on them; encouraging curiosity; being interested in the child's activity; and allowing freedom. One teacher stated that "All children are playful, it just needs to be encouraged by the adults."

Everyone emphasized the importance of giving the children choices. Although teachers daily set up a variety of opportunities and play materials from which the children chose, they did not influence the children's choices.

The teachers also spoke about the importance of the family in influencing playfulness. When the parents fostered play behavior and were interested in the child's activity and accomplishments, the child tended to be more playful. When teachers noticed a child who was not playful, they usually cited familial influences. Typical of the comments were, "Her home environment sometimes dictates how she acts out," and "What's going on in the home . . . affects the child." Similar conclusions were reported by Howes and Stewart[11] in their study of family and child care influences on child's play. They found that family characteristics, child care quality, and degrees of stress and restrictions were important influences on play and resulted in differences in the child's social competence with peers.

Issues of Credibility and Plans for the Future

In qualitative research, questions arise as to the value and soundness of the particular research. Marshall and Rossman recommend four criteria on which to evaluate the soundness of a study: credibility, transferability, dependability, and confirmability.[12] Credibility means that the study was conducted in such a manner as to ensure that the subject was accurately identified and described. In this study, children of a variety of ages were observed for at least 1 hour each time in indoor and outdoor settings. Therefore, within a particular observation period, many different activities were observed for each child and in their entirety. Because play episodes often last a long time, the richness of a variety of observed activities was not jeopardized by shorter observation periods. Nevertheless, the play of children in this setting was not compared with their play in other settings.

Transferability means that the findings can be applied to another context. Because this study involved detailed observations at only one setting, it may not offer a representative sample. In-depth observation at a variety of settings would be necessary to reveal ethnic and socioeconomic differences and varying amounts of caregiver encouragement or structure.

Dependability accounts for changing conditions in the phenomenon. Play behavior is inseparable from the culture within which it occurs. Therefore, it is very susceptible to changes in conditions. This study speaks only to these particular children in this particular setting at this particular time. Even small changes, such as a change in staff, would probably alter the data somewhat.

Confirmability addresses objectivity. A commitment was made to look at the full continuum of playfulness. When choosing to interview teachers and teachers' assistants with varying viewpoints, theoretical sampling also was undertaken. The researcher's perspective as a pediatric occupational therapist favors children having choices and being active participants in their activities. Therefore, this particular setting and the philosophy of the teachers were similar to that of the researcher. For this reason, other settings with differing philosophies need to be examined. All of these issues pertaining to credibility, transferability, dependability, and confirmability will be addressed more fully in the continuation of this research.

Conclusions

In summary, the study of children's play behavior and of playfulness is important for occupational scientists. It can yield rich and valuable information to further our understanding of the importance of play as the child's primary occupation. When examining a daily activity that is so varied and all-encompassing, qualitative methods are most useful. This study accordingly used extended observations and interviews to examine playfulness in preschool children in a child care center. Children were described in terms of playful characteristics, while their play was described in terms of categories or types, with particular emphasis on those types that tended to foster playfulness. Also described were play settings and caregivers in terms of factors that evoke or inhibit play and playfulness. Although the results are preliminary, these factors have important implications for planning child care. Most fundamentally, factors that foster playfulness, such as child-directed activities and opportunities for choice, need to be valued and encouraged.

Discussion Questions

1. What "weight" should occupational therapists place on eliciting and supporting playfulness in children with disabilities relative to the more traditional focus on helping to develop actual play skills?
2. Is there a competition between these dual concerns in that attention to one necessarily detracts from attention to the other?

References

1. Lieberman, J: Playfulness: Its Relationship to Imagination and Creativity. Academic Press, New York, 1977.
2. Barnett, L: Playfulness: Definition, design, and measurement. Play and Culture 3:319, 1990.
3. Barnett, L: The playful child: Measurement of a disposition to play. Play and Culture 4:51, 1991.
4. Barnett, L, and Kleiber, D: Concomitants of playfulness in early childhood: Cognitive abilities and gender. J Genet Psychol 141:115, 1982.
5. Barnett, L, and Kleiber, D: Playfulness and the early play environment. J Genet Psychol 144:153, 1984.
6. Truhon, S: Playfulness, play, and creativity: A path analytic model. J Genet Psychol 143:19, 1983.
7. Glaser, B, and Strauss, A: The Discovery of Grounded Theory. Aldine de Gruyter, New York, 1967.
8. Corbin, J, and Strauss, A: Grounded theory research: Procedures, canons, and evaluative criteria. Qual Sociol 13:1, 1990.
9. Knox, S: Observation and assessment of the everyday play behavior of the mentally retarded child. Unpublished master's thesis, University of Southern California.
10. Knox, S: A play scale. In Reilly M (ed.): Play as Exploratory Learning. Sage Publications, Beverly Hills, 1974.
11. Howes, C, and Stewart, P: Child's play with adults, toys, and peers: An examination of family and child care influences. Develop Psychol 23:423, 1987.
12. Marshall, C, and Rossman, G: Designing Qualitative Research. Sage Publications, Newbury Park, CA, 1989.

Dimensions of Occupation

Human occupation occurs in a matrix of time and space and is more apt to be repeated under certain conditions. Just as history focuses on events in time and geography is the study of place, particularly as it affects human activity, occupational science focuses on the study of occupation. It then draws from disciplines such as history, anthropology, geography, and social psychology to gain a sense of how time, place, seasonal changes and cycles, and other factors influence occupation. It is fascinating, for example, to learn from anthropology and sociology that, whereas !Kung San people devote only 2.5 days per week (6 hr/day) to work, "overworked" Americans spend far more time on this occupation, with one fourth spending 49 or more hours per week on the job.[1] Is this difference in quality of life due to the constraints of place, cultural demand and traditions, or ethics? Questions like this are generated and sometimes answered by searching interdisciplinary literature that illuminates aspects of human occupation. This section includes papers that begin to address the question of how time and place influence occupation and under what conditions occupations are apt to be repeated.

In the first paper of this section, Alexander Moore describes the activity spectra of band (hunter-gatherer) communities from an anthropologic perspective. Just as Goodall documented activity patterns in chimpanzees, Moore draws from the scholarly work of his colleagues to present a coherent picture of the daily, annual, and generational cycles of occupation of band communities. What is the day like for hunter-gatherers? Moore illustrates that the daily activities of such groups are regulated in part by organismic requirements, by the necessity to maintain social harmony with others, and by seasonal and climatic changes. As already stated, the "work weeks" of such groups are more relaxed than those of more technological civilizations. On a typical day, hunter-gatherers do their work, which may include hunting and gathering, housework, fetching firewood, tool manufacture, cleaning up, or drawing water, but they also have a considerable chunk of time left for play or leisure. Routinely, the daily cycle closes around the hearth or campfire, where "talking" or story telling is central for synchronizing or entraining all activities.

In addition to daily cycles, Moore describes the annual and generational cycles of activity. Groups change and move around in synchrony with the seasons and weather. Moreover, the geography associated with their migrations molds the activity patterns of hunter-gatherers. Finally, generational cycles are punctuated with rites of passage, which help to move individuals into new situations and redefine human bonds.

Moore's perspective is of particular interest to occupational therapists for two reasons. First, it illuminates the central place that ordinary occupations have in maintaining social order. Just as grooming in chimpanzee communities helps assure the stability of harmonious social relations, talking and storytelling around the campfire in !Kung communities are a powerful means of social control and of managing conflict. This occupation also is the means through which their daily and seasonal activities and the rites of passage associated with generational cycles are entrained. Can Moore's work sensitize therapists to the need to uncover the potency of certain daily activities in the lives of patients? Can it inspire therapists to ask not only what their patients do each day, but also what the overt and less obvious, but perhaps more important, functions of those activities are? Can therapists begin to see as one of their key roles the unpacking of the full meaning of daily activities as they are embedded in the cultures and experiences of their patients?

Secondly, Moore's paper alerts us to the importance of thinking about the lives of patients in terms of daily, seasonal, annual, and generational cycles. Just as a puberty ritual effects a transformation of state in a young girl, so does rehabilitation move a patient from one stage of life to another. Understanding this aspect of rehabilitation may help therapists effectively aid patients in making the transition into the next phase in which they will find themselves: leaving the hospital, usually re-entering the world from which they came but in a new status.

Dear's paper, "Space, Time, and the Geography of Everyday Life," encourages us to think about the ways in which place constrains or encourages human occupation. The paper begins with a glimpse of what a day might be like were it not bound by time, space, and resources. In such circumstances, one could spend the morning skiing in the Alps, followed by a swim in Barbados, and then dinner in Paris. However, as Dear points out, in the real world, the time-space prism rapidly constricts. "Society may be conceived of as a time-space fabric, on which the biographies of individual lives are engraved." He then describes how the time-space fabric imposes limits on the daily activities of homeless people.

What if therapists broadened their view of activities of daily living to include a focus on the time-space prism in which their patients must function? A key challenge for people with physical disabilities is trying to adjust to the fact that simple activities may take so much longer, and distances seem to elongate. One patient described the experience of walking 50 feet with her walker from her condominium door to the main gate as comparable to that of a 2-mile hike in her former able-bodied state. Dear's ideas reinforce the practice of therapists who may include in their assessment process the geography with which the patient must contend—the settings of their homes, assuming they are not homeless; floor plans; surroundings; the characteristics of neighborhoods; service and travel options; and so on.

The influence of place and time on human occupation also is addressed in Primeau's paper on human travel. The concern is not so much with place and time as separate dimensions of activity but with the occupation of traveling that enables movement from one locale to another within a given time frame. Efficient travel enables us to move about with a minimal expenditure of time and energy. With the increased suburbanization of America, people are having to spend more time on the occupation of travel. To cope with the drain on daily time available, "polysynchronicity" of occupation is becoming more and more common. While people commute, they now make cellular phone calls, listen to books on tape, enter the talk radio dialogues, and so on. When activities are polysynchronized, several are performed within the same time frame. In such situations, movement through space in time (the occupation of travel) becomes enfolded with other occupations. On the other hand, when one is on vacation, the trip itself may be enjoyed as much as the destination, and getting there may be more than half the fun.

Trip chaining, a concept discussed by Primeau, is a variation of the notion of the polysynchronicity of activity. The emphasis is on space rather than time in that the routes of several activities are overlapped to gain more than one purpose out of a trip. Occupational therapists have traditionally thought about energy conservation with respect to activities of daily living. An occupational science perspective suggests that they also should think about ways to help their patients conserve time and energy in their orchestration of daily occupations through strategies like polysynchronicity and trip chaining. Further, in chimpanzee communities, Goodall documented that increases in aggression were correlated with increases in the amount of territory males chimps had to travel to find food.[2] One wonders whether daily time spent and distance traveled by humans also are related to aggression. It would seem that assessing the daily travel requirements and styles of patients constitutes a logical application of occupational science to occupational therapy.

How do time, space, daily cycles, and other aspects of daily living affect personal productivity? In her qualitative study of the work patterns of scholars, Pierce addresses this issue, choosing as her informants scholars who seem especially able to articulate the way they orchestrate their daily activities to stay productive. Her work gives us a glimpse of the complexity of this enterprise, which involves concerns that Pierce categorized into the following five dimensions: personal definitions of a scholar, spaces, emotions, temporality, and sociocultural context. The first category addresses how the scholars conceive of their occupation. This category includes their definitions of scholarship, the criteria by which they judge its worthiness, the images and analogies that they use to describe the work, and how they perceive the relationships between teaching and scholarship. Interestingly, Pierce found that the scholars tended to describe their work through analogies with other work, with farming the most frequently appearing. Pierce's work gives us important insights into how the scholars approach their work, where they perceive tensions, and what they find most challenging and satisfying about it. The second category called "the spaces of scholars' work" addresses the physiology, tools, and offices that were used by the scholars. Physiologically, the scholars felt they could execute no more than 5 hours of demanding scholarship per day. They then needed to switch to less demanding activity. They also had developed various routines incorporating other occupations that conditioned them for working. Books, offices, and tools, such as the computer, also were necessary. Once again, we can infer that in doing occupational assessment, it may be important to consider how one occupation can be used as a warm up for the next and how spaces and tools can foster engagement in occupation.

The third category that emerged from this study has to do with the emotional experiences of the scholars, which ranged between highs and lows that were tied to their work. This aspect of occupation, that is, its emotional impact and the ways in which emotion fuels occupation, is seldom addressed in the occupational therapy literature. Florey's work, later in Section VIII, emphasizes the devaluation within occupational therapy of the psychosocial aspects of occupation. Pierce's work suggests that during certain occupations, people go through intense emotional experiences; for example, they can agonize about a task or feel ecstatic while working on certain projects, particularly, it seems, when those occupations have a central place in the framework of their lives.

Temporal rhythms also were key to the productivity of scholars. Just as Moore described daily, annual, and generational cycles in the activity spectra of hunter-gatherers, Pierce found that the scholars orchestrated their activities in accord with daily, annual, and personal temporal strategies that enabled them to be disciplined in their work. They talked about phases of work and the difficulty of entering and exiting their scholarly projects.

Finally, the sociocultural context had an impact. The productivity of the scholars was tied to having colleagues available to them, even though most of their work was done in isolation. Although Pierce's study focused on only one occupation, the categories she extracted may have broad relevance. Can we begin to probe how our patients define and experience the occupations in which they engage; what daily, annual, and career cycles their work follows; what personal temporal strategies they use; and how physiology, place, tools, and the sociocultural context impact on their productivity and satisfaction? These are creative avenues that future practitioners may begin to explore. Further, occupational temporality, in which the experience of time is shaped by occupation, may become a vital concern in the treatment process. This study begins to give us important insights on how time is organized, held, and made productive.

Another approach to the study of occupation is represented by Carlson's paper, "The Self-Perpetuation of Occupation." Drawing from the social psychological literature, he provides a synthesis of factors that is likely to enhance the probability that a person will persevere in a particular occupation. Carlson considers this repetitional phenomenon extremely important because "by choosing to engage in a given occupation at the expense of other occupations," the person initiates "a process of prolonged involvement over time that simultaneously both shapes and defines our existence and negates potential alternate expressions of our personhood."

For therapists who have difficulty tapping patient motivation to engage in occupation, Carlson's paper may be particularly helpful. He argues that the "act of participation per se in an occupation often tends to increase future involvement with the same or similar occupations." He uses the term "occupational perseverance" to refer to "prolonged engagement in an occupation that is directly or indirectly related to prior engagement with the occupation in question." Although sometimes it is difficult to initiate, once started, an activity "captures our enthusiasm and renders inscrutable our former procrastination." Carlson suggests that a powerful key to promoting motivation is helping the patient to get started. Once started, further perseverance, according to Carlson, is apt to have its own momentum. Toward the end of the paper, Carlson presents a model of several factors that he has identified that seem to influence occupational perseverance, which therapists may want to consider in their efforts to promote investment of their patients in activity. As Carlson points out, through their knowledge of occupational perseverance, therapists may be able to help patients avoid a syndrome of occupational incoherence, in which they pursue occupations in a "haphazard, inconsistent, or self-defeating manner."

The papers in this section cover dimensions of occupation that therapists may want to emphasize in practice: time, place, daily rhythms, social context, emotional intensity, and the factors that are apt to promote persistence. Therapists will be able to enhance practice by broadening their understanding of occupation as it finds itself embedded in culture, geography, individual lives, and diverse environments.

References

1. Schor, JP: The Overworked American: The Unexpected Decline of Leisure. Basic Books, New York, 1991.
2. Goodall, J: The Chimpanzees of Gombe: Patterns of Behavior. Belknap Press of Harvard University Press, Cambridge, MA, 1986.

by Alexander Moore, PhD

10

The Band Community
Synchronizing Human Activity Cycles for Group Cooperation*

* This paper has been published as a chapter in Moore, A: Cultural Anthropology. Collegiate Press, San Diego, CA, 1992. It has been reprinted by permission and modified only as necessary to match the style of this book.

The Human Community

In biology, community means "breeding population," the unit of the species within which members of the two sexes come together for procreating the next generation and, if necessary, nurturing them to maturity. As biological creatures, human beings also have breeding-population communities. As in the natural world, our community is the unit that orchestrates individual movements in space over time. In our cultural world, community is the setting in which, from one generation to the next, human beings learn how to be fully human. It also is the unit within which culture changes. In short, the community is the unit not only of procreation, socialization, and survival, but of cultural creativity and innovation. It thus is a unit with historical depth in time.

The band is the basic unit of human social life. All other human communities derive, ultimately, from band beginnings. Thus, the band contains, if only in trace forms, foreshadowings of all human future potentials. It also is built on primate antecedents. Like the primate troop, the band includes two sexes, three generations, men in leadership positions, a range over space, and functional interrelations among activities. However, these elements are put together quite differently, in conjunction with others that are wholly lacking, among nonhuman primates.

In contrast with apes, human beings have kinship systems, marriage and the family, social paternity, fully developed ritual complexes, an advanced tool kit, and the most advanced tool of all, language in the form of speech, our extragenetic code. These traits, our culture, made our species the successful hominid, replacing earlier hominid forms.

However, apes exhibit territoriality. They seem genetically programmed to stake out a home area and defend it against neighboring groups. Such territoriality does not apply to bands. Human beings quarrel, but they do not fight over territory. Rather, human beings in band organization tend to flee conflict. It is flight, not fight, for them.

Bands do, like chimpanzee communities, exhibit fission and fusion, whereby the wider community splits into smaller units much of the year and comes together in larger units at given times. Unlike apes, however, human bands assemble as the entire community on certain occasions—the fusion process is much more complete. Moreover, again unlike chimpanzees, human beings also assemble with people coming from other communities on certain other occasions.

Spatial Organization

Thus, there are three levels of spatial organization in human bands. First are the areas of local residence and day-to-day land use. These change in the course of a year as the group splits into its smallest constituent units, which then move out to the furthest reaches of its range. Second, there is the wider area of the community proper, usually named a "country" or band, whose population gathers at some time during the solar year. Third, there are broad circles of overlapping and interacting bands, the areas of foreign relations. No band is closed; all are open to visits and émigrés from other bands.

Within the band, human beings bond into characteristic groupings. The elementary human bonds are first, those of household and family, characterized by a common hearth. Several such households may camp together, forming the local group or constituent camp of the larger band at least part of the year. A circle of campfires or hearths is the first major cultural architectural rendering of space.

Men form hunting parties throughout the year. The constituent hunters vary with time. These are ephemeral coalitions of convenience; hunting parties have never been observed to have hard and fast, invariable, and consequently ritualized memberships. In large hunts, women and children form auxiliary hunting groups, often as "beaters," who beat sticks and drive the game animals toward the men. Women from the same camp likewise form ephemeral hunting-and-gathering parties in the company of their infants. These loose bonds reflect the ubiquitous and pan-human division of labor by sex.

Human juveniles, like all primate juveniles, form play groups whenever the opportunity presents itself. These cut across household and kinship identities and are the prototypical age grade from which much successively differentiated human social organization derives (such as ritual fraternities, age-graded regiments, police forces, guilds, and voluntary associations). At the end of their lives, elders, numerically far fewer than juveniles, also associate with each other, men and women together, and engage in speech rather than play. Elders talk. They reminisce, tell stories, recite myths and genealogies, and chant or sing songs.

Cycles of Activities

Social life among human beings has its local kinetics, that is, its characteristic motions. These form cycles of repetitive activities, processes organized in space and time. From the perspective of ecology, these activities can be seen as composing a factory, which moves materials from the environment to each station. These activities occur in cycles or rounds, the "factory day," after which the sequence of completed actions is ready to be repeated. There are rounds of processing activities for individual human beings (most of them physiologic and internal) and other rounds for human groups.

For example, food enters the mouth of every individual for biologic processing, beginning with chewing. Food is transformed and expended as energy and work or is absorbed as materials to build the body, while waste and by-products are eliminated. The individual must ingest food on a daily basis. This is only one such time-delayed cycle of consumption and transformation of matter and energy.

Similarly, the group is a unit of production and consumption, gathering materials from the environment, processing them, and consuming them in the wider processes of maintaining mature adults, rearing children, and producing offspring. Human beings are produced and passed from station to station, like material goods. As with all living creatures, we, as a group, reproduce ourselves. Finally, at death, our mortal remains must be disposed of like any waste item. In fact, in the early paleolithic period, human beings ceased to treat cadavers as mere discards and began to inter them with grave ornaments and goods. Cadavers became not waste, but products. This is one hallmark distinguishing human beings from all other animals.

Social and Cultural Cycles

Human individuals as factories run through cycles: Communication and perception cycles move neural impulses at 0.1 second and 6 seconds, cycles of ingestion and digestion occur at 3.5-hour intervals, and whole-body cycles occur over 24-hour periods.[1] At the end of each cycle, the "factory day" is over, and activity starts again.

Individuals must perform their own characteristic activities and coordinate them with the activities of others on similar scales. Human beings are characteristically social. Solitary lives as hermits, typical for some primate species, are atypical of human beings.

Individual cycles are entrained, or synchronized, with those of others. This synchronization is visible in typical solar days, in seasonal variations through the year, and in typical life cycles. Anthropologists must take into account generational maturation time (from 20 to 25 years) and lifetime scales (up to 90 years) for those who survive to become elders. Three to five successive cohort lifetimes form the cycles of particular cultures, at which point we can assume that the repertory of repetitive activities may have changed significantly, and in content if not in form, the culture shall have changed.

Thus, culture changes by the small-scale accretion of cultural and stylistic differences invented by particular individuals. Culture also changes in response to outside pressures and instabilities: drought, flood, famine, epidemic, and the incursions of neighboring groups. The individuals with the greatest capacity to effect culture change are shamans transformed into prophets, more specifically known as "revitalization prophets" in the anthropologic literature. In modern society, political prophets (such as Lenin) fulfill the same general creative capability, as do, as a class, intellectuals.

Let us examine the typical cycles of activities of a hunting-and-gathering band. Our discussion relies most heavily on ethnographies of the !Kung San people of the Kalahari desert[2,3] and of Australian aborigines, namely the Tiwi of Bathurst and Melville Islands.[4,5] The Tiwi exhibit greater social complexity than the !Kung, based on the same spectrum of traits. Together they represent much of the range of band societies. The Eskimos, with their extreme Arctic adaptations, differ from temperate and tropical band people by their relatively greater dependence on hunting rather than gathering.

The Daily Cycle and Cycles of Days

At dawn, a hunting-and-gathering camp universally wakes up from the sleeping positions of its various members around their campfires. A hearth is the station of a household, its gate for receiving uncooked food. This intimate use of fire is a universal trait of our species. The hearth is the crucible of family life, symbolically and energetically. The more settled dry-season villages among the !Kung San people consist of circles of huts, each with its hearth directly outside and in front of it. A wide plaza for collective life is defined by the circle of campfires.

Richard Lee tells us that !Kung San villages are surrounded by a "zone of elimination" for household trash and bodily wastes.[2,3] Presumably, eliminative behavior takes place privately and individually as each person wakes up and retreats behind the scenes, so to speak. Lee does not mention breakfast,[2,3] but Hart et al.[5] tell us that the Tiwi have a light breakfast of leftovers from the main evening meal of the previous day before setting off on their quest for food.

The gathering activities of women are daily and a constant source of food for hunting-and-gathering people, but not all women gather daily. Lee[3] measured work effort (in terms of hours per week) against calories collected for a !Kung San rainy-season village. In the 4 rainy-season weeks he measured, women were less active than men, putting in only 40 hours per week, or 5.7 hours a day. Of these, only 12.6 hours were spent on "subsistence work." Assuming that women gathered each day, their collecting activities averaged only 1.8 hours a day. In fact, neither men nor women worked at subsistence every day. Women put only about 2 days a week into gathering, while men put in 2.7 days at gathering and hunting. Men put in longer work weeks, 44.5 hours as opposed to the women (40 hours), and longer subsistence work weeks, too, 21.6 hours a week as opposed to 12.6 hours. Even so, women contributed more calories to the !Kung diet than men did, about 55% as opposed to 45%.

Housework, which Lee defined as drawing water and gathering firewood, processing and cooking food, and washing and cleaning, occupies 22.4% of a woman's hours per week. Thus, women may not necessarily gather food every day, but they certainly cook it and do other housework every day. Lee's approach illustrates some of the difficulties social scientists have in reaching a dynamic approach based on the natural history of energetics, not an imposed, rigid, yet mythical Western conceptual scheme of weeks, hours, and statistical averages. The week in this case is not an "etic" or native unit, because the !Kung San have no formal calendar, much less 6 days of work with a Sabbath day of rest, which is what the Western week is.

It is clear that the circle of !Kung households must synchronize their efforts with one another, just as members of a household must entrain their activities with one another. The result is a set of subsistence cycles forming a loose yet keenly coordinated program. Thus, the solar day is a temporal unit of food preparation at all hearths. The food preparation and consumption cycle culminates each day in the evening meal around the fire. The temporal unit of subsistence activity, on the other hand, is a 3-day cycle for any household, at least for food gathering. The male hunting cycle is perhaps more on the rhythm of a 4- to 6-day cycle. Men bring in fewer calories from hunting because empty-handed returns are frequent, even when balanced by bonanzas of larger game brought down by hunting teams.

The circle of camps is entrained or meshed through interhousehold kinship ties. Richer households that are more populous or blessed with energetic, talented "overachievers" share their bounty with importuning kinfolk, also at the evening meal. Such sharing is characteristic of the wider cycle of activities as a whole, and its relevant time scale also is the solar year.

Other activities that must go on in some household every solar day include tool manufacture and maintenance. The !Kung have approximately 28 "tools and devices" and wardrobes of animal hides. Lee's weekly averages of toolwork per individual come to 1 hour a day for men and 45 minutes for women. Once again, these tasks must be entrained differently, depending on the nature of the task and the skill of the worker, the cycle of demand, and need within the household ("Wife, will you please mend our basket"), and the cycle of such demands outside the household ("I must give that basket to your father, my father-in-law").

A typical day, then, has some individuals in a wider camp or village dispersing in the morning for the activities of gathering food, hunting, fetching firewood, and drawing water. Others remain in camp to clean up or to make and maintain tools. The day reaches its climax at the evening meal. During the day, children form play groups. Individual children, like all primates, also play with older kin one at a time. Indeed, given so much leisure time for the adults of band culture, we would expect a great many recreational activities. One of these, talking at campfires in the evenings, is of prime importance for synchronizing or entraining all activities.

A "typical" day would be one not marked by any events with cycles that fall on some other time scale. Thus, hunts by hunting parties are on some weekly to monthly scale. Among the !Kung, the size of the hunting party must vary with the size of the seasonal settlement. The large villages of the peak rainy and dry seasons have more men available for the formation of hunting teams.

The Annual Cycle

The !Kung form different settlements during the solar year based on the alteration between warming wet (spring and summer) and cooling dry (autumn, winter, early spring) seasons. From about May to October, dry-season villages form at waterholes. These groupings are identified with a "country," and the core residents are said to "own" it. In other words, this grouping is the band proper. These villages range in size from 8 to 15 huts. Populations here and in all seasons fluctuate from year to year.

Rainy-season villages are more ephemeral, only 3 weeks rather than 3 months, but may be larger (from 3 to 30 huts) because they are located near some substantial food resource that has come into season. Moreover, they may be composed of people coming from several bands.

Spring and fall camps lack huts altogether and may merely indicate stopping places as one or more constituent households of the larger band move away from the waterhole village in the beginning of the wet season or toward it in the beginning of the dry season. Overnight stops are simply hearths constructed where "the group," which can be as small as a hunting party of a few men, spends the night while ranging around.

The Tiwi in many respects exhibit internal complexity of the same patterns found among the less complicated !Kung while retaining similar overall or exterior form. Their household structure is most complex. They are polygynous. A few older men have many wives, some adult men have a few wives, and young men have no wives. Adolescent men are isolated in age grades, yet the community is still very much the hunting-and-gathering band.

We are not told much about Tiwi teams for hunting, except in the seasonal kangaroo hunts that are organized by elders, who call up all the men of several camps. They burn off grasslands in this effort, which not only yields a bonanza of meat (everyone gorges themselves for days), but clears the land for easier tracking and hunting. Tiwi boys from age 14 to their early 20s are segregated most of the year in age-graded initiation camps, which provide for their own subsistence. Thus, they organize hunts, too.

The Tiwi likewise assemble and disperse on a yearly schedule. Late in the dry season, neighboring camps unite for grass burns and kangaroo hunts before dispersing into their constituent camps of several households with the beginning of the rains in late October. Most of the households of a given named "country" (band) assemble during the late rainy season, in January and February, for the kulama yam ceremonies, which are at once initiation rites for age-graded male youths and rites of intensification for adult men, who, like the initiates, also must perform songs and dances especially composed for the event.

At the end of the rainy season in early April, Tiwi funerals commence and continue through the dry season. Bodies are interred at death, but funeral ceremonies are delayed until the dry season, when large groups of people can be assembled from many bands by kinship ties.

Thus, band societies spend part of the year dissolved into constituent camps of several households. They assemble as sections of the band on their way home for the !Kung and at kangaroo hunts for the Tiwi. They assemble as the entire band, more or less, at kulama rites for the Tiwi and at the waterhole dry-season village for the !Kung. Finally, they assemble at gatherings that bring in kinfolk and visitors from the wider field of neighboring bands at rainy-season food source villages for the !Kung and at dry-season funerals of elders for the Tiwi.

The Generational Cycle: Coming of Age and Procreating a New Generation

Solar yearly time, with its changing seasons, is entrained with human generational time through ritual: life crisis rites, called rites of passage, are observed on a seasonal schedule. These rituals define units of assemblage in the Tiwi band proper assembling for male initiation rites and in one band hosting others at a funeral.

Rites also redefine human bonds. Among the !Kung, a male youth is initiated into manhood after he kills a large game animal. He is tattooed on one arm. After his second kill, he is tattooed on the other arm and is redefined as someone who can marry. He is probably given a child bride shortly thereafter in a marriage arranged by his and her parents. He is then obliged to live with her parents and work for them ("perform bride service") for the next 8 to 10 years. He frequently marries outside his natal band. When his bride service is over, he and his wife may or may not remain with his in-laws ("affines").

Among the Tiwi, things are more complicated. Male initiation is repeated every year for 6 years in the seasonal kulama yam ceremonies. Ideally, the 14-year-old boy is carried away from his parents by a "mother's brother" contracted by his father. The youth forms a special debt to his ritual sponsor. He also is bonded to his age mates, both his own cohort and those 1 year above and below him.

After full initiation, the Tiwi man also starts bride service, but he is bonded to a putative "mother-in-law" at the latter's puberty ceremony. After her first menstruation, the young woman is segregated for a time in a special hut. Her father thrusts a spear through the young girl's legs and hands it to the young man with the promise of the young woman's first daughter as his wife! The young woman herself, having been promised in marriage before her birth, has already taken up residence with her husband. (No woman among the Tiwi is ever unmarried; each infant girl at birth already has a husband, who does not take her to live with him until she is around 9 years old.)

The point here is not to tell bizarre anecdotes of strange customs, but to illustrate that life crisis rites, even those of initiation, help to move people from station to station in the group and define the generational cycle. Age grades are a factoring out of the juvenile play group into a more pronounced spatial segregation than is the ordinary primate condition. Tiwi initiates move away from home for 6 years. When they are reincorporated, now as potential husbands, they may take up residence where they can perform bride service. It matters not that the bride is unborn in this case, nor that the ritual bonding him to a new unit is his mother-in-law's puberty ceremony rather than his marriage. The principle is the same. He has been passed along to a new station. Moreover, female puberty, with its first menstruation, must inevitably precede marriage, pregnancy, and childbirth.

Thus, one human cycle, that of coming of age and procreating the next generation, is on the order of 25 years, averaging for both sexes. The cycle is faster, generally, for women in band societies. They marry earlier than men and bear children early. This disparity is pronounced among the Tiwi, where girls marry men much older than themselves while still little girls. Tiwi men marry after age 30, and their first wife is usually a widow older than themselves.

The Life Cycles of Elders: The Scale of Cultures

Funerals among the Tiwi are not only life crisis rites restoring the survivors to society, but also rites of intensification defining different bands and debts across bands. Half the kindred of the deceased are defined as "mourners"; the other half are defined as the latter's "employees." The employees do all the menial work of the mourners, even feeding them by hand as if they were infants. They bring fine ceremonial posts. In return, at the end of the ceremony, the employees are repaid with gifts of foodstuffs and valued goods, such as bricks of paint, feather balls, and ceremonial spears. At a funeral, moreover, all the widows of a polygynous householder are remarried, bestowed on new husbands. They, too, are moved from station to station at these ritual events.

Kinship

We now have the materials for seeing the 90-year lifetime cycle. Here, language comes into play again in its subset: kinship systems, which are systems of nomenclature overlying biologic relations. Human beings have these naming systems, which are capable of extending relationships into the distant past and, by tracing common descent, giving us "kin" among distant strangers. Kinship systems reckon descent and provide formal rules for marriage: exchange of partners, alliance of affines, who may marry whom, and who goes to live with whom. Basic to kinship systems is the incest tabu, that forbids people related in the first degree to marry each other.

Kinship, then, is a mechanism to propel individuals from one camp to another and from one band to another in band societies. Over the course of a long lifetime in band societies, certain individuals build up kin ties within any given band. They may well come from outside bands, having married in or sought refuge. They have attracted relatives and in-laws. Eventually, all the people in the in-groups are their kinpersons by blood or marriage. These key elders have attracted people to their bands and bonded them to the in-group through rituals, reinforced by campfire talks and storytelling.

Power

The sources of power, or hierarchical authority, in band society are several. Power rests first of all on consent. Those who do not consent simply leave to join a more congenial band. Leaders recruit dissidents from elsewhere and expell their own dissidents. Leadership in this sense resembles the ideal type of domination Max Weber called rational. Just like the alpha animals in a primate dominance hierarchy, human leaders understand where to lead their group in terms of food resources. They also understand whom to welcome and whom to reject and with what concrete rewards they can entice others to them. Second, the nature of their recruitment hinges most on kinship and the giving of partners in marriage. Band leaders are invariably elders, who occupy a grandparental position among many households. This resembles Weber's traditional mode of domination, which he saw to reside archetypically in patriarchs. Finally, influential elders also are ritual experts. Some may be talented in these activities from the start; others may simply have to officiate at rites by default, being the most senior individuals. !Kung elders are usually expert trancers, magical curers in campfire ceremonies exorcising the ghosts of the dead. Tiwi elders are proficient at song and dance in initiation rites and at funerals. Here we have Weber's charismatic domination, that is, power resting on claims of having charisma, "the gift of grace."

Daily Speech Events: Managing Culture

Language is a set of catalytic messages that govern how systems go about processing matter, energy, and activity to maintain themselves. Language, then, governs the factory days of organisms and of their societies. A catalyst in chemistry is an agent that speeds up or even effects transformations in other matter without itself being affected. Human speech is such a catalytic language. It has been theorized that it arose as a means of organizing the labor of children and adolescents for the benefit of that uniquely human group, the married couple, their parents. Some highly speculative linguists imagine an original speech community of Homo sapiens speaking the first or UR language comprising at most 300 words. That remains speculation, which may or may not be better established by subsequent research. It does seem to fit with the facts known today, however.

Talking Around the Campfire

We do know that human speech not only surrounds all the activities of hunters and gatherers, it becomes *the* activity at one time of the day. In the typical day of hunters and gatherers, the activity that most entrains, that is, synchronizes the activities of any particular day with those of the seasons and with generational cycling of coming of age and growing old, is talk. Hunters and gatherers usually gather around fires at night to talk. No other primate does that. (No other has fire or speech.) Chimpanzees, for example, make individual nests in trees and go to sleep. Human beings, in contrast, always spend some time in the evening speaking to each other: going over the events of the day; telling jokes, stories, legends, and myths; and singing songs, which themselves may be stories. Thus, from our perspective, such speech events are a new activity in primate evolution.

What is spoken at these campfire talks? We are told that the !Kung spin stories and recite myths. We also can assume that the kind of retrospective look at daily activity helps human beings improve their skills. Although speech is not necessary for cooperative behavior, because other mammals are highly cooperative without speech, speech and retrospective story telling, by tapping into the collective memory of the group, no doubt greatly improve human cooperative skills.

Like the !Kung, the Tiwi tell stories in the evening, but we are told that elder Tiwi men rail against young unmarried men at these campfire sessions, accusing them of philandering with their young wives. In a society in which most women are married polygynously to a few old men, in which no man marries before he is 30, and then most likely to an old widow, such speech events, "gerontocratic diatribes," are a logical means of social control.

At the level of vocabulary, speech provides human beings with words for roles. Thus, a man has names for some of his activities conducted with others. Among the !Kung he is son, then hunter, then husband, then father, then (probably) trancer (one who cures by confronting the spirits of the dead in trance) and lover (one who engages in extramarital affairs, sometimes recreational, sometimes serious enough to result in divorce and remarriage). Finally, he is grandfather and elder. These roles become the characters for story telling. It seems to me that the form and structure of "stories" and folk tales are likely to borrow much from the recounting of real life "social dramas." Campfire stories, when they deal in gossip, are likely to take on the character of an ongoing soap opera.

Social Drama: Talking About and Managing Disruptive Activities

This brings us to conflict, or agonistic behavior. Like all other mammals, human beings often experience "the fight or flight response," a physiologic reaction we call "anger." The dominance competitions among chimpanzees are an example. In them, as in all vertebrates, agonistic (aggressive or conflict) sequences of behavior follow in predictable succession: threat, confrontation, flight, appeasement, and reassurance. Anthropologists have worked out a similar sequence for human beings and named it social drama, or the conflict process. It consists of anger or grievance, breach of the peace or encounter, confrontation, violence or redressive action, and flight or reconciliation. Redressive action refers to attempts to settle the conflict without violence, whether by mediating it, talking it out, or referring it to magical judgment, such as ordeals or duels. These dramas, with their beginnings, middles, and outcomes, must be the stuff of story telling at the campfires.

In band societies, agonistic behavior is channeled according to the genetic potential inherent in us as a primate species. This genetic basis is overlaid with a cultural potential derived from speech that stereotypes sequences and outcomes.

Among the !Kung, a dispute starts as a verbal quarrel, goes on to "bad words," then to hand-to-hand combat, and then to spears. At that point, the outcomes may be homicide and flight or mutual flight. Indeed, flight rather than fight is often the outcome. One party flees and takes refuge with distant friends and relatives in another band.

At any stage, the dispute may pass into the court of public opinion and be talked out in a noisy palaver among everyone who happens by. This mechanism is not available to other primates. While the wider chimpanzee community can observe a quarrel and communicate about it nonverbally, they cannot do so verbally. Frequently, the outcome of palaver is determined by some influential elder, who may change the subject by bringing up something—even a story—about which they all can agree, thus diverting the dispute and allowing it to simmer along.

The Tiwi elder who rails most evenings at philanderers may, if sufficiently angered, call an emergency gathering of neighboring camps, and hold a public duel, a redressive ritual that channels or contains conflict, not allowing it to spread beyond the two disputants. Here, decked out in full battle regalia, the elder denounces his junior "rival" in a wealth of insulting detail and then hurls his spear at the younger man. The latter's part, in turn, is to stand in silence, deny nothing, and simply dodge the spears until, when the crowd has been greatly entertained, he allows a spear to strike and draw blood. That is the end of it; the old man's honor has been vindicated, his opponent shamed. It resembles nothing so much as a ritualization of a chimpanzee male dominance display.

Summary and Conclusions

Bands are the elemental human communities of hunters and gatherers. They are the prototypical community for Homo sapiens. In them, we see a pattern of behavior emerge that is quite different from those of other primates: the division of labor by sex. Adult men hunt for meat, gather plant foodstuffs, make and repair tools, play, sing, dance, and, at times, quarrel violently. Adult women also hunt smaller game or join male hunting teams. Women gather foodstuffs; process and cook food, including meat received from men; hand out food at meals; make and maintain tools; clean house; fetch water; play; sing; dance; and, at times, quarrel, although usually not violently. Like all adult primate women, they bear and nurse young as well. Old men and women tell stories. Men and women, young and old, then cooperate with each other, and share food as a result. These activities are synchronized in kinetic cycles.

The following summarizes the kinetic cycles of repetitive activities in band societies of hunters and gatherers: First, the solar day is composed of a round of repetitive activities of eating, eliminating, working, playing, talking, and sleeping, which comes to a climax in the evening meal; second, a food-gathering cycle lasts approximately 3 solar days, and a hunting cycle lasts 4 to 6 days.

Anthropologists had first imagined that the subsistence of hunters and gatherers was precarious, that they often verged on starvation, that they were always anxious about food, and that they had to work very hard to scrounge a living from the environment. Nothing could be further from the truth. We find hunters and gatherers working rather easy "work weeks" when we impose our measure of time on them. They work considerably less than tribal horticulturists, for example, and have plenty of time left over for play, story telling, singing, and dancing.

The annual round of the solar year is marked by the regular dissolution of the population into its constituent units of households and camps and their regrouping at key food and water sources according to the seasons, usually welcoming guests from other bands. These regroupings are attended by rituals that, although often life crisis rituals, tide groups over through the solar year. The generational cycle also is marked by rituals of birth, initiation, and marriage, whereupon the cycle repeats itself in the birth of a new generation. An entire life cycle, 90 years or so, flows around the life histories of strategic long-lived individuals in band societies, who use the kinship and ritual structure to recruit others to their band, often fleeing conflict (social drama) in other bands. At the death of elders, others must emerge in their footsteps to build up the next core clientele band population.

When we look at bands, we see several uniquely human institutions fully factoring out: language and speech; kinship, marriage, and the family; and ritual. In contrast, politics, justice and law, and economics are only prototypically foreshadowed by actions in the other three institutions. The broader field remains the permeable band community in a field of such communities, through which the individual human actors flow with much greater ease than has ever been reported for their primate cousins.

Discussion Questions

1. Moore describes activity cycles over the course of generations and their influence on maintaining cultural stability in hunting and gathering societies. Is this chapter truly occupational science, or is it purely an anthropologic analysis? Is it occupational anthropology or anthropologic occupational science?
2. Must the pursuit of knowledge of humans as occupational beings be involved with drawing boundaries between disciplines?
3. In what ways does Moore's paper support and expand on occupational science's contention that engagement in occupation is the fundamental means by which humans adapt?

References

1. Iberall, AS, and Wilkinson, D: Dynamic foundations for complex systems. In Modelski, G (ed): Exploring Long Cycles. Lynne Reinner, Boulder, CO, 1987, p 542.
2. Lee, RB: The !Kung San: Men, Women, and Work in a Foraging Society. Cambridge University Press, Cambridge, MA, 1979, p 543.
3. Lee, RB: The Dobe !Kung. Harcourt Brace Jovanovich, New York, 1984, p 540.
4. Goodale, JC: Tiwi Wives: A Study of the Women of Melville Island, North Australia. University of Washington Press, Seattle, 1971, p 540. American Ethnological Society Monography No. 51.
5. Hart, CWM, Pilling, AR, and Goodale, JC: The Tiwi of North Australia (3rd ed). Harcourt Brace Jovanovich, Fort Worth, 1988, p 541.

by Michael Dear, PhD

Time, Space, and the Geography of Everyday Life of People Who Are Homeless

The Geography of Homelessness
From Knowledge to Action
A View From the Future

There is a moment in the novel *Guerrillas* by V. S. Naipul[1] that beautifully encapsulates my themes of time, space, and everyday life. One character asks another to describe her vision of a "perfect day." She proceeds simply, even predictably, to construct a day that consists entirely of a juxtaposition of the familiar with the favored. She would rise late in the day, forget the obligations of work, indulge in a leisurely lunch followed by a beach walk, perhaps an early movie, and so on. Her interlocutor interrupts, urging her to eschew the familiar, her embellishments of the commonplace, and to imagine a day unconstrained by time, space, and resources. She becomes animated and invents a lavish, liberated hedonism that includes jetting around the world so that the sun never sets on her perfect day.

Real life is, of course, remarkably tightly constrained. In feudal England, for example, the size and distribution of agricultural settlements were limited by the ability of the farm laborer to walk to and from the most distant fields and still put in a full day's work. Even in our era of supersonic travel, most people's lives remain principally limited by the discipline of the daily journey to work.

In more general terms, we can think of an individual's life as being bound by a "prism" of time and space. Both axes of time and space are strictly finite. Human well-being and potential depend on the resources a person may readily access within his or her limited capacity to overcome the daily frictions of time and distance. Thus, in resource-rich environments, individuals may flourish without hindrance; in resource-deficient environments, however, access to the means of advancement is inhibited. Needless to say, not only do the characteristics of places limit human potential but also the experiences of individuals themselves matter. For example, even in a resource-rich environment, limitations on schooling, experiences of racial or gender discrimination, and extreme poverty can effectively prevent advancement.

For the poor, disabled, and immobile, the time-space prism rapidly constricts to become a time-space "prison." Here, personal deficits and environmental deficiencies limit human development and power to escape from disadvantage. It is easy to understand how people come to wear the "imprint" of an environment like a scar and how daily life acts to transmit privilege or poverty. Recall, for instance, how frequently the sons of coal miners join their fathers down the mine shafts, how daughters follow mothers into textile mills, or how many Hollywood stars have Hollywood parents.

We can extend our thinking about time and space to encompass the whole of human society. Society may be conceived as a time-space "fabric" on which the biographies of individual lives are engraved.[2] The consequent tapestry is rich and complex, encompassing the full panoply of social, cultural, political, and economic aspirations. One goal of social science is to unravel the structure of this time-space fabric, from the highest level of abstraction to the level of detailed individual lives. Understanding the time-space fabric is an explicit focus of many social sciences, including the sociology of Anthony Giddens,[3] ethnographers George Marcus and James Clifford,[4] and the new cultural history as codified by Linda Hunt.[5] The glimpse of a "common ground" between these disciplines is, in fact, one of the most exciting developments in contemporary social thought. However, social science also is about the relationships between knowledge and action. Hence, we try to imagine and forge new time-space configurations for the betterment of humankind.

Geography's role in this undertaking is to explain how sociocultural, economic, and political processes are concretized, or localized, in particular places. Its epistemologic status is analogous to that of history. Just as history claims special insight into the time dimension of the time-space fabric, so geography privileges its spatial dimension. In terms of social action, geography opens up the potential of *manipulating* space for human betterment.

The Geography of Homelessness

The sidewalks of downtown Los Angeles are cluttered with homeless people[6] (Fig. 11–1). They are a mixed bunch. White and black people; women and children, young and old, and veterans and mentally disabled. They share the streets with other disadvantaged people: mentally retarded, physically disabled, exoffenders, or the "underclass." The group as a whole is sometimes called the service dependent. Its membership has two things in common: 1) they are disabled or disadvantaged socially, physically, or mentally and 2) they need the vast array of human

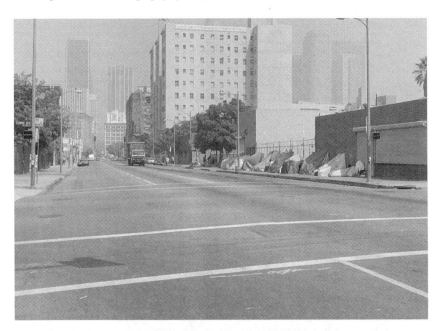

Figure 11–1. A row of makeshift homes constructed by homeless people in Los Angeles against a background of upscale urban redevelopment. (Photo by John Wolcott.)

services available on skid row (including health care, social welfare, emergency shelter, and job training). When compared with the rest of the city, skid row resembles an enormous "ghetto" of human-service agencies and the people who need their help. How did this ghetto develop? What were the processes by which this localization, this clustering of people and services, occurred?

Look more closely at the individuals on the sidewalk, and one answer to this question swiftly becomes clear.[6] They are relaxing after the day's work, talking with friends, planning cultural events, or perhaps sweeping the sidewalk around the cardboard boxes in which they sleep. Many are still busy working, panhandling, or engaged in subsistence prostitution. For these homeless, skid row is their community. It is a place where friends gather, work is offered, shelter and provisions are available, and socializing and recreation are possible. Skid row is a "coping mechanism" for the homeless. It is a support network: a well-defined time-space prism that is often the last thing standing between a homeless person and death.[7] Why here? Why skid row? Why not elsewhere in the city?

In my view, part of the answer to this question is that the "homed" communities elsewhere in Los Angeles have refused to shoulder the burden of caring for the homeless. This is the action of what is called the NIMBY syndrome for "not in my back yard." In too many neighborhoods, the objections of residents have effectively blocked the introduction of many services to assist disadvantaged populations, including homes for the mentally disabled, shelters for the homeless, and AIDS hospices. In principle, opponents typically support the concept of community-based care, although they prefer that the facilities themselves be located in more distant neighborhoods. In practice, Los Angeles area communities have responded with arson, abuse, and antipathy.[8]

Those responsible for securing sites for shelters, group homes, and hospices have found it remarkably difficult to anticipate community response. In one Massachusetts case,[6] a small-town community rejected a group living arrangement for four elderly women on the grounds that they would not be supervised after midnight! Service planners have responded in a predictable manner, searching for noncontroversial sites that tend not surprisingly to be in downtown neighborhoods already saturated with helping agencies.

Not only are individuals (homeless and homed) implicated in the localization process but institutional practices also have intensified ghettoization. Public welfare offices and mental health clinics in Los Angeles have recently undergone a "rationalization" process, referring to cutbacks in human services.[6] Many smaller scale, local offices have been closed, so services are now offered from fewer, larger centers. People in need are consequently referred to more distant, often less accessible places; the alternative is to go without assistance. Once an individual gains access to service, a host of institutional rules bind that person to a single locality. For instance, the time commitments necessary for keeping welfare agency appointments and maintaining eligibility for scarce shelter beds usually prevent the homeless from taking jobs any significant distance beyond the skid row area. In addition, many people prefer sleeping on the sidewalk to agencies that impose intrusive routines on its clients as a condition of shelter, such as attending religious services or submitting to a gynecologic examination.[9]

Deeply seated structural forces also have been associated with the ghettoization of the homeless. Principal among these has been the intense economic restructuring that has been occurring during the last decade or more, typically called "deindustrialization." The characterizations of "sun belt" versus "rust belt" or "snow belt" vividly capture the important geographic variation in the impact of the associated plant closures and layoffs. To be sure, the American economy has simultaneously been creating new jobs at a remarkable rate. However, as the work of economists Bennett Harrison and Barry Bluestone has shown,[10] almost half of these jobs pay only minimum wage levels and are typically to be found in the service sector of the economy.[11]

Unemployment and underemployment associated with economic restructuring have created an alarming increase in the "demand" for social support in this country. At the same time, however, the American welfare state continues to undergo a profound retrenchment. These changes are subsumed under the general rubric of "privatization," but they go far beyond this. Here are two brief examples.

The case of "deinstitutionalization" is perhaps the most dramatic.[12] During the 1960s and 1970s, a massive drive was launched to reduce the population of mental hospitals. Nationally, the number of patients fell from more than half a million in the mid-1950s to just over 100,000 at present. Unfortunately, the planned community-based mental health care system (intended to replace the hospitals) never fully materialized. Most of these expatients are now on the streets or (increasingly) in jail.

Equally important in the restructuring of the welfare state have been widespread cutbacks designed to eliminate or reduce government support for dependent populations. During the Reagan years, for example, the budget for assisted housing dropped from 7% to 0.7% of the total federal budget. One consequence of this has been the crisis of affordable housing common to most American cities.[13] For too many people, the "housing market" has been reduced to abandoned cars, cardboard boxes, rooftops, and even tree dwellings.

In many ways, the crisis of homelessness in American cities was entirely predictable. Recessions in the economy increased the need for social support just at the time that the social welfare network itself was being dismantled. The effect of more demand plus less supply has been an excess of human tragedy and suffering.

There is a clear, if sometimes tenuous, connection between the geography of global economic restructuring and the appearance of a homeless person on the streets of Los Angeles. These connections have to do with the inter-relationships of time and space, of global-scale and local-scale processes, and of structure and human agency. These more formal connections are discussed elsewhere.[14]

From Knowledge to Action

The link between place and power is a persistent theme in the work of Michel Foucault.[15,16] The powerful are those who are able to manipulate space for their own ends, inserting the tentacles of social control (Foucault's "micropowers") deeply into the interstices of everyday life. Foucault's archetypal examples were, of course, the prison and the asylum. In both cases, individuals are enclosed, stripped of their autonomy, and subjected to the most intense, constant surveillance. Somehow, however, hidden in the darkest recesses of everyday life, the possibility of autonomous action remains. Precisely because of the complexities of human geography, transcendental social action is always imminent. Space, then, is an expression of power. It enables and constrains. Those who do not control their geography forever remain threatened, unsure of their security.

Thus, the patterns of everyday life are deceptively simple. People sleep, eat, work, and love. Routine activities converge to build routinized lives. Aggregations of human lives give expression to geographic form, such as cities, social movements, and wars between nations. However, behind the quotidian and the local geography lies an intricate tapestry of power and control. Geography's task, as I have explained, is to understand the relationship between society and space.

What about forging new time-space configurations? Can thinking geographically help us suggest solutions to important human problems? In conclusion, here are some of the approaches being developed under the auspices of the University of Southern California-based Los Angeles Homelessness Project.[17]

1. Service hubs. For the past several years, the Community Redevelopment Agency (CRA) of Los Angeles has exercised a specific "containment" policy with respect to skid row. Its intent has been to limit the geographic spread of the "blight" associated with the row and even to eliminate it altogether. This policy is related to the CRA's desire to promote downtown redevelopment schemes (including Bunker Hill and Little Tokyo), yet in the absence of alternatives, I advocate the preservation of skid row as a vital resource for the homeless. In

fact, a principal inference from our analysis is that we should attempt to replicate the positive features of the skid row ghetto elsewhere in our cities.

The concept of a service hub assumes that the supportive social networks on skid row can and should be reproduced in other neighborhoods. Many hubs can be created simply by grafting onto existing community infrastructure the basic elements of a homeless support network. Such add-ons would typically occur in established communities where levels of existing services are high, for instance, a local shopping mall with good transportation links. The area could be transformed into a service hub for the homeless mentally ill through the simple addition of a clinic and counseling center plus some supervised housing units. The purpose of the hub is to provide the necessary level of support and choice in housing beyond the skid row locale so that the homeless are able to regain independent living.

2. NIMBY. In dealing with the NIMBY syndrome, we have witnessed many examples in which simple design architectural modifications have led to the withdrawal of community opposition. These have included an enlarged waiting room so that clients did not need to congregate on the street outside, a rudimentary screening wall, and an entrance on a different side of the offending building.

3. Sociospatial networks. We should not confine our spatial interventions solely to physical structures. One striking finding of our recent surveys[9] on skid row is the degree of disconnection between the informal networks of the homeless and their peers and the formal networks of human service providers.[7] This is undoubtedly related to the fact that more than half the homeless population are homeless for the first time and have been on the row for less than 1 month. Although the formal and informal networks are geographically coterminous, in the lives of many, they remain discrete and unattached. To overcome such a dysfunctional separation, special outreach is required to assist the homeless in accessing the formal networks. In Los Angeles, the Homeless Outreach Project is run by formerly homeless people and was created specifically to merge these two networks.

A View From the Future

What does the future hold? The present crisis of homelessness has taken 2 decades to create. It is unlikely to disappear overnight. Indeed, one skid row service provider or entrepreneur refers to homelessness as a "growth industry." I want to emphasize that we are not short on prescriptions to solve the problem: emergency shelter provision, a reconstituted assisted housing program, housing plus services for those in need, and adequate levels of welfare support for those waiting for new job opportunities to emerge. Moreover, there is no shortage of public support for the homeless. National and local polls suggest that 75% to 80% of the population are willing to spend more tax dollars to help the homeless. Why, therefore, has there been so little concrete action to solve the problem?

I recently read Alain Corbin's essay in volume four of the monumental *A History of Private Life*.[18] Writing about the secret life of the individual in rural France, Corbin observes:

Unfortunately no comprehensive study exists of the spread and various uses of the mirror. But many signs point to the fundamental importance of self-regard. In nineteenth-century villages the barber was the only person who possessed a full-length mirror, whose use was limited to men. Hawkers sold small mirrors that women and girls could use to examine their faces, but full-length mirrors were all but unknown in the countryside, where peasants still discovered their physical identities through the eyes of others and relied on intuition to control their facial expressions. Veronique Nahoum wonders how people could "live in bodies they had not seen" in intimate detail.[19]

In contrast to the *bourgeois gentilhomme* with his full-length reflection and the peasant lacking a self-image, the late 20th century is beset by a profusion of mirror images. Unable to locate our "true" original self in the collage of reflections, we embrace a convenient proximate image, uncertain of the substance that backs it. Uncertain of self, we become pathologically distrustful of the galaxy of reflections associated with our companions in the (postmodern) maze of mirrors. Who is friend? Who is foe?

Historians have already dubbed the 1980s the "me" decade. Narcissistic fascination with self has eclipsed our commitment to community and directly contributed to the manufacture of homelessness in the United States. When someone next asks you to imagine a perfect day, I hope you will find time and space to conjure a vision in which we no longer require a geography of cardboard boxes, of street encampments, and of sidewalks filled with devalued human beings.

Discussion Questions

1. Dear's paper embraces a social ethic of care for the dispossessed and disenfranchised by those who are more fortunate. In what ways has occupational therapy historically shared or not shared this ethic, beyond our traditional concern with those who are disabled? Is this an ethic that the science of occupation ought to embrace explicitly?
2. How might Dear's understanding of the potentially constricting influence of geography be applied to other identifiable groups of people, such as the well and not so well elderly and, of course, people with severe disabilities?

References

1. Naipul, VS: Guerillas. Random House, New York, 1990.
2. Dear, M: The postmodern challenge: Reconstructing human geography. Transactions, Institute of British Geographers NS 13:262, 1988.
3. Giddens, A: The Constitution of Society. University of California Press, Berkeley, 1984.
4. Clifford, J, and Marcus, G (eds): Writing Culture: The Poetic and Politics of Ethnography. University of California Press, Berkeley, 1986.
5. Hunt, L (ed): The New Cultural History. University of California Press, Berkeley, 1989.
6. Wolch, J and Dear, M: Malign Neglect: Homelessness in an American City. Jossey-Bass, San Francisco, 1993.

7. Dear, M, and Wolch, J: Landscapes of Despair: From Deinstitutionalization to Homelessness. Princeton University Press, Princeton, NJ, 1987.

8. Dear, M: Taking Los Angeles seriously: Time and space in the postmodern city. Architecture California 13:36, 1991.

9. Rowe, S, and Wolch, J: Social networks in time and space: Homeless women in Skid Row, Los Angeles. Annals, Association of American Geographers 80:184, 1990.

10. Harrison, B, and Bluestone, B: The Great U-turn. Basic Books, New York, 1989.

11. Phillips, K: The Politics of Rich and Poor. Basic Books, New York, 1990.

12. Dear, M and Wolch, J: Landscapes of Despair: From Deinstitutionalization to Homelessness. Princeton University Press, Princeton, NJ, 1987.

13. Wolch, J, and Dear, M: Introduction. Inside/Outside: Homelessness in Los Angeles. Jossey-Bass, San Francisco, 1994.

14. Dear, M: Gaining Community Acceptance. The Robert Wood Johnson Foundation, Princeton, NJ, 1991.

15. Foucault, M: Madness and Civilization. Vintage Books, New York, 1973.

16. Foucault, M: Discipline and Punish: The Birth of the Prison. Pantheon, New York, 1977.

17. Dear, M, Wolch, J, and Wilton, R: The Service Hub Concept in Human Services Planning. Pergamon Press, New York, 1994.

18. Corbin, A: The secret of the individual. In Perrot, M (ed): A History of Private Life, IV: From the First of Revolution to the Great War. Harvard University Press, Cambridge, MA, 1990.

19. Corbin, A, p 460.

by Loree A. Primeau, PhD, OTR

12

Human Daily Travel
Personal Choices and External Constraints

The Occupation of Daily Travel

Human Travel Behavior

The Role of Cognitive Maps in Travel Behavior

Personal Choices and External Constraints on Travel
Behavior

An adage attributed to theologian Romano Guardini states, "Most people don't know where they want to go, but they want to get there as quickly as possible."[1] The act of travel in the everyday life of the individual is rarely valued for the act itself but as a means to an end, to get to where the individual wants to go.[2] Today, daily travel consumes a greater amount of time than in the past, especially in large urban environments. Daily travel is not only a bridge or link between occupations but also an occupation itself. Although daily travel is a cross-cultural phenomenon, this paper focuses on daily travel within urban centers in industrial societies.

An analysis of individual travel behavior, as an occupation, must consider not only personal choice and freedom, but also external societal constraints and the relationship of each of these factors to other occupations within the individual's daily life. Goodall,[3] in her rich description of chimpanzee ranging patterns in the natural habitat, states that "group-living animals share an area of land within which they forage, sleep, raise their young, and go about their other daily activities."[4] She too discusses the influence of personal choice and external societal factors on the individual's travel patterns. A description of human travel behavior may be enriched by the inclusion of information and knowledge that emanate from primatology, social and economic transport research, geography, and cognitive psychology.

An interdisciplinary synthesis of literature pertinent to the human occupation of traveling as a component of daily life provides a perspective on the role of human information processing in occupational behavior. This paper begins with a definition and description of daily human urban travel behavior. Parallels between chimpanzee and human travel patterns are demonstrated. Next, drawing on theory and research in the disciplines of geography and psychology, the phenomena of cognitive mapping and cognitive maps, as mechanisms of information processing that contribute to the ability to engage in travel behavior, are explored. Finally, this paper discusses the role of personal choice and external constraints in making decisions about daily travel.

The Occupation of Daily Travel

Daily travel is consistently defined in the literature as a derived demand activity, meaning that travel is motivated, not from a need for travel for its own sake, but by the need to participate in an activity at the destination of the trip and in a place outside of the home.[5–6] Travel has been described as "a mediating activity between the needs of the individual, both internal and social, and the sources of their satisfaction, which are distributed in space."[7] The fact that travel is a link between activities requires that individual travel choices and behavior be studied within the context of the individual's daily activity pattern.[7–9] An activity pattern consists "of a sequence of events set in space and time."[10]

The spatial aspect of travel behavior requires an understanding of the territorial range or ranging patterns of the individual and of the group. Interesting parallels may be drawn between chimpanzee and human daily travel behavior. The home range of a community of chimpanzees living in the natural habitat is the area of land in which they carry out their daily activity patterns.[3] A core area of the home range may be identified as the area that is used extensively by group members. In a similar manner, studies of urban movement patterns have demonstrated the existence of a person's action space defined as "that area with which the individual has contact and within which his activities take place."[11] The action space of the group would include the entire city. Knowledge of, and behavior in, the urban environment is limited by the individual's action space, indicating a spatial bias toward the area surrounding the home location and frequently used paths of travel. Ranging patterns of chimpanzees and humans have a similar developmental pattern, in which there is a dramatic expansion of range from infancy to adulthood followed by range contraction with the aging process.[3,12]

The distribution of chimpanzee daily ranging patterns depends on the seasonal supply of food, health, weather, consortships, and travel activity of the previous day.[3] Generally, the sole purpose of travel behavior in chimpanzees is to forage for food. An exception occurs during consortships, when a male and female may travel to establish a consortship range. Ranging patterns of male chimpanzees typically differ from those of female chimps in terms of distance traveled and extent of range.[3] Male chimpanzees average a daily distance of 4.9 kilometers, while female chimps average 3.0 kilometers per day. Male chimpanzees frequently travel to boundary areas of the home range to conduct frequent border patrols, while female chimps tend to remain in core areas. Female ranging patterns are additionally affected by reproductive status and the age and sex of offspring.[3]

Human Travel Behavior

Human travel behavior may be studied with the use of activity approaches. Activity approaches are methods of investigation in which the role of travel in daily life is the focus.[8] Similar to chimpanzee travel, human travel enables the individual to meet physiologic and social needs.[7,8] The units of analysis in activity approaches include the individual and the household, in recognition of "the significance of the coordination of the interweaving daily timetables of individuals interacting with one another."[13] Modes of travel most frequently reported in travel behavior research are by foot, car, public transportation, and less often, by bicycle.[1,9,14] Common descriptors of travel behavior found in the literature are trip purpose, transport mode, daily trip frequency, travel time, and travel distance.[14]

To provide an overview of human travel behavior, descriptive findings of three studies using data collected in British and German urban centers in 1975 and 1976 are presented.[1,9,14] Using an activity approach to look at the reasons for travel, seven main purposes were identified according to the activity carried out at the trip destination.[1] The purposes were: 1) home; 2) work; 3) personal business, such as trips to the bank, laundromat, post office; 4) education; 5) service, including, chauffeuring passengers; 6) shopping; and 7) leisure trips, that is, trips that are made to a destination where one engages in a leisure occupation rather than trips made for their own sake.

Work and education trips were regular trips made on weekdays usually to a consistent location. Trips made for shopping and personal business had more flexibility on a day-to-day basis. More than half of all travel was for work, education, and shopping purposes. Work trips accounted for 41% of total trips made by fully employed adults, and school trips made up 43% of school children's total trips. Thirty-eight percent of trips made by housewives and 36% of those made by the elderly population were for shopping purposes. Service trips, or chauffeuring, constituted an additional 15% of housewives' total trips. Leisure trips accounted for 20% of young adults' travel and 17% of adolescent travel.

Trip frequency, travel time, and travel distance per day of various groups add to the description of human travel behavior. Full-time employees made approximately four trips to travel 27 kilometers in 77 minutes.[14] Housewives had a daily trip frequency of 3.5 in which they covered 14 kilometers, spending 54 minutes to do so. Approximately three trips per day accounting for 59 minutes were made by retired people, in which they traveled 11 kilometers.[14]

The data reported here, from three separate studies, were collected in 1975 to 1976. The data were quantitative and descriptive in nature. To move beyond the level of descriptive statistics to a level of greater understanding of the meaning of travel in daily life, current research efforts are aimed at describing the choices and constraints on individual and household travel. Prior to a discussion of the external constraints on decisions made about travel, the information processing mechanisms thought to play a role in human daily travel are presented.

The Role of Cognitive Maps in Travel Behavior

The process of cognitive mapping is thought to be a subset of the general cognitive process. As such, "cognitive mapping is a construct which encompasses those cognitive processes which enable people to acquire, code, store, recall, and manipulate information about the nature of their spatial environment."[15] Similar to other cognitive processes, a cognitive map changes with age and experience or with development and learning. The spatial behavior of an individual is based on his or her cognitive map of the spatial environment. Through a cognitive map, environmental behavior strategies are developed, thereby facilitating everyday environmental interaction, adaptation, and survival.[15]

Two questions are answered by a cognitive map: 1) where something of need or desire is located and 2) how to get to it. A goal is an integral element of a cognitive map. Downs and Stea[16] state, "We believe that a cognitive map exists if an individual behaves as if a cognitive map exists. Normal everyday behavior such as a journey to work, a trip to a recreation area, or giving directions to a lost stranger would all be impossible without some form of cognitive map."

The ability to travel around in the environment and to obtain desired goals may be observed in very young children and in many different animal species.[17] Toddlers are capable of successful movement in familiar spaces and finding favored objects, such as toys and food. The chimpanzee demonstrates the use of cognitive maps in traveling, often using several different routes to get to the same food source.[3,17] Free-ranging chimpanzees have been noted to prepare a termite fishing tool while still out of sight of the termite mound, a behavior that indicates spatial knowledge, memory, and anticipation.[3] The evidence of cognitive mapping processes in young children and animals suggests that cognitive maps are formed, not through verbal abilities, but through perception of and action in the environment.[17]

Neisser believes that perception or pick-up of information from the environment is enhanced when the perceiver is moving.[17] The act of movement produces information through two kinds of optical processes. The first of these processes is motion parallax, which occurs due to reception of different visual stimuli from different environmental points. The change in eye position during movement causes a new visual pattern. The differences between consequent patterns result in the visual perception of shapes, positions, and the physical layout of objects.[17] Because human eyes are set in different positions in the head, humans have the benefit of binocular parallax, a process through which environmental depth information is provided without actual movement.

The second process involves the creation of flow patterns as a result of the continuous change in the visual stimuli impinging on the eye while an individual moves around in the environment. Varying aspects of objects are viewed and perceived as undergoing visual changes as the individual moves, thus the objects are seen in three dimensions and in their real physical layout.[17] During movement, information is picked up about the individual who is moving and about the environment. This information includes perception of movement itself, the direction of movement, and body position, and the relation of that position to objects in the environment.[17]

Perceptual information about spatial relationships between objects, the individual, and the environment are incorporated into cognitive maps, which are used to guide movement and exploration in the external world. Of specific interest in this paper is the urban environment. Urban knowledge is a multimodal representation of a city, developed through varying perceptions of environmental features. To understand human travel within the urban environment, urban perception, as a special case of general perception and cognition, must be recognized. Three types of urban perception have been identified: operational, responsive, and inferential.[18]

Operational urban perception involves the selection of various environmental features for their role in facilitating the completion of tasks. An example of this type of perception is the use of a landmark to note a change in direction of a travel route. Operational perception is thought to be the basis for planned, goal-directed travel and is characteristic of automobile travel.[18] Visibility and personal movement, as a prerequisite for operational perception, leads to the memory of parts of a city as actions or in terms of the activity conducted in a particular location.

Responsive urban perception is usually a passive perception of a distinctive element of the environment that evokes the creation of an image in the perceiver. The stimulus may be visual, auditory, tactile, or olfactory, but its perception depends on its intensity and uniqueness in a specific context. Examples of stimuli apt to be perceived by responsive perception include billboards by the side of the road, airport noises near the airport, and chemical smells surrounding a factory. The ability of a stimulus to evoke an image is required for responsive perception and lends itself to recall as an image.

Inferential urban perception is seen as a cognitive decision-making process, consisting of the categorization of stimuli according to their functional and social uses.[18] Placement of stimuli into categories results in a personal coding system that can be generalized to each new city encountered, thus facilitating the acquisition of new urban knowledge. An example of inferential perception is the recognition of universal signs for restrooms or public telephones. Stimuli perceived by inferential perception are frequently remembered as symbols.

As Appleyard states, "a particular building can thus be recalled by the activity a person engages in when he is there, by an image, or as a name, category, or graphic symbol learned through social communication, from a map or sign."[19] The urban environment is predominantly represented through direct experience, although verbal, graphic, and other symbol systems have evolved for communication of indirect experience, such as information from friends, maps, and travel brochures.[18] Therefore, two information processing systems, one for direct experience and one for indirect experience, must exist to translate, collate, and synthesize the action events, images, and symbols arising from urban perception into a framework of urban knowledge. To do so, learning in the form of experience is essential. A lack of experience is frequently manifested by the fragmented urban representations of people who are passengers in cars or who travel only by public transportation.[18]

Urban perception and knowledge are schematic and as such, are incorporated into the schemata of a cognitive map.[17–18] To organize and categorize the volume of environmental experience, information may be simplified, structured, and reduced to fit into an existing cognitive map.[18] Cognitive economizing, or reduction of the amount of information to be recalled, is a strategy used to schematize information within a cognitive map. Thus, schematization, while fundamental in the representation of urban knowledge, necessarily results in a disjointed picture of a city.

Information is not processed purely and completely; some environmental features may assume disproportionate significance as possessors of survival value, while others are screened out or fade into insignificance.[18] The difficulty inherent in the organization of discontinuous experience frequently results in environmental errors, such as becoming disoriented at a familiar intersection when approaching it from a new direction. Although urban perception and knowledge in the form of cognitive maps may be disjointed and incomplete, it is clear that cognitive maps constitute the basic information processing component underlying human travel behavior. The influence of personal choices and external constraints on travel behavior are now discussed.

Personal Choices and External Constraints on Travel Behavior

According to the literature, decisions made about daily travel are constrained by temporal, spatial, and sociocultural factors.[20-22] Space and time constraints arise from within the urban environment and reflect the fact that objects required to satisfy an individual's needs are separated in space and time.[20] Temporal limitations are closely related to social dimensions of urban behavior. Participation in a certain occupation requires compliance with its temporal expectations. For example, work or school occupations have specific temporal expectations that set a daily schedule and routine.[21] The spatial dimension of activity patterns creates an individual action space that is determined by the individual's needs and wants; the size, structure, and location of physical facilities; the location of the individual's home; and social and temporal constraints.[21]

The phenomenon of particular interest to occupational science is the individual's participation in daily occupations and how this participation may be influenced by social and cultural expectations and by the individual's own values and personal meanings. An individual's daily orchestration of work, play, and self-care occupations, in accordance with social and cultural expectations, results in a unique set of travel choices and constraints. Rosenbloom, in her study of trip-chaining behavior, provides evidence of how differing social and cultural expectations affect travel behaviors and orchestration of daily occupations.[22]

Trip chaining is the combination of more than one purpose into one trip. Mothers in dual-career families, single working mothers, and fathers in dual-career families reported combining trips to work with trips for other purposes more often than other women and men. They tended to combine work trips with dropping off or picking up children from day care, going to the bank, or grocery shopping. Rosenbloom concludes that dual-career families with children and single-parent families have more complex activity patterns and travel behavior than do other family configurations.[22] Other researchers have found that changes that occur throughout the natural course of an individual's or family's life cycle, such as setting up an independent household, having children, making a career change, or retiring, also have a significant effect on travel behavior.[9,23,24]

Language and communication, belief systems and morals, and human emotion are frequently used by an individual to assess the value of an occupation. These factors interact to bring their own set of personal choices and external constraints to the occupation of daily travel. Choice of mode of travel may be influenced by the individual's values and morals. In Western societies, the automobile appears to have become a type of embodiment of the individual. The large numbers of BMWs, Porshes, or Mercedes-Benzes found on Southern California's freeways speak to this phenomenon. In a similar way, an individual's choice to use public transit or a bicycle for daily travel may exemplify his or her values and concerns regarding the environment or personal physical fitness, while also having a marked effect on his or her orchestration of daily occupations.

Given that the occupation of daily travel is a mediating occupation, often motivated by a need to participate in an occupation at the trip's destination rather than by a need to travel for its own sake, individuals frequently make personal choices that provide meaning to their participation in daily travel. While external constraints may leave no room for choice in the need for daily travel, individuals may make choices about how to use their time spent in travel. Some people, while traveling, may choose to sleep, read, or talk with friends. Others may choose to conduct business over a cellular phone or work on a portable computer. Daily commuting has been called a way of life, and stories abound among Southern California freeway travelers about the use of travel time for eating, listening to audiotapes of the latest novel, and applying makeup or nail polish (Fig. 12–1).

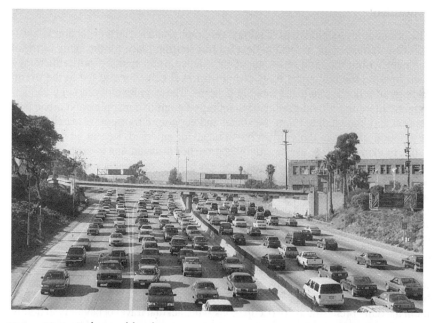

Figure 12–1. Daily travel has become a time-consuming occupation in many cities. During morning commutes, drivers have learned to use this time more efficiently by enfolding occupations such as managing business on cellular phones or listening to talk radio or books on tape. (Photo by John Wolcott.)

Richter found that women made an abrupt shift in thinking about the home domain to thinking about the work domain during their morning commute, while men made a more gradual shift in consciousness that began before leaving home.[25] The women's use of travel time to change their focus of attention was attributed to their morning domestic responsibilities. This example also demonstrates the interaction of personal choices and external constraints on the occupation of daily travel, resulting in a particular use and meaning of women's daily travel.

Discussion of the personal choices and external constraints demonstrates that frequently there may be little personal choice in daily travel decisions. As Kutter states, "It stands to reason that much more of the variety in travel behavior is determined by the objective constraints than is left to the discretion of a person or group."[26] Personal factors do enter into the decision-making process in the form of cognitions and perceptions about the travel destination. For example, familiarity with a particular shopping mall increases the likelihood that the individual will return there, rather than explore an unfamiliar mall, to meet future shopping needs. Often when faced with recurrent decision situations, an individual will develop habits and routines to reduce the requirement for conscious decision making.[24] Personal choice and freedom in travel behavior are most often manifested by the individual's personal meanings of occupations and their daily orchestration.

Conclusion

The primatology, cognitive psychology, geography, and social and economic transport research literature proved to be a fruitful starting place for the study of travel behavior within the field of occupational science. Information from primatology shed light on the biological roots of human travel behavior and led to the useful analogy of a home range and ranging patterns. The cognitive psychology and geography literature provided an understanding of cognitive mapping and urban perception and knowledge. From the social and economic transport research field, a description of human daily urban travel behavior emerged. Recent advancements in this field involved the use of activity approaches in an attempt to explain the wide variations in human travel behavior. Inherent in these approaches is the belief that activity patterns are the key to understanding travel behavior. Occupational science would also hold that belief to be true. What gives rise to an incongruence between the fields of occupational science and transport research are the reasons behind the study of travel behavior. Transport research is aimed at gaining information essential to transportation planning, traffic management, and the establishment of social and economic policy regarding urban transportation and land use.

The focus of occupational science is on the occupation of daily travel and its role in the establishment of daily schedules and routines. Through its action as a link between activities within an individual's activity pattern, travel may be a crucial factor in the daily orchestration of occupations. The fact that travel behavior is so tightly constrained by external factors makes it a key area for investigation of quality of life issues. The role of values, belief systems, and personal meaning on occupational choices, with their consequent effects on travel behavior, has been overlooked by the transport research field. An occupational science perspective has much to offer, and to gain, from an interdisciplinary approach to the occupation of human urban travel.

Discussion Questions

1. How might the concept of "trip chaining" expand occupational therapy's traditional focus on energy conservation and work simplification, particularly with respect to issues of community reintegration following the onset of a disability or chronic disease?
2. What is the relationship between cognitive mapping ability and the overall range or territory that one might reasonably be expected to cover or "tap into" as a daily resource?
3. Is traveling an occupation that can be therapeutically applied to develop an individual's capacity for cognitive mapping?

References

1. Cerwenka, P: Assessment of society's transport needs: Mobility of people. In Ninth International Symposium on Theory and Practice in Transport Economics: Transport Is for People. European Conference of Ministers of Transport, Madrid, 1983, p 7.
2. Levin, IP, and Louviere, JJ: Application of a psychological process theory to transport research. In Yerrell, JS (ed): Transport Research for Social and Economic Progress (Vol 3). Gower, Aldershot, England, 1981.
3. Goodall, J: The Chimpanzees of Gombe: Patterns of Behavior. Belknap, Cambridge, MA, 1986.
4. Goodall, p 207.
5. Daly, AJ: Some issues in the application of disaggregate choice models. In Stopher, PR, Meyburg, AH, and Brog, W (eds): New Horizons in Travel-Behavior Research. Lexington, MA, 1981.
6. Ruhl, A, Baanders, A, and Garden, JM: Assessment of society's transport needs: Mobility of persons. In Ninth International Symposium on Theory and Practice in Transport Economics: Transport Is for People. European Conference of Ministers of Transport, Madrid, 1983.
7. Michaels, RM: Future transportation: Organization of the design process. In Altman I, Wohlwill JF, and Everett PB (eds): Transportation and Behavior. Plenum, New York, 1981.
8. Jones, PM: Activity approaches to understanding travel behavior. In Stopher, PR, Meyburg, AH, and Brog, W (eds): New Horizons in Travel-Behavior Research. Lexington, Lexington, MA, 1981.
9. Town, SW: Non-transport influences on travel patterns. In Yerrell, JS (ed): Transport Research for Social and Economic Progress (Vol 3). Gower, Aldershot, England, 1981.
10. Jones, p 256.
11. Briggs, R: Urban cognitive distance. In Downs, RM, and Stea D (eds): Image and Environment: Cognitive Mapping and Spatial Behavior. Aldine, Chicago, 1973.
12. Barker, RG, and Schoggen, P: Qualities of Community Life. Jossey-Bass, San Francisco, 1973.
13. Cerwenka, p 20.
14. Hautzinger, H, and Kessel, P: Mobility opportunities and travel behavior. In Yerrell, JS (ed): Transport Research for Social and Economic Progress (Vol 3). Gower, Aldershot, England, 1981.
15. Downs, RM, and Stea, D (eds): Image and Environment: Cognitive Mapping and Spatial Behavior. Aldine, Chicago, 1973, p xiv.
16. Downs and Stea, p 10.
17. Neisser, U: Cognition and Reality: Principles and Implications of Cognitive Psychology. W. H. Freeman, San Francisco, 1981.
18. Appleyard, D: Notes on urban perception and knowledge. In Downs, RM, and Stea, D (eds): Image and Environment: Cognitive Mapping and Spatial Behavior. Aldine, Chicago, 1973.
19. Appleyard, p 112.
20. Hanson, S, and Burnett, KP: Understanding complex travel behavior: Measurement issues. In Stopher, PR, Meyburg, AH, and Brog, W (eds): New Horizons in Travel-Behavior Research. Lexington, MA, 1981.

21. Kutter, E: Some remarks on activity-pattern analysis in transportation planning. In Stopher, PR, Meyburg, AH, and Brog, W (eds): New Horizons in Travel-Behavior Research. Lexington, Lexington, MA, 1981.
22. Rosenbloom, S: The growth of non-traditional families: A challenge to traditional planning approaches. In Jansen, GRM, Nijkamp, P, and Ruijgrok, CJ (eds): Transportation and Mobility in an Era of Transition. Elsevier Science, Amsterdam, 1985.
23. Daniels, PW, and Warnes, AM: Movement in Cities: Spatial Perspectives on Urban Transport and Travel. Methuen, London, 1980.
24. Heidemann, C: Spatial-behavior studies: Concepts and contexts. In Stopher, PR, Meyburg, AH, and Brog, W (eds): New Horizons in Travel-Behavior Research. Lexington, Lexington, MA, 1981.
25. Richter, J: The daily transition between professional and private life. Dissertation Abstract International 44:3231, 1984.
26. Kutter, E: Some remarks on activity-pattern analysis in transportation planning. In Stopher, PR, Meyburg, AH, and Brog. W (eds): New Horizons in Travel-Behavior Research, Lexington, Lexington, MA, 1981.

by Doris Pierce, MA, OTR

13

The Work of Scholars

We know very little about what it is like, these days, to live a life centered around, or realized through, a particular sort of scholarly, or pedagogical, or creative activity. And until we know a great deal more, any attempt to pose, much less to answer, large questions about the role of this or that sort of study in contemporary society—and contemporary education—is bound to break down into passionate generalities inherited from a past just about as unexamined in this regard as the present.[1]

Why Study the Work of Scholars?

Scholars are the people on whom we depend for new knowledge and who enable our fast-changing society to continually rethink itself. Scholars carry the expertise of our culture. Popular representations of the scholar, the majority of whom

125

are academics, are conflicting. One pole describes scholars as lounging around campuses with a couple of classes to teach, tenure for life, summers and holidays off, sabbaticals, and no one holding them accountable.[2] The opposite perspective is of long hours, low pay, publication pressures, fierce competition, and isolation.[3]

In established fields of inquiry, the work practices of developing scholars are formed through active participation at lower level positions. For occupational therapy, an understanding of the work of scholars is especially critical. The present cohort of occupational therapy researchers received research training in a variety of disciplines. Therefore, their expectations regarding scholarly standards, methods, productivity, work routines, and career progressions differ. Due to this situation, little distinctive pattern of scholarly activity yet exists in occupational therapy. A model for training new scholars is not evident. Without a common background, disciplinary discourse is fragmented. This examination of the occupations of scholarly work can offer insight contributing to the formation of patterns of scholarly activity in occupational science.

Analogous to that well-known axiom, "Physician, heal thyself," this research brings the unique perspective of the emerging science of occupation to bear on the question of how the occupations of scholarly work are experienced. It offers established and aspiring occupational therapy scholars a window through which they may gaze to gain a fresh perspective on their own experience of scholarly activities.

A Background of Nested Debates

To examine the doing of scholarly work, it is important to acknowledge pertinent background issues. As is often the case in scholarship, it is not on an open field that we build our contribution, but a pitted and obstacle-strewn landscape. For this study, three questions are especially problematic. What is work? What is the mission of higher education? How has occupational therapy historically responded to the mission of the university?

Definitions of Work

What is work? Indeed, this is a theoretical question too complex to be settled here. However, popular understandings of the term usually emphasize activities, production of goods and services, and valuing of that product by others.[3] What then, is the work role of a scholar? The popular perception of what the scholar produces seems relatively vague. Whether these products are valued is relatively vague. It may be that much of the controversy reflected in such books as *Profscam*,[1] which lays the problems of the universities and society in general at the feet of lazy professors, are grounded in this unclear image of the work of the scholar and the relatively weak value of scholarly products in popular culture.

The work of scholars is an especially interesting case of work, due to the relative autonomy that derives from the tenure system. How is this autonomy managed within the round of activities of the scholar? Does the apparently self-directed nature of the work make it more enjoyable? Is it truly a reclusive and solitary endeavor? For occupational science, examination of the constellation of activities in such independently organized action as scholarship may provide a significant contrast to other studies of work in more structured settings.

The History of Higher Education: Conflicting Missions

The debate about the relative success of the scholarly endeavor that is reflected in *Profscam*[1] may be partially grounded in the history of higher education. The English university model is of a collection of liberal arts colleges serving a wealthy elite, preparing them for a life of proper culture. In contrast, the Teutonic model is dedicated to the generation of knowledge through science, research, and writing. In the development of American universities and colleges, the undergraduate programs followed the example of the English model, putting primary emphasis on teaching and educating students. More recently grafted onto these undergraduate liberal arts curricula are the American graduate schools, emphasizing scientific enterprise and specialization.[2] Academics must continually negotiate between these divided missions, attempting to prioritize goals of teaching and scholarship. How this conflict is managed is evidenced in their descriptions of their scholarly work.

Occupational Therapy Education: Predominance of the Teaching Mission

The historic focus of occupational therapy education on the undergraduate training of service professionals has channeled the efforts of faculty firmly toward the teaching mission of the university to the neglect of scholarly work.[4] Occupational therapy faculties are built from individuals with significant practice records, rather than from those socialized predominantly to the patterns of scholarship. Insertion of considerable service periods into the early career of faculty members shortens their scholarly potential, compared with disciplines in which direct entry from graduate school into academia is the norm. The normal pattern in occupational therapy is that established researchers just entering their prime also are just entering retirement. An understanding of the work of scholars may contribute in part to redress of this problem.

Methods

Clifford Geertz[5] argues for the importance of understanding the experience scholars have of their work, envisioning a microcosmic study of modern thought in the unity and diversity of thinking in the social sciences. He speculates that the unity of social science thought is in its process, and the diversity is in its content. Therefore, this study used Geertz's[5,6] interpretive approach, developing multidimensional, thick descriptions of the commonalities in individual experiences of scholarly work.

Design of the Study

The intent of this initial study was to gain a perspective on the primary dimensions of the work of successful scholars. Because the scholars regarded observation of their primarily solitary work as intrusive, data collection was primarily through interviews. Some observations of events at which scholars gathered were included to illuminate the sociocultural context of scholarship.

The study used an exemplar design by selecting participants who demonstrated successful scholarship. Ten full professors in the humanities and social sciences, currently on the faculty of the University of Southern California (USC), who had recent book publications were recruited. There were eight men and two women. The earlier and later career cohorts were examined in limited depth through one full professor's distinguished emeritus rank and inclusion of an additional male associate professor.

Interviews

The interview structure was relatively open. Initial interviews with two full professors, who were not primary participants in the study, were used to shape the interview questions and selection strategies of the study. Interviews usually had a relaxed and conversational air to them and ranged from a half hour to 3 hours in length. All the professors were asked for curriculum vitae. They often referred me to related books. Overall, the participants seemed quite articulate about their experience, seemed to enjoy considering the question of how they do their scholarly work, and were more open than I had anticipated.

Observations

Because direct observations of activities that professors identified as scholarly work was not possible, observations of two sites where scholars gathered around the values of scholarship were used. The Seminar on Social Thought, a small group of social scientists sharing presentations and discussions about postmodernism, was observed twice. The second observation site was the Academic Convocation, a spring university ceremony that honors outstanding members of the faculty and some students.

Analysis

Data were analyzed using the guidelines of grounded theory[7] and open and axial coding.[8] The categories first emerged in the initial interviews. From there, analysis of each interview transcript and observation generated theoretical notes and memos regarding evident and new categories. Coding groups were reorganized several times and can be considered to be just transcending open coding and entering axial coding. Coding was not as dense as it should be in the overall study, and some categories could be fruitfully developed further. These problems of analysis can be considered a product of the limited scope and time constraints of the study and would be better addressed in a fully developed qualitative study.

Limitations

The primary limitations of the study are the limited number of participants, the potential observer effects on the setting, and the difficulty of accessing direct observations of scholarly work. The ability to generalize the study to other universities, other disciplines, or scholars at other points in their careers is necessarily limited.

The Setting of the Study

To make use of the study, readers require some sense of the university context within which the scholars are working and how that may differ from their own institutions.

The participants viewed USC as unique in several respects. It is a "university on the make," intent on becoming one of the top 10 research universities in the United States. It positions itself as an emerging pacific rim school and has a large group of international students. Unfortunately for older faculty, a career centered on the earlier teaching mission of USC leaves them unpromotable to full professor and ill fit to the new university strategy. Some professors find USC pleasantly "entrepreneurial" and a good place to pursue their own research interests. Others criticize it for its reputation as a sports, party, and Hollywood school.

USC also seems to be responding to the "reactionary" political climate. Federal research funds for social science research have declined remarkably in recent years. *Profscam*[1] is a cry for reform and an announcement of the failure of the social sciences and humanities to have any effect on the general literacy, competency, or economic prosperity of American society. Recently, following Berkeley's lead, USC's President's Commission on Undergraduate Education released a report calling for improvements in teaching. Some of the scholars expect teaching competencies to acquire increased weight in tenure decisions now, but others are cynical of the call for improved teaching in view of the emphasized research mission of USC.

Doing the Work of a Scholar: Five Subjective Dimensions

The following synthesis of the experience that this articulate group identified as scholarship falls under the following headings: personal definitions, spaces, emotions, temporality, and sociocultural context. The intent of the study to retain the multidimensionality and subjectivity of the findings posed considerable challenge. However, it is this "willingness to examine and live with complexity"[9] that ensures the thick description that is the hallmark of the interpretive approach.

Personal Definitions of a Scholar

The 11 participants in the study, all full professors except one, were receptive to the interviews once they started. Their strong response to the idea of my observing them at their work conveyed an impression of the nature of their activities as personal, private, and perhaps even sacred. They expressed some doubts about the usefulness of their comments or whether it was possible to understand scholarly work in any other way except through experience. This conceptualization of certain practices as common, self-evident, or difficult to analyze in any depth is typical of the cultural systems of common sense described by Geertz.[5] One participant even seemed a bit worried, reciting a rhyme about a centipede who could not walk any longer after a frog asked him which leg he moved next.

How do you drive? . . . I do it so automatically. And that would apply to what we're talking about as to everything else. . . . Just as a runner, for example, if I were a coach, I wouldn't say this is how you must do it. You must lift your legs in this way and put them down that way. . . . You have to find out your own method . . . so for me to tell them this is how I have done my work, that might not really be much help at all. . . . When people say how do you go about writing a book? I reply, you sit down, you take out a pen, you put the pen on the page, and you write (Participant #11).

The first question of the interview was intended to bring out the participant's definition of a scholar. The answer most often referred to producing new knowledge. "Somebody who has put careful study into some body of knowledge and has also generated something original about whatever their body of knowledge is." "Making conceptual advances . . . that's the core of it all." Another aspect is that a scholar is part of a discourse in a specific area. One participant used a four-point definition: being part of a continuing dialogue, finding a particular part of that dialogue interesting, using an approach of curiosity and self-discipline, and being willing to contribute where it will be useful. Some said you could know a scholar by how many books they have published, whereas others did not buy that as a measure of anything except whether one was an academic. Another said you could recognize a scholar because "People carry their credentials with them and wave them, their curriculum vitae." Another said, "I go into the bar and Jerry the bartender says, 'Hey, how's the book coming?' . . . [it] makes you realize that people expect you to play a role and fulfill things. People expect you to produce."

The interviewees used different types of descriptors for the relative valuations of scholarly work. However, the most often used criterion was originality. The opposite of originality was boring work, resynthesis of former works, "turning the crank," or "racketeering" to publish the greatest possible quantity, often by rewriting the same project in several forms and publishing it in different places. "Fifty percent of what goes on in [a discipline] is just crap." This was often attributed to structural pressures on assistant professors facing tenure review. The emeritus professor described the historic changes in standards yet still emphasized the importance of originality, saying "You can use the bang up-to-date methods without having any great originality." Many mentioned that it was hard to judge the scholarship of other disciplines, due to a distance from the discourse in that field.

Another dimension that was considered important was whether the knowledge was useful and worthwhile. It was especially on this point of relevance and impact in the world that the professors were most critical of their own work, relating periods of anguish and self-doubt about whether their life's work had been well chosen to benefit others. Two of the participants hesitated to call themselves scholars: the associate professor because of filling a role in the department as more of a "strategist" and another because it seemed like an old-fashioned term. However, all the informants described engaging in similar groups of activities that, for them, defined the role of scholar.

The Activities of the Scholar

A typology of activities marks the role of scholar. The "modal" activity is reading: constant reading within the field and the building and use of personal libraries. Thinking and conceptualizing were emphasized, although they were challenging to describe. The phases of doing research were often cited: data gathering at the research site, the "hustle mode" of library work, and writing grants, results, more theoretical papers or books, and revisions. Many of the scholars suspected disciplinary differences in the activities of scholarship. Often, scholars mentioned the need to share and get their work out to the discipline through presentations, panels, and other avenues. They also recognized a portion of the work of scholarship that they considered "donkey work" or "drudgery": that detailed clean-up work of tracking down references, proofing manuscripts, and answering correspondence. Those who were involved as editors of journals considered it a more "social" case of scholarly work.

Images and Analogies

Clifford Geertz[5] speculates that the metaphors that scholars use are shifting from mechanistic, hard science origins to more humanistic representations, such as the game, the text, and the drama. Actually, this study showed that scholars tend to describe their work in terms of other work. The most frequently used analogy was that of farming.

> The land will absorb any amount of labor you are willing to give it, without any visible return. Fix fences, keep up sheds, drive fence, cut undergrowth. You know that at some future point there will be some payoff, but at no time can you not think of something to do. It's a system of complex prioritizations. There's always something to do. Sometimes you can just go round and round, doing things . . . should you use a rail to fix the fence, or use wire, or go milk, or if you let the cows into the pasture after you milk, they'll get through the hole. There are infinite tasks that will repay your efforts. It's like scholarship, there are always more books and thinking to do until you reach an integration of a field (Participant #10).
>
> So, unlike most other kinds of occupations, to use your words, this one has incredible flexibility. In American history, I mean one of the reasons the American dream was being a family farmer despite the incredible difficulty of that life was in fact, you have a certain amount of control over your time. Whereas, if you work in a factory or punched a clock, somebody else controlled you. Being a scholar is somewhat going back to that older image, of basically you are your own boss. There are constraints and there are rewards and penalties and all of that. But on a day-to-day basis, you regulate your own life (Participant #4).
>
> If you're a good scholar, then you don't cheat even to yourself. . . . As in gardening, you know, you take the weeds out by the roots, you get the whole thing, you don't just take the scissors to them or whatever (Participant #11).

Other such terms as "cultivating scholarship" and discussions of assistant professors who "die on the vine" for lack of effective guidance raise the question of the origins and significance of this farming terminology.

All of the farming analogies were provided by male informants. Female informants were the only ones to speak of scholarly work in terms of cooking, love, and the work of the housewife.

> When I'm through with that [book], these other kinds of [projects] come cooking along. . . . I don't have a million ideas cooking for that. . . . That [book idea] is like a fantasy. . . . It takes me quite a while to commit to what I will do next . . . reading around trying to decide. . . . I find it like choosing a marriage partner, maybe not quite as serious, but sure it is a commitment for quite a few years. . . . I published something in [a journal] and they always have . . . a blurb about the author . . . "at work on a new book" . . . and its sounds like a wedding announcement or an engagement announcement (Participant #7).

The obsessiveness is the thing, a real pleasurable obsessiveness though, like when you fall in love. . . . It has its problems. You know, like if I have to shut it off and go out to dinner and be social, it's not easy for me, to just cut off that obsessive involvement and just switch over into a whole other mode and a whole other mood. When you think about this schizophrenic state our profession is, between teaching and doing scholarship and seeing students and doing committees and it's not unlike the housewife situation where you're trying to get a whole bunch of things done (Participant #8).

Three of the professors referred to the work as a puzzle. "It's like the crossword puzzle. I don't want to have two crossword puzzles going. I've got to finish it, complete it, send it off, and then start the next project." A wide variety of other forms of work were used to demonstrate the dynamics of scholarly work in different ways: yuppies working 80-hour weeks as a more demanding work week; architects dealing with the drudgery of permits and zoning; the plumber singing at his work, showing individual work style; the demanding performance required of a musician; the creativity of a writer of detective novels; and the contrasting fixed schedule and physical exertion of the construction worker. References were often made to great scholars of fame and fiction.

The Relation of Teaching and Scholarship

None of the participants identified teaching as one of the activities of doing scholarly work, yet their attitude toward teaching was largely positive when they specifically explored it. Many of the professors found uses for teaching that related to their scholarship, such as using research in classes or editing chapter drafts through feedback from a seminar. Almost all found the graduate classes more useful for this than the undergraduate classes. They found teaching and scholarship "mutually inspiring" and "integrally linked." Teaching is "fun," but no one mistook teaching for their primary role in the University.

The whole reason of being in the academic world is to write, and teaching is simply an interlude, like just in the way that running around the block is good exercise and is also a nice change, it's exhilarating and so forth, but it's not what one would normally count as pursuit of one's general goals (Participant #11).

I believe in teaching. . . . You pay your way. . . . I wouldn't want to load myself down that I couldn't work, but I think we all should pitch in at USC, it's tuition supported, we should all make our own way (Participant #6).

There also was a general consensus that the best teachers were those who were productive scholars. They saw the vitality of teaching as dependent on involvement in ongoing research.

One participant found teaching unpleasant and a burden. Another professor said, "It can be depressing to see really poor quality teaching. . . . Most professors don't have any training as teachers. . . . They rip off their students every time they walk into the classroom and it's very depressing." Others noted that the problem with teaching is trying to schedule scholarship around it.

See, this is what's so schizophrenic about our profession, is that you teach, and that is why you can't just fit writing in around the edges. One is highly social and highly interactive with other people and the other is extremely isolated and requires solitude and a whole mental involvement that is diametrically opposed to the teaching mode. And that's why you have this thing of the absent-minded professor. . . . You get your mind going on this one mode and then you're supposed to switch into this other mode where you're remembering people's names and you're trying to bring them all together in discussion and it's very hard (Participant #8).

The Spaces of a Scholar's Work: Bodies, Tools, and Offices

The Physiology of Scholarship

It seemed to be the consensus that, unless some conceptual breakthrough had just occurred or a deadline was looming, 5 hours of really productive writing was exhausting. After that, one switched to "junk work." All scholars spoke of writing first thing in the morning as most preferred, and some had built strong routines around that preference. For some, their energy level is consistently high during their scholarly work, and for others it is more variable. Some spoke of 10-minute naps, limiting coffee and alcohol, and using swimming and taking walks to keep in condition during periods planned for major writing projects.

The Tools of Scholarship

The influence of the settings in which scholars work was easily seen in the interviews. The personal computer is the most evident tool of scholarship. Many of the professors do their writing on computers. The older scholars use it only to do revisions. Those who handwrote drafts spoke of the pleasure of that experience. One informant had specific preferences in writing utensils for different types of written work. All referred often to the importance of their books, and their offices were always lined with shelves of books related to their disciplinary interests.

Offices

The spaces in which the scholars worked included university offices, home offices, libraries and research settings, and occasionally third offices on campus for hiding away to accomplish specific tasks, such as grading (Fig. 13–1). Quietness was imperative, yet they could adapt to some noise if necessary. The political issue of space was central to the competition for resources within the university. Most had home offices where they did the bulk of the creative work because of frequent interruptions in their university offices. As one scholar put it, on campus, one might be "nibbled to death by ducks." Many regarded the aesthetics of the work space as important, and attainment of a satisfactory home office seemed to be a relished career milestone for many of the interviewees.

Emotional Experiences of Scholarly Work

The gamut of emotions in doing scholarly work run from "oceanic highs" when it is going well to "agony" when it is not. The emotions are directly tied to the work. Just engaging in the work of scholarship seems to require special attitudes of highly developed motivation, described as "naive optimism"; a pressure "to move from this conceptual level to that conceptual level"; an "appetite for the work"; and "a sort of obsessiveness." "I think there was a time when I had to make myself do it

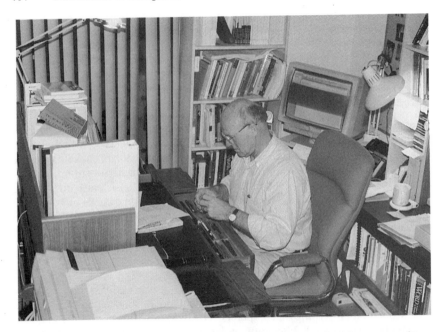

Figure 13–1. The physical space that surrounds a scholar when he or she submerges into his or her work seems to be critical for productivity. (Photo by John Wolcott.)

and now I find myself really desiring to do it." The emeritus professor said, "Some of these characters are a bit astonished when they find a person of my age engaging in writing. Now, other people will say, well, what else would one do?"

The positive end of the emotional scale includes the pleasurable engagement of solving puzzles, loss of one's self in the writing, and sense of accomplishment. Some articles, such as those that analyze and discuss statistics, are considered easier than more theoretical pieces and seem almost to write themselves. Seeing people use the work, influencing public policy in a positive direction, or being officially recognized for scholarship through awards or citation analyses also are rewarding.

The less pleasant experiences of scholarly work seem to revolve around tough points in projects and feeling unappreciated. One participant described working right into a hole, working into a "frenzy," and, in the days of typewriters, being able to tell a bad day by the trash piling up. There are certain points in a project, first sentences and first chapters, that seem especially anxiety provoking.

> Even though there are times that I am in total despair and I think I'll never be able to do it again, they're a lot less often [now]. They last a lot less time and probably I don't really, really believe it. I see people just starting out writing, it's just so hard and you really have to develop confidence through doing, but if you feel so, so afraid of it, you may not be able to work to that point where it gets easier (Participant #8).

Many of the scholars expressed extreme frustration with the effort required to go in and out of the writing phase and how much time they lose getting back into it after having to stop to do something else. They found themselves preoccupied and oblivious to interactions at times. Others described painful periods of reassessment of their work, when they doubted its value and direction. Because most of the professors are productive within their fields but are only marginally aware of others' standings within their disciplines, many are left feeling unappreciated within their own university. The most distressing emotional experience of the work of scholars seems to be writer's block.

> I know some people who really have a block, about getting a book together. . . . Even though they have enough, to sort of do it, they can't quite do it. And I think it's connected to quite deep psychological issues about completion and success, and so on. . . . I do have friends that basically, for reasons that have very little to do with their ideas or their ability to express their ideas, have been unable to come up with the sort of major scholarship that will enable them to pursue a career. And I do think it's owing to other issues, things that are more personal (Participant #8).

> There can be times when I can go for 6 or 8 weeks and not have any productive scholarly work come out of me because I get blocked or frustrated or internally bound up by, you know, some problem I can't solve or sometimes I'm just bored with it. And you can get a real sense of almost panic out of that, about how am I going to break this and get back to a mode that I like and enjoy, and sometimes those interludes can be weeks in duration (Participant #5).

Temporal Rhythms: Personal, Project, Daily, Annual, and Career

Personal Temporal Strategies

The relatively unstructured nature of the work of scholars makes the skills for prioritizing and maintaining control over the distribution of work time critical. Poor skills in this area can result in overcommitment, inability to preserve the large blocks of time required for scholarly productivity, and constant traveling, sitting on university committees, or doing departmental administrative tasks. The key concept most of the participants cited was self-discipline. "The most productive scholars make or find lots of time to write, and they do it in a very disciplined way."

> My statement is, there's not enough time. . . . Now, the obvious thing is to say that it is because there's meetings, telephone calls, machinery. Has all this machinery devoured time? . . . There's a very profound question at the core of . . . occupational science. . . . Issues that are deeply theoretical about how we organize our time, hold it, make it seem productive, or do we let our time get away from us? (Participant #6).

The different strategies the scholars use are instructive. Devices include calendars, forward planning charts, and answering machines. They structure their time. "If I sit down and win the day, I have seven typewritten pages. If I win the day 10 times, I have a 70-page chapter. . . . Twelve times more, I have the book." "I must get so much writing done every day. . . . More or less, whenever the spirit moves you, but see you keep tabs on the spirit." Others find that their productivity is more variable, that there are "seasons of work," that they can work 15 to 18 hours if they are really rolling, and that it is tied to the phases of the project more than any daily rhythm.

Some participants admit to difficulties "guarding my time," being a "bad time manager," and saying yes to things just because they have said no so many times before. Some respond to deadlines or the rhythms of collaborators. They express a lot of frustration about the time that can be devoured by responsibilities to sit on committees and work with graduate students and resentment of those who do not do their share. Those who are department chairs or graduate directors feel the pressure on their scholarly work time to an even greater degree. Arrangement can sometimes be made to shift teaching responsibilities away from a period of focused work or to "bank" teaching by doing extra one semester.

Scholars "routinize" their work in creative personal ways. They use tricks to get right back into the work, like stopping in the middle of a sentence, discontinuing at natural topic breaks, noting the next 18 things they were thinking of writing about, avoiding getting into junk work during productive work time, limiting writing to specific blocks of time, doing other things when getting tired, and moving to a space that is identified with a particular mode of work. They accept the need for breaks and let themselves settle into the work as quickly as they can.

Time Structures in the Project Sequence

The phases and lengths of scholarly projects impact the subjective experience of the work. Lengths vary greatly, from a 3-day turnaround in newspaper editorials, to a 70-year project. A book could take 6 or 7 years, and publication of an article, once it is submitted, can take 2 or 3 years. Most thought of their work as going in repeating cycles of several years. Ideas for projects could come from serendipitous meetings, careful selection within a disciplinary interest, availability of grant funding, or a notebook of potential ideas. Some have overlapping projects, whereas others prefer to work on a single project in a focused way. They speak of phases of gearing up for the project, reaching saturation in the literature, data gathering, the sequence of chapter writing, and a series of revisions. Most described the tough initial parts of different phases and places where conceptualization breaks loose. Following a major effort, there is often a "fallow" phase or "reassessment" and the beginning of transitioning to a new project.

The impact of the phases of the work on the subjective experience of the participants cannot be overstated. The emotional dimension is strongly tied to the temporality of the project sequence. The acquisition of the ability to identify and accept the emotional conditions of different portions of a project is essential to the mature scholar's ability to persevere through difficult periods and attempt increasingly larger undertakings. Looking back over a career, the scholars tend to think in terms of a series of accomplished products. In this study, activity was not shaped by time so much as the experience of time was shaped by the activities that occupied it.

Daily Temporality

All the participants reported being best able to work first thing in the morning and being more tired in the evenings. Some have strong routines that organize their time around that realization. They use later times of the day for other activities. Often, these routines continue through the weekend. One participant worked in the evenings until the first child joined the family and then switched to early morning writing. They note a difference in the ability to do productive scholarly work once they leave the house and interact with others.

> I find it almost impossible to go out and come back and get to work. . . . I don't know, there's a sort of connection almost to dreams or something, to nighttime, to dream-

ing. . . . I mean, once I go out, I just can't imagine getting up and going out to a gym and coming back, it just sounds appalling to me (Participant #8).

I like getting up, absolute get up in the morning and get there. Total pig look. No shave, no shine, nothing, just a beast. . . . You come down [to the office], you meet personalities, people, then you're in a different mode. So up and at a desk and get to work (Participant #6).

Annual Rhythms

Because being a scholar, for these academics, occurs in tandem with being a teacher and administrator, the work has annual variations shaped by the academic calendar. The scholars seem best able to have the long blocks of time necessary for creative work in the summers and holiday vacations. This schedule becomes an expected work period, and they look forward to it each year. The semesters have their own schedules also due to the demands of administrative work, admissions, and grading.

The Temporal Experience of the Career

The changes the scholars recognized throughout the time spans of their careers were in attitudes and skills. They spoke of graduate school as fraught with demands to meet the expectations of others, an orientation that took many years to overcome. Some said that one finds one's "voice" or "persona" in the dissertation process, while another is finding it now as a senior professor.

The interviewees remember the experience of assistant professorship and recognize it in their departments as one of "structure pressures" from tenure, "gatekeepers breathing down your neck," the "great ritual of the dossier," being tested against "national standards" in publication, and worrying too much about the long-term directions and importance of their work. Self-doubts and rejections seem to be the hallmark of this period. Guidance is critical at this stage. One professor was thankful that he had heeded some advice not to publish certain strong opinions in early papers, which would have embarrassed him now, and not to become a department chair, which would have destroyed his scholarly work.

Once tenured, work does not let up, but scholars seem to feel more free to steer their own course in selecting topics. Some noted strong theoretical or methodological shifts and even midlife changes in career directions. At this point, the full professors feel that they have gained several critical perspectives on scholarly work. They expect the tough parts of a project and are not as distressed at the difficulties. Most have moved from collaboration to more sole-authored works. They are more interested in broad theoretical issues now and want to have an impact on the directions of their field. They also have established reputations that lead to more invitations to speak and publish than they can fulfill. They have to learn to say "no." Most noted an increased freedom from rules and conventions, more creativity, and even a playfulness in their work, which they had not had before. Their skills are sharper, making projects easier to accomplish. They feel the pressures of a finite amount of time left in their careers. "Now I am absolutely a . . . prose machine. . . . I will not live to unleash the amount of things that I want to." They choose the remaining projects more carefully. One noted the lack of guidance that professors receive in the middle career years. The overall picture is of competent and confident scholars at the peak of their careers who see the importance of the choices and influence they now have in their disciplines.

The Sociocultural Context of the Work of Scholars

The ivory tower image of the scholar, writing alone in a garret or mountain retreat is probably based on the conditions that the study participants described as crucial to productive work. They spoke of the importance of becoming accustomed to solitude and a "lonely discipline." One interviewee estimated the amount of time spent alone in scholarship as 60%. Some attributed the proliferation of meetings, colloquia, and national associations to the scholar's need for face-to-face interaction.

The preoccupied state of the scholar can make family life difficult. Examples of stress resulting from the interaction of family and scholarly roles included working in shared spaces, fending off children while working, sitting at the dinner table and not hearing, having a spouse demand a choice between a reasonable amount of family participation or a divorce, and having intense work periods "come out of my family's hide." Usually they design some type of schedule to try to accommodate both realms. Women with children appear to have the greatest difficulty with this situation.

Colleagues, coworkers, and collaborators are the primary intersection of a scholar with his or her discipline. Despite the image of solitude and isolation, scholars are intimately tied into the current thinking in their field through constant reading, shared work, and formal and informal exchanges of views. Doing research with students may guide a project choice but is usually focused on fostering the scholarship of the student, rather than that of the mature scholar. The primary connections are with colleagues within and beyond their own university departments.

All of the scholars reported having trusted friends to whom they sent manuscripts for first reviews, criticism, and support. These were absolutely central relationships for their work. Some meet regularly with a friend of similar interests during the writing phase of a book to talk about the project. Occasionally, they depend on the more informal support of friends outside academe.

More formal and interdisciplinary networks exist for working on theoretical issues, such as seminars, study groups, and colloquia. Two observations of the Seminar for Social Thought seemed to indicate that it was being used to process the concepts of postmodern theory and bring them to bear on the disciplinary interests of the participants. The atmosphere of the seminar was one of quiet, attentiveness, civility, respect for others' views, and scholarly debate. One interviewee termed it a "community of scholars." For others, such groups were writing groups, groups organized around editing a journal, organizers of a particular interdisciplinary curriculum, or interuniversity groups focused on a topic. For some, the people with whom they collaborate and those they study provide important colleagues.

The atmosphere of university departments can range from congenial to highly charged and polarized. Participants shared horror stories of departments split into opposite camps, usually disputing along theoretical lines, which then become struggles about hiring assistant professors to strengthen one side of the battle or the other. This can result in massive resignations and a department losing much strength. Sometimes full professors take advantage of assistant or associate professors by loading them down with an unfair amount of responsibilities when they need to be publishing. Most departments have faculty load profiles, which usually distribute percentages of teaching, research, and service along a 40/40/20 division. Some departments have informal quotas for the numbers of publications expected each year. The annual merit review also can be a point of "disputatiousness." Some of the professors used a strategy of just avoiding the conflicts and trying to concentrate on their own work, but it was difficult to do. One said that the people who cultivate scholarship are crucial in a scholar's life, primarily chairs and deans. Another scholar complained that, after being recruited because of a reputation for writing, the teaching load and committee load were preventing writing. Three informants quoted different versions of a statement by Henry Kissinger, to the effect that the conflict in academia was so intense because the gains to be made are so small.

> If you put together 15, 20, 30 people with incredible autonomy, the [possibility] that they could build any kind of intellectual community out of that is pretty limited. . . . A new issue comes up, the same old speeches are trotted out. . . . We're all predictable. . . . Imagine yourself sitting around an old people's home sixteen years (Participant #4).

Departments that are not productive and do not form a collective effort can be at a disadvantage in the competition between departments and divisions for their share of the "zero sum" resources of the university. When a department gets a reputation for conflict and impaired productivity, it can be "cannibalized" by resources being channeled into another of the Dean's departments. Although faculty members may resent differences in merit increases, the faculty of cohesive and active "departments on the move" make better salaries overall. The interdisciplinary nature of tenure and promotion review committees highlights differences in expectations for productivity. Expectations for publication from different departments vary greatly: quantities of single-authored quantitative articles, single major theoretical works, prolific creative writing, and a mix of books and articles.

Conclusion

This study of the multidimensional, contexted experience that scholars have of their work offers a mirror to the aspiring scholars of occupational therapy, an unraveling of an interesting case to those who want to understand better the occupational nature of human existence.

This description may be useful to occupational therapy scholars in the emerging discipline of occupational science. The combination of the scholar's striving for original work in "a lonely discipline" and their complete contextualization in a disciplinary network of reading and collegial relationships seemed to drive and regulate the cutting edge of scholarship at its best. The dimensions described in this early interpretation outline evident facets in the underlying structures of all occupations: personal conceptualizations framing an activity, physiologic and material space, emotional experience, temporality, and sociocultural context. The relative autonomy of these scholars also provides a glimpse of the patterns occupations take when less constrained by our industrialized society's fascination with the synchronized work day. There is a rhythm in the tasks of scholarship, of difficult slow starts, highly charged long hours in the creative center of projects, even-tempered rewrites and revisions, and short periods of the drudgery of clean-up work. The specific temporality that is tied, not to physiologic or social rhythms, but to phases of the work and submergence and surfacing from engagement in that work, highlights the powerful regulator that activity is in shaping subjective experience.

Exploring Occupational Experience to Strengthen Intervention

The question of how such studies as this will contribute to occupational therapy's concern with improving therapeutic assistance to people with disabilities is a difficult one to answer at this early stage of occupational science. However, some indications of the basic dimensions of occupations that a therapist could consider when strengthening his or her selected interventions are provided by this study.

The strongest of these potentially important dimensions of occupation is the task rhythm that was evident in these relatively autonomous workers: the anxiety of beginning points, the frustration and inefficiency of stopping for other activity when submerged in concentration, the drudgery of the closure phases of the project. Perhaps we should be giving therapy in short initial sessions with lots of breaks for the stress of start up; then longer treatment times for the exciting productivity of the main body of the project; and then, short bouts for finishing off and cleaning up? Do some patients have trouble with one phase and not with others? Could we gain more in one 3-hour activity session than three 1-hour activity sessions by cutting out submersion and surfacing time, letting involvement in the task reach a central peak? The scholars imposed personal routines and strategies on this task rhythm. Do some patients have trouble generating and enforcing these personal routines? At this time, these are not much more than provocative questions, yet if only in our internal dialogue, a question can be a valuable springboard to insight.

As a beginning, this study of the work of scholars has been illuminating. I will close with this quote from the distinguished emeritus scholar.

> The most important thing of all is not to talk about writing, but to write. . . . This is the great merit that the old monastic orders had. They had the rule of silence. . . . It's not merely that you keep the convent nice and quiet and peaceful, it's that you get time to do some work, and then the focus comes to be on what you do (Participant #11).

For occupational therapy and its emerging science, the most important thing will always be not what we say about occupation, nor even what we write about it, but what we do with it.

Discussion Questions

1. Does the fact that scholars assume a rather elite and usually privileged position in society make generalizations about their primary occupation any less relevant or applicable to the "general" population?

2. How might the phases of the occupations of scholars (gearing up, reaching various points of saturation, feeling fallow or reassessing) bear clinical significance with respect to scheduling constraints on the kinds of activities that might realistically be pursued, given short lengths of stay? What are creative ways that occupational therapists might address some of these constraints so that richer and more complex occupations can be therapeutically pursued?

References

1. Sykes, CJ: Profscam: Professors and the Demise of Higher Education. Regnery Gateway, Washington, DC, 1988.
2. Lewis, LS: Scaling the Ivory Tower: Merit and Its Limits in Academic Careers. Johns Hopkins University Press, Baltimore, 1975.
3. Rothman, RA: Working: Sociological Perspectives. Prentice-Hall, Englewood Cliffs, NJ, 1987.
4. Yerxa, EJ: Occupational therapy: An endangered species or an academic discipline in the 21st century? Am J Occup Ther 45:680, 1991.
5. Geertz, C: Local Knowledge. Basic Books, New York, 1983.
6. Geertz, C: The Interpretation of Culture. Basic Books, New York, 1973.
7. Glaser, BG, and Strauss, AL: The Discovery of Grounded Theory. Aldine, New York, 1967.
8. Corbin, J, and Strauss, A: Grounded theory research: Procedures, canons, and evaluative criteria. Qual Sociol 13:3–21, 1990.
9. Reilly, M: Play As Exploratory Learning. Sage, Beverly Hills, 1974, p 26.

by Mike Carlson, PhD

14

The Self-Perpetuation of Occupations

From childhood to old age, most of our waking hours are spent performing personally meaningful, goal-directed activities. Whether gardening, cooking, playing tennis, driving a car, watching television, or working on a personal computer, we almost continually engage in purposeful pursuits that collectively and sequentially structure our existence, lending meaning to our lives. Culturally defined "chunks" of purposive activity, as exemplified in the above instances, have been termed "occupations."[1,2]

By virtue of their existence in the cultural lexicon, occupations represent conceptual gestalts that are considered by members of a given society as potentially filling a given unit of one's time to achieve one or more desired goals. A key attribute of occupations is their salience within our everyday awareness. Occupations commonly exist at the forefront of our conscious attention because they are the subject of decision-making processes prior to their overt initiation on a given occasion; typically demand concentration and engender an awareness of what one is doing during their enactment; and represent observable, concrete, personally meaningful indicators of personality and life-style. Given their fundamental place in our everyday awareness, it is not surprising that the choice and patterning of participation in occupations is linked to health,[3,4] happiness,[5] personality development,[6,7] and life satisfaction.[8,9] Also underscoring the importance of occupations is the additional finding that the outcomes of daily life occurrences predict psychological health to an even greater degree than do major life events.[10,11]

In this paper, I argue that occupations are important not only because they fill our waking hours and sequentially structure our lives, but also because they often possess an important self-perpetuating property, which I term "occupational perseverance." I suggest that this principle of perseverance can operate within any of four hierarchically related levels of occupational involvement and present a tentative typology of factors that can foster its operation. Finally, the relevance of these ideas to the practice of occupational therapy is addressed.

Occupational Repetition

Occupational participation is important because it undergirds much of our temporal sphere of existence. However, in addition to the ubiquity of occupations in a broad sense, people's tendency to repeat engagement in the same or similar occupations can magnify significantly the overall impact of occupations within our lives. The term "occupational repetition" refers to the phenomenon whereby an individual's participation in a given occupation is continued. To the extent that occupational repetition occurs, a person's sequential pattern of occupational selections is less variable, and the overall impact of occupational involvement is likely to be enhanced relative to what would be the case if successive occupational choices were relatively independent of each other. As an illustration, consider a 25-year-old man who chooses to go out drinking with friends on four successive evenings. Such a situation, which exemplifies occupational repetition, is likely to be associated with a greater overall degree of impact of occupational activity than would be present if, on the four evenings, the man had chosen to go out drinking with friends, stay home and read a book, attend a movie, and go bowling. In the former case, for example, the cumulative effects of drinking with friends might lead the man to redefine his social identity or might contribute to the development of an alcohol problem. In the latter instance, the different occupations, being diverse, may to some extent mutually cancel each other's effects and therefore be less likely to play a confluent, lasting role in shaping the man's future.

The repetition of a specified occupation can produce potent effects, for better or worse, on human personality and achievement. Much human greatness has obviously resulted from sustained involvement with particular occupations, as exemplified by Einstein's work in physics or Michael Jordan's basketball skills. Likewise, the repetition of relatively unfulfilling occupations, such as television viewing, snacking, or sun bathing, may, over the long term, indirectly lead to wasted talent and personal mediocrity.

It is hard to overestimate the importance of this repetitional phenomenon because its operation substantially determines the fabric of our being. Often by choosing to engage in a given occupation at the expense of other occupations, we initiate a process of prolonged involvement that simultaneously shapes and defines our existence while also negating potential alternate expressions of our personhood. However, the importance of occupational repetition in a given individual's life does not necessarily correspond in a simple way to the objective number of times that an occupation is performed. Rather, the manner in which an occupation fits into one's overall life-style, in light of time constraints and other limiting factors, must be taken into consideration in any evaluation of the impact of whatever repetition occurs. For example, going on a semiannual boating trip to a serene lake may be significant if such an activity is highly meaningful to a person. However, the role of a specific occupation within a person's life generally will tend to loom more important in terms of its self-judged meaningfulness, its impact on health and psychological well-being, and its diminution of alternative occupations that could instead fill the time spent, when it is engaged in more frequently.

Many different considerations may potentially promote repeated engagement in a specified occupation. For example, external rewards or pressure, genetically based physical predispositions that promote certain types of activities, need satisfaction, personality-based activity preferences, and social role requirements may, in given cases, foster continued participation in an occupation.[12–16]

Occupational Perseverance

In this paper, I argue that in addition to factors such as those noted above, the act of participation in an occupation often tends to increase future involvement with the same or similar occupations. The term "occupational perseverance" refers to prolonged engagement in an occupation that is directly or indirectly related to prior engagement with the occupation in question. The operation of occupational perseverance is analogous to a snowball effect. Once rolling, the snowball, by virtue of its past movements, gathers a momentum of its own that perpetuates the continuance of the roll. In a similar vein, much occupational involvement tends to perpetuate itself. Akin to the potentially colossal effects of self-perpetuating physical phenomena, such as landslides, tidal waves, or tornadoes, persevering occupational activity can produce significant results, for better or worse, within our lives. The high school graduate who decides to attend college instead of entering the full-time work force, the adolescent who begins to participate in gang activities after school, and the alcoholic who goes out for a social drink after abstaining for several years have each set out on a journey that, due largely to the operation of self-perpetuation processes, is likely to shape the subsequent course of their lives. Although not all occupational choices have as much potential impact in their consequences as these examples, I would argue that the phenomenon of perseverance is fairly ubiquitous and typically important.

Perhaps the most clear-cut evidence of occupational perseverance consists of cases in which a chosen occupation becomes a constant source of attention and excitement for a person but only after initial engagement in it. All of us can think of times in which we greatly enjoyed and continued to participate in an activity (and perhaps even felt like dropping everything else in its pursuit), despite the fact that it was perhaps difficult or even distasteful to initiate. In such cases, the pronounced shift in the occupation's perceived attractiveness following its initiation is evidence that actual participation critically mediated the occupation's continuance, as other factors, such as long-term personality characteristics or external pressure, are not likely to have produced such a profound, short-term leap in our esteem for the occupation. The excitement that often accompanies writing a paper that had been previously put off is an example of this. Although difficult to initiate, the activity, once started, captures our enthusiasm and renders inscrutable our former procrastination. In such a case, the actual performance of the occupation is largely responsible for its continuation. As noted previously, occupational perseverance has not occurred when factors other than previous participation are exclusively responsible for repeated engagement in an occupation. Thus, the social psychological finding that individuals' recreational activity patterns remain relatively stable over time,[6] while potentially based in part on occupational perseverance, may primarily result from the tendency for individuals to select situations that are consistent with their long-term personality traits.[7,13,17]

Four Levels at Which Occupational Perseverance Can Occur

Occupational perseverance could be enacted within any of at least four levels of generality. From most specific to least specific, these levels correspond to a particular occupational performance enacted on a single occasion; a specific occupation engaged in on different occasions; a broad occupational category, such as work, rest, or leisure; and activity in general.

At the lowest level, the phenomenon of perseverance is exemplified by the case in which a person plans to view only a few minutes of a television movie but becomes enthralled with the plot and as a consequence watches the entire show. At the next higher level, particular occupations can perseverate by virtue of being enacted repeatedly across different occasions, such as when a person views a soap opera every day to keep abreast of its latest developments.

Beyond specific occupations, higher order occupational categories, like work, rest, or play, may be subject to perseverance. A potential illustration of perseverance at the higher order occupational category level concerns the child who continuously plays instead of doing homework. Although distinct, specific occupations within the larger category "play" may or may not persevere individually, the higher order category perseveres in its own right. Likewise, the adult "workaholic" who feels compelled to engage in psychologically interchangeable varieties of busyness exhibits the perseverance of a higher order occupational category.

In a broader manner, it is possible that a person's general activity level may exhibit persevering properties. In this sense, any activity, if initiated, may possibly breed further activity and thereby disrupt the perpetuation of inaction.

Whether occupational activity perseveres at the level of individual performance, occupational type, higher order occupational category, or activity in general may depend in part on the level of action identification that the performer adopts. As Vallacher and Wegner[18] have pointed out, while performing an activity, an individual at any given moment tends to define his or her action in terms of only one of any of a number of different levels. An artist, for example, may think of himself or herself as moving their brush, creating a beautiful work of art, or finding personal fulfillment, but due to the unidirectional nature of human attention at any point, he or she is likely to define their action at only one level. It seems reasonable to speculate that an attention focus on higher order categories (e.g., work, rest, or play) will facilitate perseverance at the higher order level, while attention to the specific occupation will produce a persevering sequence at that level.

Differentiation From Habit

While the concepts of occupational perseverance and habit both involve the phenomenon of repetition, they differ in at least two critical respects. First, occupational perseverance is specific to the initiation and continuation of occupations, while habits, as they have been variously defined, are more general and can refer to such things as nervous twitches, punctuality, smoking cigarettes, cussing, and obeying the speed limit. A second distinction is that habits generally refer to relatively automatic, nonvoluntary, or unconscious actions, while occupational perseverance stems largely from active, volitional choice processes (for example, an individual actively chooses to continue in his or her current line of employment so that they do not "waste" their previously gained experience and expertise).

Kielhofner's[19] use of "habit" within the habituation subsystem of the model of human occupation illustrates the difference between habit and occupational perseverance. He defines habits as "images guiding the routine and typical ways in which a person performs"[20] that "function largely without conscious intervention."[21] Thus, according to Kielhofner, habits are broader than the occupational selection process and are primarily automatic. Habits rather blandly reproduce response patterns in the face of relevant stimuli. In contrast, I construe occupational perseverance as the outcome of a dynamic process in which volitional, active decision making interacts with whatever automatic processing is present. This posited dynamism reflects an acceptance of the purposeful intentionality of occupational involvement, along with an acknowledgment that selected situational and personal factors can influence the occupational selection process.

Differentiation From Flow

The construct of "flow" refers to the experiential state that occurs when an individual is engrossed in an occupation that provides challenges that are approximately equal to his or her level of skill.[22,23] Flow is an intrinsically rewarding psychological state that is accompanied by such features as clarity of goals, heightened concentration, a merging of activity and awareness, and a distorted sense of time.[23] Thus, flow represents a certain quality of experience and as such, differs from occupational perseverance, which relates to the frequency or persistence with which an activity is initiated and that may be enacted by numerous considerations other than flow, as is described subsequently.

Although flow may promote the perseverance of a given occupation, as when through repeated engagement if one seeks to reinstate a pleasurable flow experience, it is neither necessary nor sufficient for occupational perseverance to occur. The perseveration of nonflow-inducing occupations (such as sun bathing) and the generation of flow in nonrepeated occupational endeavors (such as a man with a "macho" image who experiences flow while cooking for his sick wife but who refuses to cook after she recovers) illustrate this principle. Thus, flow is one of many factors capable of affecting occupational perseverance.

Theoretical Rationale for the Notion of Occupational Perseverance

Within psychology, a good deal of classic theoretical work is consistent with the notion of occupational perseverance. For heuristic purposes, relevant considerations are somewhat arbitrarily grouped into cognitive/perceptual and affective/motivational categories in the ensuing discussion.

Cognitive and Perceptual Factors

Priming

Studies of human memory have shown that information is stored in hierarchically interrelated networks.[24,25] As a consequence of this organizational memory storage principle, the act of mentally attending to a given thought or idea increases the ease with which similar, semantically related cognitions will surface in consciousness, as when a person accesses a series of interconnected memories when reminiscing about the past. This phenomenon, which is termed the "priming" effect,[26] suggests that occupational participation may stimulate future thoughts that direct attention toward key aspects of the same or similar occupations. For example, participation in weight lifting may temporarily enhance the salience of thoughts related to the importance of keeping fit, physical strength, and one's body image at the expense of cognitions related to other concerns, such as nature or art appreciation. Because, in this example, the former types of thoughts predominate as a result of the priming effect, the likelihood of subsequent participation in weight lifting will be enhanced to the extent that occupational selections are influenced by one's psychologically salient cognitions.

Cognitive Set Effects

A second cognitively based consideration that may contribute to occupational perseverance is that of "cognitive set." In discussion of human problem solving, a cognitive set refers to a fixed, repetitive problem-solving strategy that is based on past efforts in solving the same or similar problems. Luchins[26] classic problem-solving investigations exemplified the cognitive set phenomenon. In this research, subjects were asked to solve a series of simple mathematical problems, the first several of which could be completed by the use of a common algorithm (B – 2C – A). Luchins found that after completing the first few problems, subjects tended inappropriately to continue using the initially used algorithm when confronted with new problems that could be solved with much simpler strategies for solution (e.g., A – C). The repeated engagement of a specifiable strategy led subjects to form a cognitive set and thereby overlook alternate problem-solving methods. Related to the cognitive set notion is the observation of "functional fixedness"[27,28] in which commonly used tools are overlooked in terms of their potential to be used in a nonstandard manner to solve a problem.

Cognitive set effects are relevant to the study of occupation in that a person's occupational choices can be construed as an active problem-solving effort to adapt to and master his or her environment.[29] Thus, as in the case of the businessman who continues to jog because he believes it is a good way to reduce stress and consequently fails to consider alternate strategies, persistence of particular occupations may be promoted to the exclusion of other occupations due to perceptual blinders stemming from ongoing occupational selection strategies.

Self-Perception

To an important extent, individuals rely on their own observations of their behavior to make judgments about themselves.[30,31] Thus, one's self-concept and other personally relevant cognitions are influenced by self-made observations of what one is doing or has done. Because people generally strive to act in a manner consistent with their self-concepts, occupational perseverance may occur as people attempt to match their future occupations to their self-concepts, which mirror their past occupations. Thus, a high school soccer player may be likely to participate in other sports-related occupations to achieve consistency with his self-definition as an "athlete," a label which is to a significant extent based on his prior occupational involvement.

Increased Appreciation

In a manner not unlike the development of a taste for a new food or wine, an individual may better appreciate an inherently worthwhile occupation by virtue of participation in it. Although it may seem boring or senseless when viewed at a distance, a given occupation may take on a new world of meaning when it is personally experienced or explored. Often, this occurs when new differentiations that pertain to an occupation are noted. For example, a person who initially viewed basketball as a nonsensical waste of time in which people merely run back and forth and toss a ball around may come to enjoy watching the sport when he or she learns the identity of the individual players, the rules and strategy, and other aspects of the game. Thus, increased appreciation can result from learning new facts that pervade an occupation. However, the placement of increased appreciation in the cognitive/perceptual category is somewhat arbitrary, because in principle, a heightened appreciation that is primarily affective also could occur. A person might potentially cultivate an enjoyment of classical music, for example, that is not directly linked to any increase in knowledge.

Affective and Motivational Factors

Personal Investment

In many cases, involvement in an occupation increases the likelihood that future participation in the same, as opposed to another, occupation will be more profitable for an individual. For example, skill and knowledge commonly increase following a series of occupational performances. As a consequence, the particular occupation will generally prove to be more rewarding than other occupational selections on subsequent occasions. By repeated engagement in a particular occupation, a person capitalizes on experience, acquires an area of specialized competence, and avoids the wasted effort that would result from incoherency in occupational selections. However, this principle is limited by the capacity of the occupation in question to provide continued satisfaction. For example, in playing tic-tac-toe, most people will achieve mastery quickly and move on to another occupation due to boredom.

Functional Autonomy of Motives

Allport's notion of functional autonomy refers to "any acquired system of motivation in which the tensions involved are not of the same kind as the antecedent tensions from which the acquired system developed."[32] In this view, an activity may persist despite the fact that its original motivating forces are absent. The intrinsically motivated computer buff who spends 10 hours in front of a terminal but whose original reason for working with computers was merely to fulfill a course requirement illustrates the principle of functional autonomy. Because particular occupations commonly are capable of satisfying multiple needs, they may be subject to perseverance as a person uncovers new motives for continued engagement as a result of prior occupational performances.

Although related to the category of increased appreciation noted previously, the notion of functional autonomy is nevertheless conceptually distinct from it. For example, although an increased appreciation for an activity might stimulate a new motive for engagement in it, enhanced appreciation also may generate increased participation in the absence of the development of novel motives, as would be the case if one learned to play chess because it was perceived as mentally stimulating and continued to play for the same reason after discovering that chess is even more intellectually challenging than was initially supposed.

Social Motivations

Many occupations, such as bowling, police work, furniture moving, working as a member of an auto-racing pit crew, or singing in the church choir, feature an important social element. Typically in such cases, the attitudes of the coparticipants will favor continued participation with the occupation in question. When a person becomes part of a group by pursuing an occupation, he or she becomes subject to the group's shared ideas and norms. Consequently, and especially to the extent that the other participants are part of one's "reference group,"[33] conformity pressures and other social influence processes may engender the perseverance of such occupations.

Alteration of the Physical Situation

In addition to occurring for psychological reasons, occupational perseverance can potentially result from physically based considerations. First, the acquisition of physical materials necessary to engage in a particular occupation for the first time may stimulate future participation in the same occupation relative to other occupational possibilities for which the necessary equipment is unavailable. Thus, when choosing whether to purchase a motor boat or a piano, it is likely that the outcome of one's choice will proliferate participation in the occupation that is consonant with what is bought, that is, either boating or piano playing. A second physical factor conducive to occupational perseverance is geographic. It can be hypothesized that people will choose living environments that promote continued involvement with a favored occupation, as would be the case with a herpetologist moving to the desert or a blackjack player migrating to Las Vegas. Once in the new environment, the occupation can be more readily performed and is likely to be engaged in more frequently. Finally, occupational perseverance may result from bodily changes in an individual, as in the case of an elderly woman who is able to engage repeatedly in aerobics because of the physical changes produced by prior involvement or an alcoholic whose prior drinking sprees have led to a physiologic addiction.

Relation of Occupational Perseverance to Intensity of Involvement

While occupation perseverance applies to the dimension of frequency of participation, each of the proposed contributing factors may additionally enhance the vigor or excitement with which the occupation is performed. Thus, for example, altered self-perceptions or increased personal investment in an activity may elevate its importance in the life of an individual and thereby generate increased effort during its engagement. Occupational perseverance is therefore typically expected to be associated with enhanced intensity of the underlying performances relative to nonpersevering occupations. This correlation between perseverance and intensity can occur independently of the enactment of flow. For instance, a maintenance man whose self-concept incorporates the notion that he is an excellent, dedicated worker who takes pride in his work may approach his job with great zeal, despite the fact that it doesn't offer a level of challenge equal to his self-perceived skills. Further, the intensity of an occupation can rise as a result of external reinforcement. Therefore, even in the absence of flow, a persevering occupation may be performed with great intensity and psychological involvement. However, to the extent that flow is enacted, it will likely contribute to the intensity, mental concentration, and enjoyment of participation.

Summary of Theoretical Factors Promotive of Occupational Perseverance

Figure 14–1 summarizes the previous discussion of the mediators of occupational perseverance. Within the figure, occupational perseverance is represented as a feedback loop in which, once perseverance is underway, the occupation and the internal changes that are connected with performing the occupation are simultaneously antecedents and consequences of each other. Note that in the model, the cognitive, affective/motivational, and physical changes that may accompany participation in an occupation are presumed to influence each other. Thus, for instance, occupation-promoting cognitive and affective/motivational changes enhance the likelihood that an individual will choose to relocate as a means of fostering continued participation (a physical factor). In most cases, not all of the proposed internal mediators are expected to operate; further, the set of included factors is not presumed to be exhaustive.

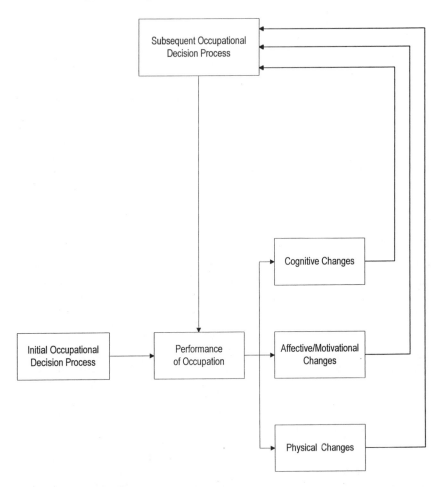

Figure 14–1. Feedback loop of occupational perseverance.

The persevering portion of the figure is analogous to a self-sustaining electrical feedback circuit. Using such an analogy, the frequency or intensity of the enacted occupational performances can be equated with the luminance of open wires that connect the different relay points within the circuits (and that correspond to the arrow-lines in the figure). An active or intense persevering sequence would thereby produce a hotly glowing circuit. To the extent that the degree of perseverating intensity waxes and wanes with time, the circuit will exhibit a flickering pattern. Following a series of disappointing experiences with the occupation, the circuit's luminance will diminish, and if occupational engagement is terminated completely, the electrical circuit shuts off altogether.

The feedback loop pictured in Figure 14-1 is similar in terms of underlying process to the "model of the human subsystems that influence occupation" that has been proposed by the faculty of the University of Southern California (USC)

Department of Occupational Therapy.[29] In the USC model, internal human subsystems (transcendental, symbolic, sociocultural, information processing, biologic, and physical) interact with each other to produce occupational behavior, which in turn feeds back to alter the individual (and his or her environment) and thereby affect future occupational behavior. The feedback loop presented here represents a specific version of the more general USC model in that it emphasizes the importance of the tendency for occupation to sustain itself, as opposed to documenting the more general effects of participation in a given occupation on future occupational behavior, as in the USC model.

Although in Figure 14–1 the cognitive, affective/motivational, and physical processes that influence occupational selections are clearly distinguished for heuristic purposes, they are nonetheless assumed to be complexly intertwined in their actual operation. Thus, instead of conceptualizing occupational perseverance as either primarily cognitively or affectively based, the inherent interdependence of cognition and emotion is emphasized. This view is consistent with theories of motivation and emotion, which posit the complex interplay of affective and cognitive factors.[33]

Occupational Termination

To comprehend fully the processes by which occupational activity perseveres, it is necessary to additionally understand the factors that make people less likely to continue participation. Occupational termination can be defined as the phenomenon whereby participation in an activity reduces or eliminates the possibility of subsequent participation. Occupational termination is an important consideration insofar as its underlying processes compete against, possibly in a push-pull fashion, the set of factors that facilitate occupational repetition. Although it is not the purpose of this paper to describe in depth the mediators of occupational termination, several factors that may promote withdrawal from further participation in particular occupations are listed in Table 14-1. Occupational termination may potentially occur at any point in a person's history of involvement with an occupation, including a prior persevering sequence. Also, occupational termination could occur at any of the four levels of occupational perseverance previously postulated: specific performance, particular occupations over time, higher order occupational categories, or activity in general. For example, with respect to higher order occupational categories, a chronically unemployed individual might harbor powerful negative expectations surrounding work in general. It is likely that occupational perseverance and occupational termination interact in complex ways. Further study is needed to understand better the nature of this interrelation.

A Preliminary Study of Occupational Perseverance

To gather preliminary documentation of the occupational perseverance effect, a pilot study was performed in which USC occupational therapy master's students who were enrolled in an independent study course reported on their pattern of engagement in thesis writing throughout the spring 1991 semester. Of 19 students enrolled in the course, 18 filled out a brief questionnaire, which included, among other items, the following question: "When you worked on the project (i.e., your

Table 14-1   Factors Promoting Occupational Termination

Factor	Example
Unpleasant experience leading to negative future expectations (e.g., disappointment, frustration, physical pain, embarrassment)	A man develops severe blisters on his feet during a hiking trip and vows never to go hiking again (e.g., physical pain). A woman decides to quit her career as a novel writer after being unable to find a publisher for her work (disappointment, frustration).
Lack of resources or physical accessibility necessary for continued participation	A deep sea scuba diver moves from California to Kansas (physical inaccessibility). A girl is forced to discontinue taking flying lessons because her family can no longer afford the instructional fees (lack of resources).
Reduction in psychological fulfillment (e.g., boredom, perceived mastery)	A youngster masters the game of tic-tac-toe and becomes bored with it (perceived mastery, boredom).
Completion of an externally circumscribed task or activity	After assembling his own small airplane in his garage for 6 months, a man stops this work because the job is completed.
Presence of a more attractive or important occupation than the initial occupation	A medical student gives up chess playing because of the pressing need to devote time to his studies (more important occupation). A woman gives up tennis when she discovers that she is better suited for racquetball (more attractive occupation).
Physical incapacity or death	A man must discontinue body surfing following a spinal cord injury (physical incapacity).

thesis) during the semester, did the act of working on it tend to 'feed on itself,' that is, did it either directly or indirectly create a self-perpetuating tendency for you to continue?" A "yes" answer to this question was thus presumed to reflect occupational perseverance. Of the 18 students, 100% answered the question affirmatively, thereby supporting the notion that occupational engagement, or at least thesis writing, is commonly self-perpetuating.

After answering the above item, the students were asked to list open endedly their perceived reasons as to why their thesis writing was self-perpetuating. In classifying these expressed reasons, each of the proposed cognitive and affective/motivational changes that were previously described as potentially resulting from occupational participation, with the exception of altered self-perceptions, was listed by one or more students. Elements from the category of physical changes were not mentioned, probably as a result of their diminished relevance to the occupation of thesis writing. The most common reason stated for the perpetuation of thesis work was that immediate prior involvement with the work was reinforcing in that it signaled movement toward the goal of thesis completion and thereby motivated the student to continue. Underscoring the conceptual distinction between occupational perseverance and flow, the experience of flow or elements indicative of a flow state were mentioned by only three students as an underlying reason for self-perpetuation of thesis work. In sum, this pilot study supported the importance of occupational perseverance and provided tentative evidence that cognitive and affective/motivational changes elicited by occupational participation contribute to the effect.

Relevance of Occupational Perseverance to Occupational Therapy

Because occupational therapists foster personal growth recovery in their patients through the use of activity, a more systematic understanding and application of the factors that are conducive to the persistence of occupations in patients' lives has the capacity to enhance the potency and long-term impact of therapy. If patients engage in growth-enhancing activities that are persevering, the results of therapy are likely to be longer lasting and more beneficial. For example, to the degree that an occupation perseveres, the patient will be more likely to initiate it spontaneously outside of the immediate therapeutic context. Additionally, within the therapeutic situation, the patient is more likely to benefit if selected features conducive to occupational perseverance, such as altered self-perceptions, increased appreciation, or social motivations, are explicitly promoted by the therapist. Thus, an increased awareness of the factors that lead to the initiation and sustaining of involvement with particular occupations holds promise for enhancing therapeutic efficacy.

Knowledge concerning the perseverance of occupations also may be useful in combating maladaptive patterns of inconsistency that are exhibited in patients' occupational choices. For example, some individuals may suffer from a syndrome of occupational incoherency or a tendency to pursue occupations in a haphazard, inconsistent, self-defeating manner. The person who fails to maintain a steady line of employment by continually quitting jobs and trying new ones exemplifies this pattern of incoherency. If such an individual were able to achieve increased insight into the causes of his or her inconsistent behavior, then positive changes could more easily be accomplished. In this context, many of the special challenges associated with disabilities, such as architectural barriers or discrimination in employment settings, may reduce the ease with which the individual is able to sustain engagement in selected occupations of importance on a consistent basis. Increased knowledge of the specific interactions of these special challenges with the tendency to initiate and sustain activity would be therapeutically useful.

In summary, a recognition of the self-perpetuating sequence that often accompanies engagement in occupations is an important component to consider in the development of a science of human occupation. While further research is needed to understand better the conditions under which this phenomenon occurs, the acquisition of such knowledge is capable of enhancing occupational therapy practice.

Discussion Questions

1. How might occupational therapy practitioners take advantage of the phenomenon of self-perpetuation of occupations?
2. When might occupational therapists need to assist patients or clients with occupational termination?

References

1. Clark, FA, Parham, LD, Carlson, ME, Frank, G, Jackson, J, Pierce, D, Wolfe, R, and Zemke, R: Occupational science: Academic innovation in the service of occupational therapy's future. Am J Occup Ther 45:300, 1991.
2. Yerxa, EJ, Clark, FA, Frank, G, Jackson, J, Parham, LD, Pierce, D, Stein, C, and Zemke, R: An introduction to occupational science, A foundation for occupational therapy in the 21st century. Occup Ther in Health Care 6:1, 1989.
3. Reis, HT, Wheeler, L, Kernis, MH, Spiegel, N, and Nezlek, J: On specificity in the impact of social participation on physical and psychological health. J Person Soc Psychol 48:456, 1985.
4. Rodin, J, and Langer, EJ: Long-term effects of a control-relevant intervention with the institutionalized aged. J Person Soc Psychol 35:897, 1977.
5. Fordyce, MW: Development of a program to increase personal happiness. J Counsel Psychol 24:511, 1977.
6. Emmons, RA, and Diener, E: Situation selection as a moderator of response consistency and stability. J Person Soc Psychol 51:1013, 1986.
7. Diener, E, Larsen, RJ, and Emmons, RA: Person x situation interactions: Choice of situations and congruence response models. J Person Soc Psychol 47:580, 1984.
8. Reich, JW, and Zautra, AJ: Demands and desires in daily life: Some influences on well-being. Amer J Com Psychol 11:41, 1983.
9. Beisner, M: Components and correlates of mental well-being. J Health Soc Behav 15:320, 1974.
10. Kanner, AD, Coyne, JC, Schaefer, C, and Lazarus, RS: Comparisons of two modes of stress management: Daily hassles and uplift versus major life events. J Behav Med 4:1, 1983.
11. Monroe, SM: Major and minor life events as predictors of psychological stress: Further issues and findings. J Behav Med 6:189, 1983.
12. Crandall, R: Motivations for leisure. J Leis Res 12:45, 1980.
13. Furnham, A: Psychoticism, social desirability and situation selection. Person Individ Diff 3:43, 1982.
14. Kielhofner, G: Occupation. In Hopkins, HL, and Smith, HD (eds): Willard and Spackman's Occupational Therapy (6th ed). J. B. Lippincott, Philadelphia, 1983.
15. Levy, J: A paradigm for conceptualizing leisure behavior: Towards a person-environment interaction analysis. J Leis Res 11:48, 1979.
16. Tinsley, HEA, Barrett, TC, and Kass, RA: Leisure activities and need satisfaction. J Leis Res 9:110, 1977.
17. Emmons, RA, Diener, E, and Larsen, RJ: Choice and avoidance of everyday situations and affect congruence: Two models of reciprocal interactionism. J Person Soc Psychol 51:815, 1986.
18. Vallacher, RR, and Wegner, DM: What do people think they're doing? Action identification and human behavior. Psychol Rev 94:3, 1987.
19. Kielhofner, G: A Model of Human Occupation. Williams & Wilkins, Baltimore, 1985.
20. Kielhofner, p 28.
21. Kielhofner, p 30.
22. Csikszentmihalyi, M: Beyond Boredom and Anxiety: The Experience of Play in Work and Games. Jossey-Bass, San Francisco, 1975.
23. Csikszentmihalyi, M, and Csikszentmihalyi, IS: Optimal Experience. Cambridge University press, Cambridge, MA, 1988.
24. Anderson, JR: Cognitive Psychology and Its Implications. Freeman & Co., San Francisco, 1980.

25. Clark, MS, and Isen, AM: Toward understanding the relationship between feeling states and social behavior. In Hastorf, A, and Isem, AM (eds): Cognitive Social Psychology. Elsevier, New York, 1982.

26. Luchins, AS: Mechanization in problem solving. Psychol Mono 54 (Whole No. 248), 1942.

27. Dunker, K: On problem solving. Psychol Mono 53 (Whole No. 270), 1945.

28. Maier, NRF: Reasoning in humans: II. The solution to a problem and its appearance in consciousness. J Comp Psychol 12:181, 1931.

29. University of Southern California (USC) Department of Occupational Therapy: Proposal for a Ph.D. program in occupational science, 1989. (Unpublished manuscript).

30. Bem, DJ: Self-perception: An alternative interpretation of cognitive dissonance phenomena. Psychol Rev 74:183, 1967.

31. Hastorf, AH, Schneider, DJ, and Polefka, J: Person Perception. Addison-Wesley, Reading, MA, 1970.

32. Allport, GW: Pattern and Growth in Personality. Holt, New York, 1961, p 29.

33. Kinch, JW: Social Psychology. McGraw-Hill, New York, 1973.

Biology and Occupation

In the use of systems models of humans functioning as occupational beings, the biological aspect of our humanity is usually modeled as a lower subsystem, constraining the functions of higher levels. It is frequently misperceived in the old "soul versus material" or "mind versus body" paradigm with overtones of good and bad. That is, it is as if humans could be holier or better if not for the constraints of our material, biological nature. It is hard to imagine why a field of practice, such as occupational therapy, should be interested in a holistic approach to understanding people if all that means is that we must take the bad with the good. We believe that we reject a view that sees disease, perinatal disability, traumatic disability, and chronic disability as symbols of evil at work through demons, curses, or other evil forces. However, we encourage the individual to "rise above" disability, and in effect, we try to help people "compensate" for disability, suggesting that they can be "just like everyone else."

The world of diversity, which most of us are attempting to understand and live in today, does not suggest that people of different ages, sexes, races, and ethnicities learn to compensate for their uniqueness. Recognizing biopsychological and sociocultural forces that produce the individual, we celebrate the diversity that is a part of being human. Similarly, our biological nature need not be seen solely as constraint, keeping us from what we might be, but as enabler, providing the capacity for highest levels of adaptation. Increasingly, we see the evidence for the uniqueness of each individual, not in the interchange between a transcendent self and a material environment, but in the oneness of a biological and transcendent self. In such a view, transcendence is attained through the symbolic and subjective meaning we give the occupational behaviors with which we flexibly build beyond the biological basics of our existence.

Zemke's paper reviews the work of Nobel prize winner Gerald Edelman as an example of theory that supports the importance of biological processes as a link between the material substance of our nervous system and the development of consciousness. She identifies the key roles of activity and for the human, occupation, in this evolutionary and ontogenetic developmental process. Such theories, and the research supporting them, remind us that our biological functions are not only constraining human action, function, or occupation, but enabling it for each of us, as we build meaning as individuals, societies, and cultures.

Mailloux uses basic principles to introduce the concepts of a sensory integrative approach in occupational therapy. Most therapists are familiar with the basic principles of sensory integrative treatment, but looking at these concepts as principles for occupational therapy in general may be a stimulus for rethinking the environment in which we provide service. One principle suggests that controlled input can be used to evoke an adaptive response. Occupational therapists regularly attempt to grade activity as a therapeutic challenge to elicit adaptive psychological and physical responses, integrated into a meaningful whole through the occupation itself. Similarly, using another principle, we find that successfully meeting the therapeutic challenge of participation in occupation better prepares the individual for future environmental challenges. The more inner-directed or internally motivated activity participation is, the more meaning that activity holds for the patient and the more integrative the occupation will be. The development of increasingly complex behaviors and behavioral organization is seen not only in the sensory integrative approach within occupational therapy, but reflects traditional principles of all occupational therapy practice. While therapy may begin with the components of performance, they become linked through meaningful and contextual practice into skills, habits, and routines that form the basis of our normal daily round of occupations. The adage, "A journey of a thousand miles begins with just one step" holds true for occupational therapy when the focus is on the goal of the journey, not the step alone.

Mailloux describes an appropriately enriched environment for sensory integrative functioning; her description may lead therapists to wonder what an appropriately enriched environment for occupational integration would be. Are the clinical environments in which we provide therapy enriched for occupation? Are they less a natural environment for patient occupation than a laboratory setting, with such settings' inherent sterility and potential for meaningless stimuli? Mailloux's work suggests that occupational scientists and therapists explore, for example, contemporary urban environments or considerations of novelty, variety, complexity, and natural conditions relative to the occupations of city dwellers, inner city minority youth, and the homeless.

Arnold Chamove presents brief but tantalizing questions about the qualities of activity that may make it intrinsically motivating, based on the results of primate enrichment projects (attempts to improve the environment of captive primates). Acknowledging the effectiveness of foraging activity in replacing aggressive use of time, he notes that such activities make up a prevalent activity in the econiche of the free primate. However, the assumption that primates engage in such activities solely to provide necessary food is questioned by the finding that foraging activity takes place even when, in captivity, sufficient food is readily available. Chamove suggests that foraging, which he calls the work of nonhuman primates, may be part of a biologically driven evolutionary program that is enjoyable because it is work normally performed for long periods of time in the wild. Thus, he postulates that in treatment, occupational therapists may want to consider the effectiveness of participation of patients in occupations that include needed physical exercise or activity within a form of familiar "prevalent work" from their life outside the institution, thus tapping into a basic biological predisposition. Occupational therapists and occupational scientists similarly identify a biological disposition toward adaptive interaction with the environment through exploratory behaviors, the progressive development of skills, and competent participation in a round of daily occupations.

Hedricks' paper demonstrates a blending of research methods that is necessary for our beginning attempts to answer questions of particular interest to occupational science. Natural settings of daily occupations and experience sampling with subjective data collected about mood and activation at the time of the activity are combined with the use of biomarkers of hormonal activity. Through this type of multiple measurement, the physical and biological subsystems can be linked in a description of their interactive relationships with higher level subsystems through routine occupations. One of the major issues in Hedricks' paper is the bidirectionality of the interaction between hormones and occupation, while acknowledging the impact of environment.

Hormonal rhythmicity is noted, with its biological basis in circadian, menstrual, and other cycles. Human temporality has a cyclic or rhythmic quality, which has been frequently identified in such biorhythms. While we find a psychological stability in human perceptions of well-being, we suspect that psychorhythmic cycles produce mood variations within as yet unidentified time periods. Sociotemporal rhythms are easily identified through our work-rest expectations on a daily, weekly, and annual (holidays) basis. However, the balance of occupations so highly valued by occupational therapists has not yet been identified through any occupatiorhythmicity or cycles of occupational choice by type, inherent characteristics, or any of the other qualities we use to describe the experience of engagement in occupations. The interaction and directionality of some of these varied rhythmic influences are considered in Hedricks' paper. It should act as a stimulus for occupational scientists' research and occupational therapists' exploration in practice situations of the potential occupational rhythms providing the underlying "beat" to the orchestrations of our daily occupational rounds.

One of the most basic biological functions of living creatures is reproduction, and in primates, this is the result of mating. Human primates have, however, through their psychological, social, and cultural symbolism, invested the process of mate selection with extensive meaning, which guides the individual. Many older cultures have an extensive set of activities in which the family and individual proceed to screen potential marriage partners and the appropriate mate. Krishnagiri's paper presents a pilot study relating to the occupation of mate selection. Interviewing Indian young adults living in the United States, some raised in America and some raised in India, presents a wide range of views about the method they will or are using in their search for a life partner. Further discussion of characteristics desired in such a partner produces some intriguing findings related to previous studies of this topic. The impact of culture, in spite of differing geographic and broad cultural environments, is evident in her findings.

The questions raised and answered in Wendy Wood's paper have important implications for occupation science and occupational therapy. We need to stand back and attempt to sort out just how much of the sexual division of occupations is biologically based versus socially constructed. Beginning with questions rising out of occupational therapy's history and current headlines, Wood uses study of nonhuman primates to consider activities relating to caregiving and territorial defense. While the sexual division of work is seen, individuals within nonhuman primate groups do not all fit these stereotypes. Ecological variables and ontogenetic history affect the actions individuals undertake.

With human potential for development of the self through engagement in occupation, the interaction of biological factors with environmental needs and personal history becomes even more important. As individuals can learn to expand their behavioral repertoire and occupational skills to better use their potential, capacity, and vision, so can professional fields. Is the nurturing role of occupational therapy congruent with appropriate professional behavior designating our "turf," our special area of expertise in occupation as process and product of healthy adaptation? It would not seem so, based on Wood's interpretation of the implications of nonhuman primate work for human occupation.

by *Ruth Zemke, PhD, OTR, FAOTA*

15

Brain, Mind, and Meaning

Mind-Body Dualism

Science: Dualistic Stability or Holistic Adaptability?

Theory of Neuronal Group Selection

Memory, Concepts, and Learning

Consciousness

Occupational Science: Holism of Mind and Matter

My hypothesis is this: Occupational therapists are enmeshed in a mind-body dualism with philosophic roots and look for guidance in therapy to sciences that do not reject this dualism. With the interdisciplinary nature of the development of occupational science, we must search for and use scientific knowledge that rejects dualism and supports the complexity of the human as an occupational being. One such element of scientific knowledge is Edelman's theory regarding the biological basis for human consciousness and the mind,[1] originating from his theory of a "neural Darwinism" shaping the individual brain.[2] This hypothesis of philosophically rooted dualism is briefly explored, and then Edelman's theories are outlined, proposing one approach to ending that dualist view.

Mind-Body Dualism

Plato suggested a dualism between reality and appearance, ideas and objects, reason and sense perception, and soul and body.[3] These pairs are connected: The first in each pair is superior to the second in reality and in goodness. Thus, the distinction between mind and matter, which has become commonplace in philosophy, science, and popular thought, began as the distinction of soul and body.

Rene Descartes, considered the founder of modern philosophy and one of the creators of science, brought to fruition the dualism of mind and matter that was begun by Plato and further developed by Christian philosophy. According to Bertrand Russell, whose history of philosophy is a classic reference, "the Cartesian system presents two parallel, but independent worlds, that of mind and that of matter, each of which can be studied without reference to the other."[4] The body, or matter, was considered a machine, governed by the laws of physics. The worlds of mind and body were, however, considered parallel worlds, like two clocks running with different symbols on the dials, as if the body clock reads "thirst" and the mind clock reads "unpleasant." This type of parallelism, however, suggested a determinism in which the physical laws applying to the body were constraining to the mind. Consequently, ideas about volition and free will were difficult to handle within this view.

Science: Dualistic Stability or Holistic Adaptability?

The traditional physical science that developed from Cartesian philosophy tended to reflect the view that matter, the physical, was an appropriate topic for study, while the mind was territory for philosophy (or for the soul, theology). The physical world was viewed as a stable one needing only taxonomy and study of the parts, which had a few general rules that could explain the whole.

However, over time, biology developed as a more eclectic science, considering results at different levels of understanding as it addressed the study of living organisms, life, and the whole of life, which was greater than the sum of its parts. That which contributed to the understanding of subsystems or structures also contributed to the overall biological explanation, whereas any one of the partial explanations may have been of little interest as an isolated subsystem. In this way, biology, with its different levels of understanding, ultimately emerged as a more holistic, synthesizing science, trying to create knowledge by interpreting the integrated effects of interacting components and subsystem levels.

Darwin's biological concepts of evolution required a dynamic view of change and adaptation. From that biological approach, contemporary theorists are approaching science as having the potential for linking the mind and body and are thereby rejecting traditional dualism. The biological theory of consciousness of Gerald Edelman, 1972 Nobel Prize winner in Medicine and Physiology, is such an approach.[5] As such, it offers information and a model for consideration in the developing science of occupation.

Theory of Neuronal Group Selection

In adapting to the environment through evolution, animal species rely on natural selection acting on variance in populations of a species. However, an animal endowed with a richly structured brain also must adapt to a complex environment to govern its actions in its world. The theory suggests that this adaptation also occurs through a selection process that depends on the existence of variance within a population of neuronal groups in the individual animal.

Selectionist notions in neurobiology have, in the past, been directed mainly toward the description of evolutionary aspects of behavior or of the phylogenetic evolution of the brain and its various centers. They have not considered that neuronal selection accounts for the ontogeny and physiological function of the brain in somatic time, the time of ontogenetic development. Basic elements of Edelman's theory of neuronal group selection are consequently presented, and their relationship to his theory of higher functions of the brain, including consciousness, are described.

The general requirements of any selection theory are:

1. A source of diversification leading to variations
2. A means for effective encounter with an environment
3. A means of differential amplification over some period of time of those variations in a population that have greater adaptive value[6]

These requirements obviously are met by evolution, in which mutation and gene recombination provide major sources of diversity; function provides sampling of the environment; and heredity assures that some of the results of natural selection will yield differential reproduction of adapted phenotypes. This emphasis on adaptation as a process of interaction between living organisms and their environments was a major step for biology because it departed from the presumption of preset econiches for each biological structure.

The theory of neuronal group selection meets the three general requirements of selectionist theories by specifying that, in the nervous system:

1. Diversification of neural connections occurs in embryonic development, and experiential diversification of synaptic efficacy continues later.
2. Action leads to encounter with and parallel neural sampling of the environment with differential amplification of the synapses of neuronal groups whose interactions are adaptive.
3. Memory maintains some of the unique patterns that have been selected by development and experience.

To expand and explain these specifications further, four basic premises of Edelman's theory that pertain to primary neuronal repertoires, secondary neuronal repertoires, and local and global cortical maps are discussed. First, during development, neural anatomies form that are specific for a species but that nevertheless possess enormous individual variation. A population of millions of groups of thousands of neurons in a given brain region is known as a primary repertoire. At conception, human cells resemble each other. If no changes occurred, we would not have organs, but, while cells contain the same set of genes, each activates only a small subset. Cells divide and migrate in sheets of epithelia. Some die and others adhere to each other and begin to differentiate through protein synthesis controlled by genetic subgroups. Place and time determine which growing, moving cells form groups that then become organs.

Certain protein molecules, known as cell adhesion molecules (CAMs) and substrate adhesion molecules (SAMs), regulate movement and adhesion, thereby providing a matrix on which other cells move and modifying the way cells organize. While some of this is genetic and thus species specific, it also is individual, depending as it does on the temporal and spatial history of the cell and developing embryo. Thus, we see that an individually diverse primary repertoire of brain cells is the result of a dynamic process of developmental selection occurring in time; it is not the result of an infinitely detailed preset anatomic configuration.

Edelman's second premise is that during behavior and as a result of neural signaling, a second means of selection for diversity occurs. In experiential selection, synaptic connections and transmissions are strengthened through axonic and dendritic sprouting, and changes in neurotransmitter efficacy occur as the result of behavior, thereby providing a secondary neuronal repertoire. According to Fishbach, "synapse formation during a critical period of development may depend on a type of competition between axons in which those that are activated appropriately are favored" (p 56).[7] Thus, again, individual history has major impact on the functional effectiveness of brain structures, increasing the diversity and differentiating one human from another.

Edelman's third premise is that through action relating the individual to the environment, repertoires are arranged in local cortical maps. The prime example of neuronal mapping is in our visual system. Clear mapping is evident in adult optic tracts and within the occipital lobe. Such local maps are connected by parallel and reciprocal connections that are called reentrant signals into functional distributed systems. That is, numerous local maps receive signals from the world at the same time, and their reentry connections to each other acknowledge this sharing. According to Schatz, the specific left or right eye responsivity of neurons in the lateral geniculate body of kittens is not present neonatally, but the responsiveness of the connections into lateral groups in adults is the result of a developmental fine tuning of the circuitry. As this occurs, during critical periods in postnatal development, one might say, as does Schatz, "In a sense, then, cells that fire together wire together."[8] Similarly, maps may be stimulated by other brain maps because they are coupled by re-entry circuits. These neural processes form the functional groupings for basic cognitive processes, such as perceptual categorization, memory, learning, and "higher level" functions, such as concept formation.

According to Edelman's theory, categorization or recognition of patterns is fundamental and must occur before extensive learning can take place. Edelman's fourth premise suggests that categorization occurs because of multiple interactions among local neural maps, resulting from sensorimotor activity, producing what he calls global mapping. A global mapping is a dynamic cortical structure containing many local maps that are re-entrantly connected. The concept of a global mapping takes into account that perception is involved in action. In this view, categorization does not occur solely in a neural sensory area that then executes a program to activate motor output. Instead, the results of continual motor activity are an essential part of categorization or pattern recognition in space. This implies that neural global mappings carrying out such categorization contain sensory and motor elements. This aspect of the theory is reflected in Reed's action theory, which emphasizes that there is no sensory or motor system, but only sensorimotor action systems as humans act within, and as a part of, their environment.[9]

Memory, Concepts, and Learning

Within a global mapping, long-term changes in synaptic strengths provide the basis for memory. Kandel and Hawkins describe long-term potentiation at synapses in the hippocampus that lasted from hours to weeks and that were restricted to the pathway that was stimulated by action.[10] Memory, according to Kandel, is not a store of fixed information to be called up as needed. In this view of memory, sensorimotor performance units are intimately tied together by the global mapping. The mappings change because action and environmental change are constantly prompting recategorization.

Cortical mappings alone, however, are insufficient to deal with the temporal ordering of events and their neural signals. Cortical global maps must be linked to cerebellar structures and basal ganglia, which plan and time smooth movement sequences, and to hippocampal structures, which order sequences of maps. Initially, this temporal ordering is primarily within the present, and the primary focus is in support of the temporal linkages of ongoing units of activity.

Edelman holds that during phylogenetic and ontogenetic development, concepts precede language and meaning. Concept formation depends on a special kind of connectivity in which the brain categorizes its own activities and global mappings by type, for example, those connected to objects, those concerned with motion, or those concerned with hedonic states. In humans, the areas for these conceptual distinctions are assumed to be the frontal, temporal, and parietal lobes and the cingulate gyri. This process is viewed as an active organization of forming concepts, not a recognition of existing information in the environment. Edelman sees the world as an unlabeled place, where data are taken into the human system, and information is the result of our processing of the data.

Learning involves relating categorization and memory to species-specific functions laden with evolutionary values, such as hedonic, consummatory, appetitive, or pain-avoiding behaviors. This requires the linkage of the cortex and cortical appendages, such as the hippocampus and basal ganglia, to structures of the limbic system. While these values support evolutionarily adaptive functions, values can be altered by later synaptic changes due to consciously controlled decisions.

Such a system of neural linkages can determine the relative importance of external events according to internal values and schemes. It affects the selection of goals and purposeful action. Thus, learning becomes the link between categorization and value to yield an adaptive response that satisfies the organism's values.

Consciousness

Recombinations of categories and higher-order generalizations become possible and with them, so too do conceptual categorization and memory prerequisites for forming a model of the world. The sequencing of such conceptual states emerged from systems involved with motor plans and motor sequences. This provided a prelanguage model that is the basis for primary consciousness in animals.

Edelman proposes a continuum of consciousness from primary to higher levels. Primary consciousness requires:

1. Neuronal group selection leading to categorization and memory
2. Sensorimotor distinction between self and nonself
3. Evolutionary values for adaptive behaviors
4. Neural system for successive events
5. Interaction between #3 and #4 for memory
6. Re-entrant connections between memory system and present experience

According to Edelman, "previous memories and current activities of the brain interact to yield primary consciousness as a form of remembered present."[11] While an animal possessing this early form of consciousness generates a "mental image" determined by immediate multimodal perceptual categorization, it is still largely dependent on the succession of events of real time. Possessed with primary consciousness alone, most animals are bound to small time intervals mediated by short-term memory; they have no concept of the past. With the evolution in hominids of Broca's and Wernicke's areas, however, a means for symbolic categorization emerged. Symbolic categorization and language permitted concepts of past and future to be developed along with the time-independent abstract models of self and world. This freed humans from a dependence on the sequence of events in real time concrete experiences. Such a development must have greatly facilitated planning, which requires making distinctions between past, present, and future acts. With such time-independent models, the more developed forms of higher order consciousness became possible.

An early level of higher consciousness is the ability to distinguish between categories related to the "self" and those related to entities classifiable as "non-self," whether similar (as other humans are) or dissimilar (as all else is). With this ability, we may consider that the beginnings of higher order consciousness are in place, as may be observed, for example, in chimpanzees. In Edelman's view, however, only with the appearance of true language in a social context can this form of consciousness fully flourish,[5] because language facilitated the development of the model of a conscious self acting on things.

The entire speech system evolved by way of affective and observational learning in a social scene. The actual signs and symbols of language are arbitrary, but they link concepts to a specialized system of sound production and recognition. The development of a sufficiently large vocabulary leads to further categorization by the system. This form of conceptual categorization of symbols, independent of current perceptual input, leads to an increasingly rich set of meanings. The bases for the emergence of meanings are early, in that before language, the brain had already evolved areas that carried out extensive concept formation. With speech, however, a symbolic means of remembering and altering concepts arose, enriching meanings by symbolic connections to new values.

With higher order consciousness and language, models of the past and future can be constructed. The continuity of consciousness is not broken by this constructing; instead, it becomes possible to compare the flow of the present action simultaneously with the content of these models of the past (perhaps as cause) and the future (perhaps a result). The resultant sense of temporal duration of current activity is modifiable by sensory input, attentional and arousal states, and the nature of activity. The comparative flow of external and internal events may be emphasized or suppressed to a greater or lesser degree, but the comparison is never fully suppressed in conscious states. The parallel comments generally attributed to St. Augustine and William James, stating "I know what time [consciousness] is when I experience it, but I can't explain it," are both likely to be rooted in this curious flow of inner and outer states.

Occupational Science: Holism of Mind and Matter

The conscious mind is a process occurring separately in each individual; it is historical, changing, and linked to action. It is not a property of particles of matter or even of most biologic arrangements of matter (living things). Matter exists prior to mind, and at death, individual minds are doomed to extinction in the sense that the conscious processes and thoughts of individuals are no longer possible.

Although the world of matter is not of our making, while alive, we nevertheless may alter it and ourselves by conscious means. Those socially cooperative interactions that lead to an increasingly rich culture are the most valuable heritage we have. While primary consciousness is based on an ethologically determined set of values, the acquisition of higher order consciousness and the interactions in a culture allow us to achieve new values. Edelman suggests that a view that allows us to see the origins of consciousness in the relations between matter, evolution, and brain development "will allow an individual to see his place in the world with greater clarity—how he came from the world, and how he may contribute to his fellows while he enjoys for a brief time the privilege of consciousness and communication."[12]

Science is a communal cultural achievement and is among the highest achievements of human consciousness. However, the scientific view derives from other cultural ingredients and should not drive them. Science is only a partial experience of consciousness that, once born and developed in human culture, has a potentially endless sweep in subjective personal experience as reflected in art, literature, and music. Much in our experience is of our own making, and much of it is the most precious part of our lives. The world of traditional science and the world of human science sometimes seem like different worlds, as do the arts and the humanities. Perhaps these worlds reflect the mind-body dualism, which causes therapists to separate treatment into psychosocial and physical areas. Perhaps for all our talk of holism, we really have not developed a scientific base that truly acknowledges the integration of these human elements.

Edelman, in his research and theory, offers a view of science that acknowledges the action of the human and celebrates the evolutionary effects of environmental interaction through activity. His theory of neuronal group selection reflects a biological scientist's attempt to describe the conscious mind as the result of processes within the evolving brain interacting with the environment through activity. The strength of theories of this sort for occupational science can be tested only in the future, but the science of occupation that integrates biologic to transcendental human subsystems is one which we must develop.

In response to questions that seem to reflect the old mind-body dualism, such as "On which end of the proposed hierarchy of human subsystems should occupational science focus its studies?" we should consider this comment from Richard Feynman, theoretical physicist.

> I think that the right way, of course, is to say that what we have to look at is the whole structural interconnection of the thing; and that all the sciences, and not just the sciences but all the efforts of intellectual kinds, are an endeavor to see the connections of the hierarchies, to connect beauty to history, to connect history to man's psychology, man's psychology to the working of the brain, the brain to the neural impulse, the neural impulse to the chemistry, and so forth, up and down, both ways. And today we cannot, and it is no use making believe that we can, draw carefully a line all the way from one end of this thing to the other, because we have only just begun to see that there is this relative hierarchy.
>
> And I do not think either end is nearer to God.[13]

Discussion Questions

1. In what ways does Edelman's theory of neuronal group selection support the basic tenet of occupational therapy that adaptation occurs through purposeful action and activity?
2. How might Edelman's theory change or modify the more traditional view of biology as constraining the human ability to find meaning in daily life?

References

1. Edelman, GM, and Mountcastle, VB: The Mindful Brain. MIT Press, Boston, 1978.
2. Edelman, GM: Neural Darwinism. Basic Books, New York, 1987.
3. Russell, B: A History of Western Philosophy. Simon and Schuster, New York, 1972, p 134.
4. Russell, B: p 567.
5. Edelman, GM: The Remembered Present, A Biological Theory of Consciousness. Basic Books, New York, 1989.
6. Mayr, E: The Growth of Biological Thought: Diversity, Evolution, and Inheritance. Harvard University Press, Cambridge, 1982.
7. Fishbach, GD: Mind and brain. Scientific American 267(3):48, 1992.
8. Schatz, C: The developing brain. Scientific American 267(3):61, 1992.
9. Reed, ES: An outline of a theory of action systems. Journal of Motor Behavior 14(2):98, 1982.
10. Kandel, ER, and Hawkins, RD: The biological basis of learning and individuality. Scientific American 267(3):79, 1992.
11. Edelman, p 105.
12. Edelman, p 270.
13. Edelman, GM: Bright Air, Brilliant Fire. On the Matter of the Mind. Basic Books, New York, 1992, p vii.

by Zoe Mailloux, MA, OTR, FAOTA

16

The Occupational Therapy Center as an Enriched Environment

Five Principles of Sensory Integrative Theory

Sensory Experience

Social Experience

Environmental Complexity

Occupational therapy is steeped in a long history of concern for purposeful activity within relevant environments. Early occupational therapists, who were concerned by the idleness experienced by patients confined by hospitalization, became interested in balancing the work, rest, play, and sleep cycles of their patients. They used stimulating environments to facilitate organization, self-satisfaction, and success in daily living. Morevoer, the everyday settings of home, garden, classroom, work station, playground, and marketplace provided the challenges on which occupational therapists built their practice. According to Clark and Jackson,[1] occupational science emphasizes the human capacity to pursue and organize occupation actively in response to environmental challenges.

This paper focuses on ways in which occupational therapists use the environment for therapeutic purposes. Sensory integrative theory, an example of an occupational therapy frame of reference heavily dependent on environmental interaction, is highlighted. What research has taught us about enriched and deprived environments will be applied to what is known clinically about individuals who are unable to engage fully with the demands of their environment.

About 30 years ago, Jean Ayres, an occupational therapist, began work on a theory that had major implications for the profession of occupational therapy. In her interaction with children and adults who had neurologic disabilities, Ayres sensed that these individuals had difficulties that extended beyond muscle incoordination and poor visual perception usually seen as their major problems. During postdoctoral work at the Brain Research Institute at University of California, Los Angeles, she formulated early hypotheses regarding the role of basic sensory systems in providing information for interaction in the physical and social world. Sensory integration, commonly defined as "organization of sensation for use,"[2] is the basis for a complex theory that provides explanations of the way individuals use sensory information to organize their actions and master their environments. Ayres' research, which was so heavily based on the understanding of functional neuroanatomy, also was strongly guided by the values of occupational therapy; her theories accordingly evolved as they were enacted within the therapeutic environments that she created. Five principles of sensory integrative theory, summarized by Clark, Mailloux, and Parham[3] are used to demonstrate the neuroscience base of sensory integrative theory, the influences of occupation, and the importance of environmental interaction.

Five Principles of Sensory Integrative Theory

The first of these principles is that controlled sensory input can be used to elicit an adaptive response. Adaptive responses are purposeful, goal-directed actions that add functional meaning to motion. For example, holding onto a rope or bar for play constitutes a simple adaptive response (Fig. 16–1). For children unable to make the appropriate response, in other words, for children who cannot initiate or maintain grasp, movement or displacement of the center of gravity may facilitate "holding on." On a more complex level, the tactile sensation and feeling the movement generated as one's fingers work across a loom will probably facilitate the skill attained in weaving and generalized fine motor skills as well. When an individual is able to register and organize sensation, accurately judge the demands of an action, and execute a successful response, adaptive behavior occurs.

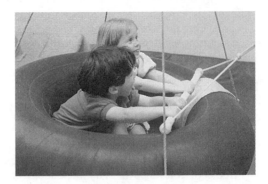

Figure 16–1. These children are engaged in self-directed activity in the enriched environment of an occupational therapy center. (Photo by Shay McAtee.)

The second principle notes that as adaptive responses are made, they contribute to sensory integration. Successfully meeting a challenge helps to organize sensation and thus better prepares an individual for future environmental demands. Mastering a climbing tower requires visual, tactile, proprioceptive, and vestibular sensory processing, as well as motor planning. A successful or adaptive response to this challenge facilitates the way these neural functions can be used in new tasks. Knowledge and skill attained through past action influence future organization of sensation for use.

A third principle is that the more inner directed a child's activities are, the greater potential of the activities for improving neural organization. According to Ayres,[4] people have a built-in drive to interact adaptively with the environment. In occupational therapy, children are seen as, and respected for, having an inner drive to engage in activities that will bring about brain organization and sensory integration. Thus, a child engaged in active, self-directed tactile exploration will probably gain more from the challenges inherent in this activity than the child who passively accepts such motion. Use of inner drive is the starting point of occupational therapy, even when this function may be compromised, as in the patient with autism or head injury. When inner drive is compromised, activation of self-direction becomes a goal.

Fourth, as primitive behaviors become more consolidated, more mature and complex patterns of behavior emerge. Simple adaptive responses provide a foundation for the complex practice, cognitive, social, and emotional functions that make up daily living. Successful interaction in an environment allows for increasingly greater generalization of skill. On the other hand, individuals who have difficulty making simple adaptive responses, such as children who cannot perceive the position of their bodies well in relation to objects and people around them, also will have difficulty mastering more demanding behaviors, such as playing a game of soccer or conducting a meeting.

A final summarizing principle of sensory integrative theory is that better organization of adaptive responses will enhance the child's general behavioral organization. Individuals learn to weave adaptive responses into complex behaviors through functions such as timing, sequencing, and reading environmental cues. The process of coordinating thought and action leads to overall organization of behavior. According to Ayres,[4] "adaptive behavior promotes personal growth."

To develop these principles and their related concepts in sensory integrative theory, Ayres built an enriched therapeutic environment that would allow for the promotion of adaptive behavior in children. Choosing appealing colors and novel pieces of equipment, Ayres created a setting that would elicit inner drive and allow a child to feel safe in experimenting with new behaviors. The setting was constructed to allow a variety of challenges and ease transition from one activity to the next. The types of activities made available to a child and the way they might be arranged entice the child toward purposeful play behavior.

Some of the concepts from research on enriched environments and how they apply to children with disability are examined next.

Sensory Experience

Research examining the effect of sensory experience on behavior includes a large body of work on sensory deprivation and sensory stimulation. Experiments altering exposure to visual, auditory, tactile, and vestibular sensory input in nonhumans and humans at varying stages of development suggest that those sensory systems cannot develop normally based purely on genetic factors, but rather, depend on stimulation during critical periods of brain plasticity.[5] In related research, Mears and Harlow[6] demonstrated the importance of self-motion play in rhesus monkeys. In a setting not unlike our therapeutic environment, they examined the importance of self-motion play or peragration, which means movement through space. Mears and Harlow believed self-motion to be a primary form of play that was a reinforcer in and of its own right. Noting that monkeys who had the opportunity for peragrations showed less rocking, huddling, and ventral clinging than those who did not, these researchers suggested that such play possessed strong psychotherapeutic benefits.

Deprivation conditions in nonhumans and humans have been associated with poor sensory registration, decreased motor skills, irritability, lethargy, and difficulty in concentration. Children with neurologic disabilities may experience conditions that could be likened to sensory-deprived states due to a number of factors, including extended illness and hospitalization, poor or absent sensory registration and perception, and lack of exposure and experience. A particularly severe example of a child experiencing sensory deprivation was reported by Ayres and Mailloux in the *American Journal of Occupational Therapy* in 1981.[7] A deaf, partially sighted, and autistic, 11-year-old girl demonstrated little ability to interact purposefully in her environment. In addition to her lack of visual and auditory experience, tactile, proprioceptive, and vestibular sensory processing input also had been severely limited due to a lack of normal physical and social play experiences. Prior to intervention, her behavior was characterized mostly by total body motions of a self-stimulatory nature; she appeared to seek desperately input from purposeful environmental interaction that was not otherwise forthcoming. Children with less severe disabilities also have signs of behavior reminiscent of research subjects in deprived or overstimulating sensory conditions. Hyposensitivity or hypersensitivity to touch, movement, sound, and visual stimuli is often accompanied by withdrawal, irritability, poor attention span, lack of motivation, and poor self-esteem.

Social Experience

Extensive work by Rosenzweig,[8] Bennett,[9] Diamond,[10] Greenough,[11] and Rosenzweig and colleagues[12,13] has demonstrated the importance of the social situation on brain development and behavior. Social experience appears to be intimately intertwined with sensory experience in relation to the effects of varying environmental conditions. For example, some studies, particularly those conducted by Rosenzweig, suggest that brain effects induced by laboratory environmental enrichment may be a product of the social stimulation inherent in the standard enriched environment. In addition to anatomic and brain chemistry changes found in animals reared in enriched environments, enhanced learning, memory, and species-appropriate social behavior have been found.

In humans, social isolation has been associated with temporal disorientation, hostility, and loneliness. Children with a disability often experience peer or self-inflicted social isolation for a variety of reasons. Segregation of children with disabilities and peer rejection may limit social experiences, and lack of skill or self-perception of inability may further inhibit opportunities for social interaction. In rats, there is an interplay between sensory and social aspects of environmental effects. It is probable that sensory processing deficits in humans are closely related to social skill development and successful role performance within varying environmental conditions.

Environmental Complexity

Exactly what constitutes an enriched environment is a matter of debate in the literature. Considerations of novelty, variety, complexity, and relationship to natural conditions are among the factors considered in these discussions. Social psychologists, such as Bruner, Sutton-Smith, and White, and occupational therapists, such as Reilly, Florey, Knox, Takata, Robinson, and Matsutsuyu, have been concerned with similar concepts in relation to play in children. Finding the optimal level of novelty, variety, and complexity was an important consideration for Ayres as she designed her treatment settings. Each of these factors proved to be relevant in relation to facilitating inner drive, "the just right challenge," and appropriate adaptive responses.

Consideration of the likeness of an environment to the natural setting elicits some interesting questions in animal research. For example, it has been debated whether change is brought about directly by objects that are added to a laboratory environment or merely by the fact that their addition makes an environment more naturally complex and variable. In some of the earliest studies in the 1940s, Hebb[14] reared his rats as pets in his home and found that animals reared as pets improved more during testing than those reared in laboratory cages. One might assume that a home setting is more similar to a natural situation for a rat than is a laboratory. The degree of normalcy in the surroundings, in conjunction with sensory and social experiences, might provide a broader perspective on how the environment affects behavior, particularly in animal studies where total living conditions are so different from natural habitats.

In treatment, Ayres[2] tried to conceive of activities that would be novel, varied, and relevant to the types of experiences children receive through normal play behavior. Thus, equipment was devised to provide a variety of self-activated sensory and practic opportunities within a social situation. Camp Avanti, a summer program especially designed for children with sensory integrative disorders, is a good example of a therapeutic and enriched environment that uses a natural setting for play and exploration. The therapeutic activities provided in this occupational therapy approach are meant to allow the child to engage in age-appropriate experiences that may not otherwise occur due to fear, lack of skill, poor ideation, decreased initiation, or social rejection.

In summary, the objective of occupational therapy is to improve function so that an individual can better interpret his or her environment, respond to it, and interact within it. This process might be summarized as facilitating adaptive behavior, and to accomplish this, the nature, structure, and function of the environment play a central role.

Discussion Questions

1. How does Ayres' theory of sensory integration link the biophysical aspects of the human engaged in occupation with "higher level" function?
2. Do you think these principles can be useful concepts at a more metaphorical level rather than only at a biophysical level?

References

1. Clark, F, and Jackson J: Contemplative occupational therapy: Thoughts on the application of the occupational therapy negative heuristic in the treatment of persons with human immunodeficiency infection. Occup Ther Health Care 6:69, 1989.
2. Ayres, AJ: Sensory Integration and the Child. Western Psychological Services, Los Angeles, CA, 1972.
3. Clark, F, Mailloux, Z, and Parham, D: Sensory integration and children with learning disabilities. In Pratt, PN, and Allen, AS (eds): Occupational Therapy for Children, C. V. Mosby, St. Louis, MO, 1989.
4. Ayres, AJ: Sensory Integration and Learning Disorders. Western Psychological Services, Los Angeles, CA, 1972.
5. Bennet, EL, Diamond, MC, Kreck, D, and Rosenzweig, JR: Chemical and anatomical plasticity of the brain. Science 10:610, 1964.
6. Mears, CE, and Harlow, HF: Play: Early and eternal. Proc Nat Acad Sci USA 72:1878, 1975.
7. Ayres, AJ, and Mailloux, Z: Influence of sensory integration procedures on language development. Am J Occup Ther 35:383, 1981.
8. Rosenzweig, MR: Environmental complexity, cerebral change, and behavior. Am Psychol 21:321, 1966.
9. Bennett, EL: Cerebral effects of differential experience and training. In Rosenzweig, MR, and Bennett, EL (eds): Learning and Memory. MIT Press, Boston, MA, 1976, p 279.
10. Diamond, MC: Anatomical brain changes induced by environment. In Petrinovich, L, and McGaugh, J (eds): Knowing, Thinking, and Believing. Plenum Press, New York, 1976.
11. Greenough, WT: Enduring brain effects of differential experience and training. In Rosenzweig, MR, and Bennett, EL (eds): Neural Mechanisms of Learning and Memory. MIT Press, Boston, MA, 1976, p 255.
12. Rosenzweig, ML, and Bennett, EL: Enriched environments: Facts, factors, and fantasies. In Petrinovich, L, and McGaugh, J (eds): Knowing, Thinking and Believing. Plenum Press, New York, 1976, p 179.
13. Rosenzweig, MR, Krech, D, Bennett, EL, and Diamond, MC: Modifying brain chemistry and anatomy by enrichment or impoverishment of experience. In Newton, G, and Levine, S (eds): Early Experience and Behavior. Charles C Thomas, Springfield, IL, 1968, p 258.
14. Hebb, DO: Organization of Behavior. John Wiley & Sons, New York, 1949.

by Arnold S. Chamove, MA, MPhil,
PhD, CPsychol, FIBiol

17

Enrichment in Primates
Relevance to Occupational Science

It may not be obvious, but the result of research on enrichment in primates is directly relevant to the work of the occupational scientist in general and of the occupational therapist in particular. Some interesting but speculative connections between these arenas have accordingly been selected for discussion. The paper's primary theme is as follows: While occupational therapists are often concerned with the "work" that incapacitated people would normally be doing, those who provide enrichment to primates are often concerned with the "work" that captive animals would normally be doing. It is my view that "work" is behavior that individuals would prefer to be doing rather than doing nothing or doing what they are restricted to doing by means of their institutionalized or captive conditions.

There have been many studies of environmental enrichment or environmental improvement in primates. In this discussion, primates refers to nonhuman primates below the level of apes, that is, monkeys and prosimians. Although few studies have compared differing techniques of enrichment in animals, two studies that have done so show that, for primates, foraging is the most effective enrichment technique available.[1,2] These studies compared toys with foraging and found that interest in a single toy is soon lost, whereas foraging maintains its interest over the duration of testing and probably for the life of the animal. The effectiveness of foraging is not surprising when you realize that primates spend between 25% and 90% (usually more than 50%) of their day foraging for food. This involves moving to new food sources, searching for and collecting food at that source, and processing the food. Foraging may accordingly be viewed as the normal "work" for primates.

One way in which the effectiveness of enrichment techniques is normally measured has been to see if subjects perform specific behaviors at all, that is, how

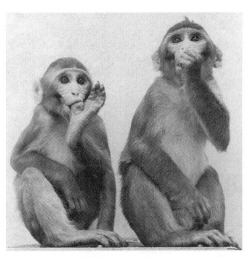

Figure 17–1. Captive monkeys without the work of obtaining food have nothing much to do. (Photo by Arnold Chamove.)

much they like to do it or are motivated to do certain kinds of activities. This technique was used to measure foraging in one species of terrestrial monkeys living in captivity. In their normal housing, the floor was bare and cleaned twice a day. Food was normally fed in hoppers twice a day and was consumed in a few minutes (about 1% of the day). The animals had the rest of the day with nothing much to do, that is, without the work they normally would have to occupy their time in a natural habitat (Fig. 17–1). The monkeys spent about 2% of the day vainly searching the floor for any food scraps that might have been dropped, while aggressive behavior occupied over 30% of their day. However, when clean woodchips were spread over the floor, thereby providing them with opportunity to work, their searching increased to 7% even though there was no food to be found in the woodchip litter (Fig. 17–2). When small items of food (bird seed) were subsequently buried in the litter, foraging time of these monkeys increased to 32% of the day (Fig. 17–3).

It appeared that the monkeys were foraging to obtain the food, yet when they were given free food consisting of containers of bird seed, they still foraged. Recall that they had worked to find food in the clean litter when day after day, there was never food in the woodchips. Moreover, they worked to find food in the litter when the same food was available in convenient buckets nearby. This study suggests that the monkeys enjoyed doing the same type of work that they had evolved to do in the wild when given a chance to work at tasks they normally perform for long periods, so-called "prevalent activities."

There were other consequences of this opportunity for potentially gainful activity. The most dramatic of these was that squabbling decreased to one third of that present in the bare-floor condition. In other words, aggression decreased when work was available. These findings have been repeated in several species of monkey housed in bare conditions in zoos and laboratories.[2] Making food more difficult to process also reduced aggression.[3]

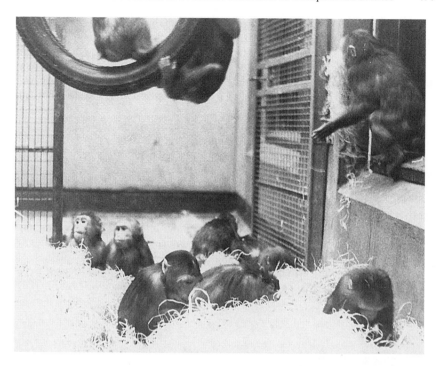

Figure 17–2. With litter spread in their cage, the monkeys foraged for food. (Photo by Arnold Chamove.)

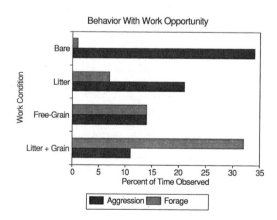

Figure 17–3. Comparison of percent of aggressive versus foraging behavior in monkeys under differing conditions of potential for normal work behavior.

Although many occupational therapy techniques have not been formally evaluated, it is clinically clear that they are useful. The techniques appear to reduce abnormal behaviors and increase well-being. The level at which they are working is unclear. Long-term psychiatric inpatients appear to improve and report that they feel better on days they exercise.[4] Some theoreticians speculate that participation in exercise leads to increased competence and self-esteem, but primates show the same behavioral effects from activity.

Could it be that the techniques used by the occupational therapist are effective insofar as they increase competence and involve physical exercise or actions? Some techniques may achieve their goals this way, but many effective occupational therapy techniques do not use exercise. Could it be that they are effective insofar as they use occupations that are common in unhospitalized people, normal work?

Few studies are evaluating these questions,[5] that is, assessing the relative effectiveness of techniques based on the component of physical exercise versus prevalent occupations, such as work, similar to foraging in monkeys. The research on primates suggests we can improve their environment and improve behavior by using prevalent activities. Perhaps occupational therapy is tapping a basic biologic predisposition for work when it focuses not just on the physical aspects of activity, but on occupations that have meaning, as do the prevalent activities of our daily routines.

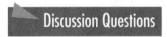 Discussion Questions

1. How valid is Chamove's basic premise that deeper understandings of human work can accrue from studies of captive nonhuman primates?
2. What are the implications of Chamove's paper for understanding the experiences of intrinsic motivation, boredom, disease, and health?

References

1. Bryant, CE, Rupniak, NMJ, and Iversen, SD: Effects of different environmental enrichment devices on cage stereotypes and autoaggression in captive monkeys. Journal of Medical Primatology 17:257, 1988.
2. Chamove, AS: Environmental enrichment: A review. Animal Technology 40:155, 1989.
3. Chamove, AS, and Anderson, JR: Examining environmental enrichment. In Segal, E (ed): The Psychological Well-being of Primates. Noyes Publications, Philadelphia, 1989, p 183.
4. Chamove, AS: Exercise improves behaviour: A rational for occupational therapy. British Journal of Occupational Therapy 49:83, 1986.
5. Brown, JI, and Chamove, AS: Mental and physical activity benefits in adults with mental handicap. Mental Handicap Research 6:155, 1993.

by Cynthia A. Hedricks, PhD

18

A Biosocial Perspective on Human Occupation

This paper explores some relationships between hormones, the social environment, human occupations, and psychological states; thus, the research presented falls within the domain of behavioral endocrinology. The hormones discussed are those classically associated with the reproductive system. The social environments under investigation are somewhat diverse and are therefore discussed within the context of the research question being addressed. Occupations studied include sexual intercourse and work; psychological states include mood and activation.

Often, progress in science is limited by available technology. In the case of human behavioral endocrinology, there are limitations in the collection and measurement of hormonal activity and in understanding how a molecular substance, such as a hormone, could actually be related to human occupation. Progress also is limited by the way many researchers in this field approach their subject matter. For example, there are at least two major gaps in this field today: failure to evaluate how the social environment relates to correlations between hormones and occupation and failure to view findings as evidence of hormone-occupation relationships that acknowledge the possibility of bidirectionality between these two factors. A majority of researchers still interpret their data as evidence that hormones regulate or determine a particular activity or occupation.[1] This viewpoint may stem from the historic roots of behavioral endocrinology and particularly from the numerous animal studies performed on rodents. However, even in rodents and nonhuman primates, there is evidence that behavior can influence hormonal activity[2,3] and that the social environment can mediate the nature of hormone-behavior relationships.[4–9]

The general questions to be addressed include the following: Are hormones related to human occupation or psychological states? Is the social environment related to human occupations or psychological states? What is the nature of the interaction among hormones, the social environment, and psychological state during human occupation? Due in part to the combination of the methodologic techniques discussed below, these questions are beginning to be addressed.

Methodological Approach

Three methodological techniques have been combined to understand better relationships among reproductive hormones, the social environment, and human occupation.

Collecting Biomarkers of Underlying Hormonal Activity

The rhythmic nature of hormonal activity lends itself to the investigation of how this natural variation in hormonal activity relates to the timing of human occupations, be they changes in sexual activity, psychological state, or work schedules. Some of the rhythms last about 1 day and are called "circadian" rhythms. Some rhythms are the length of the female menstrual or ovarian cycle; still others are seasonal. Thus, there are options regarding the time frame of observation.

All three classes of the steroid hormones of reproduction are rhythmic in their activity. These three classes of hormones are the androgens (e.g., testosterone), estrogens (e.g., estradiol), and progestogens (e.g., progesterone). Hormonal effects are mediated through the central nervous system; androgens and estrogens are typically associated with increased neural activity, while progesterone is typically associated with decreased neural activity. Not surprisingly, the general effects of these hormones on nervous system function often parallel the relationships between these hormones and behavior, for example, general activity level or sexual behavior.[10–12]

A methodologic necessity for understanding relationships among hormonal mechanisms and human occupations or psychological states is to obtain biomarkers of underlying hormonal activity. Greatest precision would be obtained by multiple collections of biologic specimens, such as blood, urine, or saliva, across some length of time. This can be done for men and women. Fortunately, with respect to women, there also are noninvasive biomarkers of underlying hormonal activity, although they are somewhat less precise than actual hormonal measurements derived from collection of biologic specimens. These include daily recordings of waking temperature (basal body temperature or BBT) or changes in cervical mucus.

Because of time and budget constraints, however, many researchers do not collect biomarkers of hormonal activity. Instead, they use published information to estimate when hormonal fluctuations should be taking place. This is particularly true of researchers who study behavioral correlates of the human menstrual cycle.[13] One problem with this approach is that there is variation in the timing of hormonal fluctuations across the menstrual cycle, both between and within individuals.[14] Thus, the failure to collect biomarkers of hormonal activity is partially responsible for the disagreement between studies on whether behaviors or psychological states change in a consistent manner along with hormonal fluctuations, such as those that characterize the female menstrual cycle.

Prospective Research Design

It is common for behavioral endocrinologists who study humans to use a retrospective method of data collection. People are asked to reach back in time and memory regarding the occurrence of activities and psychological states. This type of inquiry continues to pervade a number of fields, even though many studies have found that it is difficult for people to remember precisely how often and when some event occurred.[15-18] Exceptions would be only those salient life events.

Others, including this author, have used a prospective method to observe how often and when an activity occurs. This prospective methodology often takes the form of having study participants complete daily activity checklists for many consecutive days. For more in-depth study, and particularly to investigate relationships between the social environment and occupation, electronic pagers have been used to obtain on-the-spot measurements of activities and psychological states.

Observations in the Natural Environment

Many attempts to study hormone-behavior relationships have been in the laboratory, often a small and convenient research setting. However, this type of setting bears little similarity to the natural environment of the species under observation. Thus, some behaviors observed may be due to the use of the artificial laboratory environment and are therefore unlikely to have lawful relationships with hormonal mechanisms.[8] In the natural environment in which humans live, one is more likely to observe a behavior or occupation that has evolved in this type of setting; thus, one is more likely to find lawful and meaningful relationships between hormonal mechanisms and human occupation.

Examples of Biosocial Correlates of Occupation

The previous section is a brief overview of the problems that face researchers in this area and attempts made to reduce these problems. The remainder of this paper contains examples of how these methodologic innovations have been integrated into the complex study of hormones, the social environment, and human occupations or psychological states. The diverse social contexts studied have included the male/female dyad; the immediate social group; and the culture in which we live.

Regardless of the hormonal biomarkers collected or the social context studied, the general questions asked have been:

1. Do hormones relate to psychological states during human occupations, or are occupations and psychological states above influence from biologic factors?
2. What role does social context play with respect to psychological states during human occupations?
3. Can one simultaneously study hormonal and social correlates of psychological states during human occupations?

The Male-Female Dyad

The first research example involves the social unit of the male-female dyad. The question asked was, within this social unit, "Do changes in female hormones coincide with the human occupation of sexual activity?" More specifically, "Does sexual intercourse peak around the time of ovulation in the female, when hormones and other biologic mechanisms make conception most likely?"

The data were collected by researchers at the Carolina Population Center, University of North Carolina at Chapel Hill under the direction of the Center's director, J. Richard Udry, PhD. The couples were married, but more importantly, they lived together and thus theoretically had daily opportunity for engaging in sexual intercourse with each other. None of the women were using contraceptive methods that interfered with endogenous hormonal activity.

The methodology involved daily collection of first morning urine specimens from the women, aged 17 to 30 years, along with "yes/no" reporting of whether the couple had engaged in sexual intercourse the previous day and whether the woman had menstruated the previous day. Both the biologic specimens and the behavioral reports were picked up daily at the couple's home. Data collection lasted for about 100 days; thus, data were available for approximately three consecutive menstrual cycles of each woman.

The urine specimens were used to measure luteinizing hormone (LH), a hormone that rises significantly from baseline and then peaks approximately 14 to 16 days before the first day of next menstrual bleeding. The onset of the rise in LH typically indicates that ovulation is about to occur, which is the release of an egg from the female ovary. It has been reported that ovulation occurs ±1 day from the peak in LH.[19] Therefore, in this study, LH was used as a biomarker to estimate the timing of ovulation.

Although there is a surge in LH around the time of ovulation during most menstrual cycles, the timing of when the LH surge begins can be variable from woman to woman and even from cycle to cycle for the same woman.[14] For this reason, each individual cycle was standardized, or organized, around the day that the LH surge began.[20] The day the LH surge began (LH surge onset) was designated as "day 0." The day before this was designated as "day −1" relative to LH surge onset day, and the day before that was "day −2" and so on. The day after LH surge onset was "day +1" relative to LH surge onset day, and the day after that was "day +2" and so on.

The occupation of interest was sexual intercourse. The hormonal event of interest was day relative to LH surge onset (day 0). A plot was made of the proportion of couples having intercourse (y axis) on any given day relative to LH surge onset (*x* axis). The most interesting finding was that the peak intercourse rate coincided with the day of LH surge onset.[20] The percentage of couples engaging in intercourse on this day (72%) was significantly greater than at any other time during the female menstrual cycle (see Figure 1 in Hedricks et al.[20]; the average rate was 44% of the couples on any given day of the female's cycle). Note that when the female's cycle was organized by using nonhormonal methods to estimate the timing of ovulation, such as counting backwards from next menses onset, a significant peak in sexual intercourse at the estimated time of ovulation was not found.[20] Furthermore, although day of LH surge onset is significantly associated with length of the menstrual cycle (a gross index of underlying hormonal activity), cycle length is an insufficient predictor of LH surge onset day.[21]

This finding generated a number of interesting questions surrounding the issue of causality. For example, LH is not thought to have any properties that would stimulate sexual activity in men or women, but steroid hormones like androgen and estrogen, particularly androgen, have been linked with increases in female sexual activity. What is the steroid hormone profile around the time of peak intercourse? What role did the steroid hormones play in both the peak intercourse rate and LH surge onset (estrogen is classically considered to be the main determinant of LH surge onset and peak). With respect to possible bidirectionality, what role does intercourse play, if any, in the timing of the LH surge of ovulation?[14]

The findings of this study had meaning for the scientific community and for the evolution of our species. By observing at the social level of the couple and collecting biologic specimens, one can begin to build a biosocial model of an occupation that is related to conception in humans. Not all couples engaged in sexual intercourse on the day of LH surge onset or on the day of LH peak; thus, peak hormonal activity did not necessarily mean that the occupation of sexual intercourse would occur. This indicates that social and psychological factors play some role in this phenomenon. One advantage of some variation in when couples engage in intercourse around the time of ovulation is that it enables our species to have variation in the sex of our offspring. Inseminations a few days prior to ovulation increase the probability of having a son, while inseminations closer to or on the day of ovulation are more likely to result in a daughter. Inseminations shortly after ovulation are associated with a moderate rise in the probability of having a son.[22,23] This phenomenon has recently been replicated in male-female pairs of rats that were mating spontaneously and to satiety in a seminaturalistic environment.[9] These data suggest that the rat could be used as an animal model to investigate some mechanisms related to sex determination in humans.

The Immediate Social and Physical Environment

In this study, the goal was to look at variability in psychological states of women as they varied according to hormonal phases of the menstrual cycle and according to the immediate social and physical environment. Thus, this study could address a question that is often asked with respect to women in the childbearing years, "Does the psychological state of women vary according to phase of the menstrual cycle?" Furthermore, this study could address the role of the social and physical environment in modulating effects of hormonal fluctuations.

The study was begun at the University of Chicago by R. Breckinridge Church, PhD, Judith LeFevre, PhD, Martha K. McClintock, PhD, and me. The female participants were either married to or living with male partners. None were taking any medications, including hormonal contraceptives, which would interfere with endogenous hormonal activity. Although our focus was on women, information also was collected on how the psychological state of man varied according to the phase of the woman's menstrual cycle and according to the context of the natural social environment.

The study was presented as one on relationships between biological rhythms and psychological states. Biological, social, and psychological data were collected for 30 consecutive days on 13 couples. Women and men recorded waking temperatures (basal BBT) and filled out daily checklists of physical symptoms, many of which are typically reported as changing across the menstrual cycle. Women also recorded changes in cervical mucus and days of menstrual bleeding. The woman's BBT, changes in cervical mucus, and menstrual dates were used to categorize the data into one of six phases of the female menstrual cycle: 1) *menses 1*—the first 3 days of menstrual bleeding; 2) *menses 2*—the remaining days of menstrual bleeding; 3) *follicular*—the interval between menses 2 and the periovulatory phase; 4) *periovulatory*—a 4-day period in which the estimated day of ovulation occurred (estimated day of ovulation was derived by a concordance of BBT nadir and copious amounts of fertile cervical mucus, which usually occurred approximately 14 days prior to next menses onset); 5) *luteal*—the interval between the periovulatory phase and the premenstrual phase; and 6) *premenstrual*—the 3 days prior to onset of next menses.

The use of electronic pagers, or the "experience sampling method,"[24] to prompt data collection enabled us to assess the occupation in which the individual was engaging and psychological state, within the context of the natural social and physical environment. That is, both members of the couple wore pagers as they went about their daily lives, for example, working, going to and from places, preparing and eating meals, engaging in personal and home maintenance, or attending events in public. The pagers "beeped" on a semirandom schedule three times a day between 8:00 AM and 10:00 PM. The first beep was between 8:00 AM and 12:00 PM, the second beep was between 12:01 PM and 5:00 PM, and the third beep was between 5:01 PM and 10:00 PM. When the beep sounded, the participant filled out a short questionnaire as soon as possible. Each time the participant was beeped, he or she filled out the questionnaire (all questionnaires were identical). This particular study had the potential to generate 2340 questionnaires (30 days × three questionnaires per day = 90 questionnaires per person × 26 persons [13 men and 13 women] = 2340).

To evaluate the contribution of the social environment, space was provided for the participants to indicate on the questionnaires with whom they were and where they were when they were beeped. With whom the participant was when he or she was beeped was considered to be the social context; where the participant was when she or he was beeped was considered to be his or her physical location in the environment.

Analyses to date have concentrated on relationships between the female's menstrual cycle phase, the immediate environment (social and physical), and two psychological states, "mood" and "activation."[25-29] The psychological states of mood and activation were measured by participants' responses to 15 pairs of adjectives presented in the form of semantic differentials. The pairs of adjectives were counterbalanced with respect to which side negative and positive adjectives were placed. Factor analyses using this methodology have revealed that four pairs of adjectives embedded in the list represented a psychological construct that could be labeled "mood," and four different pairs could be labeled "activation." Although the following discussion presents the results of analyses with respect to relationships among social context, physical location, menstrual cycle phase, and the psychological state of mood, relationships among these variables and the psychological state of activation were similar.

An average mood value was calculated for each person, based on all the times they completed a questionnaire. Deviations from the mean (z-scores) were used to evaluate whether mood was increased or decreased (represented by positive or negative z-scores, respectively) across social context, physical location, and menstrual cycle phase. The same procedure was repeated for the psychological construct of activation. Female mood did vary as a function of the social context. Mood was higher than average when with others, including their partners; mood was lower than average when the women were alone. Mood also varied according to the woman's physical location in her environment. Mood was higher than average when the women were out in public and lower than average when the women were at home or at work. Thus, social context and physical location, as evidenced by this natural field study, did contribute to variability in the psychological state of mood. Psychological states of the women also varied according to phase of their menstrual cycle. The majority of women (75%) showed increased mood around the estimated time of ovulation. Although social and hormonal factors contributed toward variability in mood, the greatest variability in mood was a function of the social context or with whom the woman was when she was beeped.[27] A moderate amount of variability in mood and activation was due to physical location, or where the woman was in her environment. The least amount of variability in mood was due to hormonal factors, as indexed by phase of the female's menstrual cycle.

These findings have important scientific, political, and clinical implications. Scientifically, they speak to the importance of including multiple levels of analysis (psychological, biological, social) when studying human activities or occupations. They also indicate that although a woman's hormonal changes can contribute toward variation in psychological state, these effects are likely to be strongly modulated by the social environment. Because hormonal state (as indexed by phase of the menstrual cycle) accounted for only a small portion of the variability in mood, hormonal state is unlikely to have as dramatic a relationship to psychological state as the press would lead one to believe. These results also undermine the argument that a woman is incapable of being in situations that require decision making because she undergoes hormonal changes across her menstrual cycle.

Rather, this biosociopsychological approach, conducted in the natural human environment, suggests an interplay between these various systems. Finally, clinicians might use these findings to support their efforts to improve the mental health of patients. For example, the results of the study support the therapist's recommendation that patients spend more time with friends or try to get out of the home more often. Also because the occupational therapy clinic is a social environment, it has the potential to influence the psychological state of the patient and therefore the course of treatment.

The Cultural Environment

In the preceding two examples, interactions between the immediate social environment, hormonal factors, and human behavior have been presented. In this last example, the potential for interactions between the culture in which we live, the female hormonal system, and the human occupation of work is discussed.

There is almost worldwide demand for 24-hour services. These are primarily in areas of telephone communication, health care, air transportation, data processing, and food and beverage service. In our country, as in others, women predominantly work in jobs that require 24-hour services. Night shifts are typically defined as those in which at least half of the hours worked fall between midnight and 0800 hours.[29] Those who work nights may do so on a fixed or variable (rotating) schedule. Generally, employees with the least seniority work nights or rotating shifts that include nights. It is estimated that as high as 26% of all employed women between 20 and 64 years are engaged in night or shift work.[30] Recent surveys of female laboratory workers, nurses, and telephone operators outside the United States have reported an association between working nights (commonly referred to as shift work), menstrual complaints, and adverse pregnancy outcome, including spontaneous abortion.[31,32]

Because of the rise in shift work by women in the childbearing years, the reproductive health and well-being of women engaged in shift work may become one of the most critical issues for occupational health specialists in the next few decades. Although the associations between shift work and female reproductive function are provocative, the following question remains to be answered. Does engaging in shift work cause dysfunction in the female reproductive system?

Toward an answer to this question, a longitudinal, within-subjects pilot study was conducted that focused on shift work–related changes to a woman's menstrual function. One underlying notion of this study was that menstrual disturbances can be an early warning of environmental hazards to female reproductive function. Although surveys have shown significant associations between shift work and reproductive function in women, the direction of causality is unknown. A longitudinal, within-subjects design was chosen to determine direction of causality. This type of research design also reduces or eliminates the confounds of recall, response, and selection bias, three types of error that plague surveys of work-related effects on health, particularly with respect to female reproductive function.

Twelve college seniors in a nursing program volunteered to be unpaid participants in the pilot study. They agreed to be intensively studied on a daily basis for 5 consecutive months. Three of the 12 participants did not complete the pilot study, one because of taking oral contraceptives and two because of the commitment involved. Another participant flew part-time as a flight attendant, and her data are not included here. The remaining eight participants contributed at least 5 consecutive months of daily BBT, cervical mucus changes, physical and psychological symptoms, and sleep-wake-work schedules. Daily urines also were collected during the menstrual cycles for precise measurement of hormonal activity. A few individuals in this pilot study contributed almost 1 year of daily data. The primary focus of the methodology was to gather baseline data on the women prior to graduation and entry into the work force and then to continue to follow these same individuals as they entered full-time work as nurses.

Initial findings of this pilot study were reported to the Society for Menstrual Cycle Research.[33] One important finding was that the participants could follow the experimental protocol. Another important finding was an awareness of some of the methodological problems associated with studying women who are engaged in shift work. For example, because the women were altering their daily sleep-wake rhythms, which are linked with daily temperature rhythms, BBT when awakening could not be used as an index of underlying hormonal activity. With respect to the research question posed, the two participants who began working nights displayed longer menstrual cycles than any cycles reported prior to entry into shift work. (However, no cycles were longer than 40 days, which can be an indicator of ovulatory dysfunction.) Additionally, both of these participants reported becoming sick almost as soon as they began shift work; one was briefly hospitalized. Thus, even in this small sample, one sees how a change in the pattern of everyday activities has an impact on health. A current study is further investigating this research question with a larger sample size.

Conclusions

The field of human behavioral endocrinology is still in its infancy. To develop it further, researchers and clinicians need to focus on how the social environment in which humans live modulates hormone and behavior relationships. Toward this end, it is recommended that three methodological techniques be used, often in combination with one another. One is to observe humans in the natural environment in which they live. This approach makes it more likely that the researcher will observe a behavior, or occupation, that has evolved in this natural setting. Therefore, more meaningful theories of relationships between hormones, the social environment, and human occupation are likely to emerge. Another methodological technique used is a prospective method of collecting data. That is, study participants volunteer information on at least a daily basis concerning their current behavior or psychological state. This method reduces or eliminates errors associated with the retrospective or survey methods of data collection. Perhaps the ultimate way to gather data prospectively is by the experience sampling method, in which electronic pagers are used to signal study participants to volunteer information on their activities and psychological states within the immediate social and physical context. Finally, biomarkers of underlying hormonal activity have been collected. For studies in which time and financial resources are restricted, noninvasive biomarkers of female hormonal changes have involved daily recording of BBT, changes in cervical mucus, and dates of menstrual bleeding. When financial resources are available, hormonal activity can be more precisely measured through laboratory assays of biological specimens.

These techniques have been used in a number of diverse studies, yet the research questions addressed by the studies are similar. Each has investigated whether correlations between hormonal activity and adult occupation exist. Each study also included attention toward some aspect of the natural social environment in which humans live. For example, the studies described in this chapter have observed human occupation at the level of the male-female social dyad, the immediate social group, and the culture. Regardless of the scientific contributions of each study toward the knowledge base that is developing in human behavioral endocrinology, all studies discussed here had clinical implications for the practice of occupational therapy, for the treatment of infertility, or both.

Results of some studies suggest that relationships among the social environment, hormones, and occupation have evolutionary consequences for the human species. Results of some studies have political ramifications, such as the finding that changes in female mood are more likely due to social context than to hormonal changes across the menstrual cycle.

This is an exciting field that holds promise for young and established researchers alike. Future work in this area should include low-cost, noninvasive measures of changes in hormonal activity of men and how engaging in an occupation influences underlying hormonal activity.

Discussion Questions

1. Do you agree with Hedricks that sexual activity comprises an occupation?
2. Do you think Hedricks' methodology could be applied to a wider range of activity and life contexts, such as young children playing at school, older adults engaged in structured activity programs within nursing homes, or patients receiving divergent kinds of occupational therapy within inpatient settings? What kinds of knowledge might doing so generate for occupational science and occupational therapy?

References

1. Hedricks, CA: Female sexual activity across the human menstrual cycle. Ann Rev Sex Res 5:122, 1994.
2. Moss, RL, and Cooper, KJ: Temporal relationship in spontaneous and coitus-induced release of luteinizing hormone in the normal cyclic rat. Endocrinology 92:1748, 1973.
3. Day, JR, Morales, TH, and Lu, JKH: Male stimulation of luteinizing hormone surge, progesterone secretion and ovulation in spontaneously persistent-estrous, aging rats. Biol Reprod 38:1019, 1988.
4. Wallen, K: Influence of female hormonal state on rhesus sexual behavior varies with space for social interaction. Science 217:375, 1982.
5. Rowell, TE, and Hartwell, KM: The interaction of behavior and reproductive cycles in patas monkeys. Behav Biol 24:141, 1978.
6. Gordon, TP: Reproductive behavior in the rhesus monkey: Social and endocrine variables. Amer Zool 21:185, 1981.
7. Cochran, CG: Proceptive patterns of behavior throughout the menstrual cycle in female rhesus monkeys. Behav Neural Biol 27:342, 1979.
8. McClintock, MK: Simplicity from complexity: A naturalistic approach to behavior and neuroendocrine function. New Directions for Methodology of Social and Behavioral Science 8:1, 1981.
9. Hedricks, C, and McClintock, MK: Timing of insemination and secondary sex ratio of the Norway rat. Physiol Behav 48:625, 1990.
10. Morris, N, and Udry, JR: Variations in pedometer activity during the menstrual cycle. Obstet Gynecol 35:199, 1970.
11. Udry, JR, and Morris, N: Effect of contraceptive pills on the distribution of sexual activity in the menstrual cycle. Nature 227:502, 1970.
12. Udry, JR, Billy, JOG, Morris, NM, Groff, TR, and Raj, MH: Serum androgenic hormones motivate sexual behavior in adolescent boys. Fertility and Sterility 43:90, 1985.

13. Hedricks, CA: The methodology of menstrual cycle research: Specific relevance to women's sexual health. Submitted for publication.
14. Hedricks, C, Davis, FG, Schramm, W, and Udry, JR: Coital exposure in relationship to timing of the LH peak in human females. Presented to the Conference on Reproductive Behavior, Atlanta GA, June 8–11, 1990.
15. Yarney, D: The Psychology of Eyewitness Testimony. Free Press, New York, 1979.
16. Hornsby, PP, and Wilcox, AJ: Validation of questionnaire information on frequency of coitus. Am J Epidemiol 130:94, 1989.
17. Englander-Golden, P, Chang, H, Whitmore, MR, and Dienstbier, RA: Female sexual arousal and the menstrual cycle. J Human Stress 6:42, 1980.
18. Stone, AA, Hedges, SM, Neale, JM, and Satin, MS: Prospective and cross-sectional mood reports offer no evidence of a "Blue Monday" phenomenon. Person Soc Psychol 49:129, 1985.
19. Singh, M, Saxena, BB, and Rathnam, P: Clinical validation of enzymeimmunoassay of human luteinizing hormone (hLH) in the detection of the preovulatory luteinizing hormone (LH) surge in urine. Fertility and Sterility 41:210, 1984.
20. Hedricks, C, Piccinino, L, Udry, JR, and Chimbira, THK: Peak coital rate coincides with onset of luteinizing hormone (LH) surge. Fertility and Sterility 48:234, 1987.
21. Hedricks, C, Piccinino, L, and Udry, JR: A first attempt at estimating luteinizing hormone (LH) surge onset day at midcycle. In Taylor, D, and Woods, N (eds): Menstruation, Health, and Illness: Neuroendocrine, Sociocultural and Clinical Perspectives. Hemisphere Publishing Corp., Washington, DC, 1991, p 59.
22. Guerrero, R: Sex ratio: A statistical association with the type and time of insemination in the menstrual cycle. Inter J Fert 15:221, 1970.
23. Guerrero, R: Association of the type and time of insemination within the menstrual cycle with the human sex ratio at birth. N Engl J Med 291:1056, 1974.
24. Larson, R, and Csikszentmihalyi, M: The experience sampling method. In Reis, HT (ed): Naturalistic Approaches to Studying Social Interaction. New Directions for Methodology of Social and Behavioral Science, no. 15. Jossey-Bass, San Francisco, 1983, p 41.
25. Church, RM, Marquette, LB, LeFevre, J, Hedricks, C, and McClintock, MK: Changes in psychological state during the human menstrual cycle. In Massimini, F, and Inghilleri, P (eds): L'Esperienza quotidiana. Teoria e metodo di analisi. Franco Angeli Libri s.r.l. (Italian), 1986, p 359.
26. Hedricks, C, Church, RB, LeFevre, J, and McClintock, MK: Changes in the psychological state of couples during a menstrual cycle: "On-the-spot" sampling from everyday life. Conference on Reproductive Behavior, Asilomar, CA, June 2–5, 1985.
27. Church, RB, Hedricks, C, LeFevre, J, and McClintock, MK: The importance of environmental context in mood and cognitive changes during the menstrual cycle. In Golgert, D (ed): Proceedings from the Society for Menstrual Cycle Research 9th Conference. Mind-body Rhythmicity: A Menstrual Cycle Perspective. Hamilton and Cross, Seattle, WA, 1994, p 41.
28. LeFevre, J, Hedricks, C, Church, RB, and McClintock, MK: Psychological and social behavior of couples over a menstrual cycle: "On-the-spot" sampling from everyday life. In Dan, A, and Lewis, L (eds): Menstrual Health in Women's Lives. University of Illinois Press, Chicago, 1992, p 75.
29. Hedges, JN, and Sekscenski, ES: Workers on late shifts in a changing economy. Monthly Labor Rev 102:14, 1979.
30. Gordon, NP, Cleary, PD, Parker, CE, and Czeisler, CA: The prevalence and health impact of shiftwork. Am J Public Health 76:1225, 1986.
31. Uehata, T, and Sasakawa, N: The fatigue and maternity disturbances of night work women. J Human Ergol 11(Suppl):465, 1982.
32. Axelsson, G, Rylander, R, and Molin, I: Outcome of pregnancy in relation to irregular and inconvenient work schedules. Br J Ind Med 46:393, 1989.
33. Hedricks, C: Effects of shift work on the menstrual cycle. Society for Menstrual Cycle Research, Seattle WA, June 6–8, 1991.

by Sheama Krishnagiri, PhD, OTR/L

19

Mate Selection as Occupation

Selection of another human being as a companion or partner in marriage is a universal human tendency. However, this process is carried out in many different ways, varying from culture to culture and between and within societies. In the human species, not everyone prefers all potential partners equally. The characteristics of the individuals play an important part in the selection process. Theories about the process, whether from evolutionary biology or from social psychology, tend to emphasize resource exchange as a basis for the series of activities that make up the occupation of mate selection. The chunks of activity comprising the mate selection process are assumed to be ones that will clarify the characteristics of the individual representing the desired resources. While evolutionary biological theories tend to explain the exchange in terms of reproductive opportunity and benefits, the social psychological models generally assume that cultural or personality characteristics will be determining factors in the pattern of exchange.[1] Thus, superficial observation of subcultures within American society might suggest mate selection activities ranging from traditional marriage processes arranged by families to premarital personality and sexual exploration by the couples themselves. When people migrate from one society to another, assimilation of young members into the dominant culture may produce, within one subculture, this range of activities within the mate selection process. This first large group of migrants from the subcontinent of India to the United States came in the late 1960s and early 1970s. They tended to be highly educated professionals in the fields of engineering, medicine, or academia.[2] Many of their children were born and raised in the United States and are attending colleges or working. They also are simultaneously engaged in the occupation of selecting a mate.

Most of the Indians in the last few years (the second wave) are, for the most part, relatives of early migrants, many of whom are not necessarily professionals. At the same time, increasingly larger groups of young adults also come to the United States for their graduate education. Most of these people, raised in India, are searching for a mate. One of the ways that an individual living in this country can ensure the retention of his or her culture and values is through the bond of marriage to another within his or her own culture.

In general, in the Indian culture, particularly those following the Hindu philosophy, the tendency and desire is to marry within one's own community. For many, this translates into marrying within one's own caste (grouping with respect to occupation in ancient times), socioeconomic status, and educational level. The offspring of first-generation immigrants, who have been raised in the United States, may reflect the Western focus on the individual over the family and want to select their mate from outside the community based on personal choice. Therein lies conflict between cultural family traditions and the young adult. Young adults who were raised in India, migrating here only recently, have been exposed to rapidly changing values in India with a leaning toward Western attitudes and mores, but they may be more inclined to have their parents arrange their marriage traditionally and marry within the community.

The purpose of this pilot study is to gain insight into the views of these two groups of young adults with regard to their choices in mate selection methods and characteristics desired in potential mates. This chapter begins with some of the research questions that arise with respect to heterosexual mate selection in the Indian subculture in the United States. Then it discusses some information about mate selection from the literature. Next, the setting and subjects are described. The method used in this study is presented. Finally, the results are presented with some conclusions and implications for occupational science.

Research Questions

The following questions are addressed:

1. What are the differences and similarities between the heterosexual mate selection process of people raised in India and those raised in America?
2. With regard to preferred characteristics of potential mates, what are the differences and similarities between the two groups in terms of community (caste), religion, nationality, social status, economic status, and education?
3. How much do parental, cultural, and social expectations influence the choice of a mate?

4. What factors do these groups consider important with respect to heterosexual mate selection, and how do they compare with those found in western literature?
5. Are there gender differences within or between the two groups?

Theories of Mate Selection

Darwin proposed sexual selection, or choice of the individual with which to mate, as a second process (after natural selection) causing evolutionary change. With this concept, he was able to account for findings that could not be explained by natural selection alone; that is, he was able to account for characteristics that had no survival value and that therefore seemed to elude the forces of natural selection.[3] The importance of sexual selection depends on the nature of the mating system. For example, if the sex ratio is 1:1, random selection or panmixia[4] will provide gene pool variation for natural selection in a species. If, however, the sex ratio deviates from 1:1, then sexual selection also becomes relevant. When mates of one sex are a scarce resource, characteristics favoring the selection of certain individuals over others as a sexual partner will have a primary effect on the gene pool variations available for natural selection. That is, those with favored characteristics will be more likely to be chosen as a partner or have a choice of partners and thus increase the likelihood of these characteristics affecting the gene pool.

All human mating systems deviate from panmixia, with sexual selection producing assortative mating in monogamous societies. Assortative mating is based on nonrandom sorting or sexual selection on the basis of certain characteristics. A wide range of characteristics show positive (homogamous) assortment (both members of the couple are similar), including race, religion, social status, age, cognitive ability, values, interests, attitudes, personality dispositions, drinking, smoking, physical attractiveness, and a host of other physical variables, such as height and weight.[5] According to Buss and Barnes,[6] the pervasiveness of homogamous (mating of like with like) or character-specific assortment is one of the most well-established replicable findings in the psychology and biology of human mating. These consensually desired mate characteristics are commonly sought but are in short supply. Most individuals attain an overall "market value" based on combinations of different degrees of different consensually preferred characteristics.

A second type of assortative mate selection found in humans is one in which different attributes may be highly valued by each gender. For example, if, given cultural values, women value earning power and men value physical beauty, then penurious men and unattractive women are selected less frequently than men who are homely and women who are poor.

More recent evolutionary theorists have suggested variation in the selectiveness of the genders based on differential parental investment. Kenrick et al.[7] propose that the degree of preference in a partner is associated with the level of anticipated investment in the relationship. Their study of the criteria used for choosing partners at different levels of involvement (a single date, sexual relations, steady dating, marriage), with 93 undergraduates as subjects, showed that women were generally more selective in their criteria than men, but there also was a significant interaction between gender and level of involvement. That is, as the involvement increased, the men became more selective.

A variety of social psychological theories have attempted to explain western societal methods of mate selection relative to assortative characteristics. Winch[8] proposed that while homogamous cultural variables (race, culture, religion, socioeconomic status, education, age) are important in choosing a mate at the screening level, the actual selection of spouse occurs on psychological grounds based on complementarity of needs.

Murstein[9] proposed the stimulus-value-role (SVR) theory, which suggests that at various stages of courtship, different activities evaluate different kinds of variables in developing relationships. The cues exchanged during the stimulus or initial stage do not depend on personal interaction but on the other's physical attractiveness, voice, dress, and reputation. In the value comparison stage, the focus is on information gathering by verbal interaction. The information concerns the partner's interests, attitudes, beliefs, and needs. The stage concerned with role compatibility involves not only intimate verbalizations, but getting to know how to interact with the partner and getting to know what roles the partner can play in satisfying one's own needs. This is the only theory that suggests types of activities or occupations that might be used for evaluation of assortative characteristics at the different stages.

Assortative Characteristics

Selected studies report on some consensually desired characteristics and some that are gender specific. Buss and Barnes'[6] study of 92 married couples between the ages of 18 and 40 and 50 male and 50 female undergraduates revealed that of 76 characteristics, the most valued homogamous characteristics in a mate include the following: good companion, considerate, honest, affectionate, dependable, intelligent, kind, understanding, interesting to talk to, and loyal (in decreasing order). In gender-specific results, women generally preferred mates who were considerate, honest, dependable, kind, understanding, fond of children, well liked by others, good earning capacity, ambitious, career-oriented, good family background, and tall. What men preferred in a mate included being physically attractive, good looking, a good cook, and frugal.

Buss[10] reports on cross-cultural gender differences in preference for characteristics of one's mate characteristic preferences. Thirty-seven samples from 33 countries with a total sample size of 10,047 showed the predicted differences in the characteristics of earning potential and ambition or industriousness. That is, in 36 of the 37 samples, women valued these characteristics more highly than men. In all of the samples, men preferred mates who were younger. This preference was borne out in checks of the actual age differences. All samples showed differences in preference for physical attractiveness in the predicted direction, with the men valuing it more.

Buss and Angleitner[11] conducted a study on mate selection preferences in Germany and the United States with large sample sizes of 1094 in Germany and 1450 in the United States. Again, women in both countries ranked good earning capacities higher than men, and men preferred to be older than the women in both cultures.

Siddiqu and Reeves[12] studied the mate selection practices of Indians in India and Indian nationals in the United States. As part of a more formal system of activities for mate selection, matrimonial advertisements may be placed in newspapers, indicating interest in potential partners with certain characteristics. The authors collected their data by performing a content analysis of a systematic random sample of 956 matrimonial advertisements appearing between 1974 and 1980 in four regional newspapers in India and 947 advertisements between the same years in *India Abroad*, a US publication. The results showed that family background, religion, caste, and the region of origin in India were more important for those in India than for those in the United States. They also found that occupation, personal income, language, and color were not significantly more important among one group than the other. Shared interests were more important for those in the United States, while mutual love was not a significant criterion for either group. However, those people advertising in the United States have not necessarily been raised in the United States and vice versa. Limitations of their study suggest the need for further study of this topic.

Methods

The methods used in this study include participant observations and intensive interviews. Participant observations were conducted at social gatherings, such as dinners and dances. Each of the observations was for 3 to 4 hours. Because the researcher is of the same ethnic heritage as the subjects, there was little difficulty in gaining information from them. The study included 11 interviews of approximately 1 to 1.5 hours each. Interviews were conducted mostly at the researcher's home and occasionally at the interviewee's home. Interviewees include four men raised in India, three men raised in America, two women raised in India, and 2 women raised in America.

The subjects came from university settings in Southern California. They were either friends or acquaintances of the researcher. The age of the subjects ranged from 19 to 28 years. All were students and spoke fluent English. None of the subjects were nor had ever been married. The interview roughly followed guidelines set forth in the interview guide (Appendix A). However, the questions varied according to the dynamics between the researcher and the subject, the nature of their previous acquaintance, and the mood of the subject. The data analysis was performed using Corbin and Strauss' methods of coding.[14]

Results

Methods of Mate Selection

The activities of mate selection range from formal traditional arranged matches to dating any person of interest. Some subjects reported participation in each form of the process, and several are participating in more than one form of mate selection. Finding a mate for marriage in traditional Indian culture involved a lengthy process. In general, when a woman came of marriageable age, her father would begin looking for a suitable bridegroom within their community, that is, someone who is within their own religion, caste, creed, and usually socioeconomic level and status. The reasoning behind this was to ensure that the woman had some common cultural bonds with the man and his family and would not find it difficult to adjust in her new home. When eligible men were found, meeting times would be set up in which the potential groom would visit the prospective bride to see if he would like to marry her. If a groom consented to the match and the groom's family could agree on the dowry (an endowment or gift the bride brings to the groom), an auspicious date would be set for the engagement and finally for the wedding. This procedure varies widely throughout India, depending on the traditions of the particular region of the country and of the particular community. As one of the subjects, a 23-year-old woman raised in India, stated, if she had not fallen in love here, she would have been subject to something similar and would have accepted it. In fact, she stated that, in her community, couples sometimes do not even meet until the day of their marriages and that the

> engagement is something [of] an agreement between the parents of the two sides so they are the ones that exchange salt and specify that "On such and such a day in front of the whole town I hereby declare that I will give my daughter in marriage to so and so." [She states that] usually you have to stipulate the dowry but nowadays you don't have to say it, they are supposed to exchange salt. The guy and the girl have nothing to do with it. If they are around, then they exchange rings.

The trend nowadays, at least in the modern cities and among educated and wealthier people, is to move away from such tradition and rituals but still keep the culture and values. For example, a family can find a mate who comes from the same background but not go through the rituals of the man coming to see the woman and then sending word whether he likes her or not. Ravi, a 24-year-old man raised in India, best illustrated this:

> Me and my parents have decided that I'm not going to visit girls and you know so that she knows that somebody is going to come and see her and have to set out a cup of tea and stuff and I go without letting her know and say I'd get back to you and then say I'm sorry. Yeah. I don't like that, I'm not going to do anything of that sort. Unless I'm very sure, me and my parents aren't going to indulge in any of these things.

Ravi also stated that he was very much against dowry, as are his parents. All of the subjects in this sample were against dowry and were very unlikely to indulge in the practice unless circumstances forced them into an arranged marriage through their parents.

The mate selection method many of the subjects found to be acceptable was the semiarranged method. In this method, subjects were introduced to prospective mates by their parents or friends. If prospective mates met the families' requirements and the subjects' personal requirements, then the two individuals would talk it through and decide whether or not they should get married. An example of this is a 22-year-old woman raised in America. This woman preferred the semiarranged method because she believed that people are not who they seem, so "if my parents introduced me to a person, and they knew who he was and I knew who he was, then maybe I could go out with this person knowing that my parents know that." Another example was Vinay, a 28-year-old man raised in America, who said he would be open to someone his parents found for him and introduced to him, but at the same time, his parents would be open to someone he found on his own and introduced to them. An example of a man raised in India who would be open to this form of arrangement was Ravi, who was willing to consider someone his parents would choose. However, even he believed that his parents would be open to someone he chose and brought home, as did Vijaya, a 25-year-old woman raised in India.

Unlike the above individuals, other male and female participants in this study who belonged to either the group raised in India or the group raised in the United States stated that they would like to find their mates on their own, giving varied reasons. Sarma, a 27-year-old man raised in India and living here for the past 5 or 6 years, stated that he does not even want to consider the semiarranged method, much less have his parents involved at all:

> First of all, if I were getting introduced by my parents, I don't think I will be introduced to anyone other than people from my own caste, subcaste, whatever. So that's completely ruled out, not even a possibility. I don't want such an option because I don't think that is very important to me personally. Since I'm keeping the whole thing open, I'm meeting new friends, I'm meeting friends through other friends, not a set up meeting for other reasons. If I like a person maybe I'd ask them out.

Another 28-year-old man raised in India, who has lived here for 6 years, stated he liked the idea of dating and getting to know the woman first and that he preferred to choose his mate on his own and not necessarily from his community. Jay, a 19-year-old man, stated that he would be open to being introduced to a woman of his parents' choice but that he would have to go out with her, but he does not prefer this because it limits his choice to only Indian women.

As seen in these three examples, many of the reasons for moving away from the traditional arranged style of mate selection seem to stem from the views held by the subjects about what is acceptable in a mate. They reportedly are open to people who don't belong to their race, religion, or community, and they are unwilling to limit themselves by tradition and culture. As one individual stated, "people are people." For example, Sarma, the 27-year-old man raised in India, stated:

> I would prefer to meet this person on my own rather than being fixed up with somebody. I would rather have the happiness of choosing this person on my own. And with that thing in mind, I'm not restricting myself to any particular person. That includes nationality, race, creed you know. As long as it's a she. That would have been eliminated if I had gone through something organized through my parents or whatever.

In fact, except for one individual, a 30-year-old man raised in India, everyone else stated that they would not mind people of another community or caste. Some of them preferred someone from the same region of the country. Rani, a 21-year-old woman raised in America, said,

> I am looking for most probably an Indian, I mean I would prefer an Indian who is probably brought up here like me, not necessarily born here, and who has the same ideas and habits that I've gained by growing up in America, versus some of the traditional old ways of India which I don't think I can be compatible with. And, it would be great if he were from the state of Maharashtra, speak the same language as my family and I do . . . what I know is that basically there are four castes and it's important for Indian families to keep marriages within the caste, which I can understand as far as like older times in India but I think now it is unrealistic. I think it's very unrealistic in the U.S. to try to get a marriage within the same caste, because first of all we are so dispersed and there aren't that many of us anyway the chance of getting [someone] within our caste is even less. I don't see a big differences in my Maharashtrian friends.

For example, Devi, a 22-year-old woman raised in America, stated:

> I don't think I would have a lot of things in common [with a non-Indian], it would just be temporary if we did have something in common. This is something I've real-

ized. I have a lot of non-Indian friends, there is always a wall between us. I don't understand some stuff about them and they don't understand some stuff about me in every which way. So I don't think it would be a good idea for a marriage that would last the rest of our life.

In summary, then, both Indians raised in India and those raised in America would not prefer an arranged marriage, although the two women raised in India felt that they would have accepted it if they were in India. The question, then, is how much of an influence does the environment have on the views of the individuals? The subjects raised in India said they feel that living here (in America) has had an effect, but that they would have had similar views even in India; however, they might not have been as strong. In other words, they might have succumbed to parental and societal pressures more easily if they were living in India. One individual noted that staying away so many years from his parents has made him a bit stronger in his views.

The subjects raised in America felt that because of their exposure to Indian culture at home and in the local community, they were willing to consider arranged or semiarranged marriage, but still wanted to know the person. Therefore, one can conclude that the environment, that is, living in a different culture, does have an effect on the preference for less traditional forms of mate selection and likelihood of participating in one.

Except for the one man, none of the subjects would consider only someone from their own community, although about half said that they would prefer someone who is an Indian national for the sake of a common cultural background. The data did not indicate a difference between the groups. In fact, there seemed to be more homogeneity between the groups than disparity with respect to nationality of mate, method of mate selection, and disregard for community and caste needs. The exception seemed to be when comparing the women in the two groups. The American-raised women more strongly seemed to prefer Indian men, whereas the women raised in India were more open to marriage to non-Indians as well. Perhaps the American-raised women were more aware of the realities of such a match and with more personal freedom, are reflecting actual choices, while the women raised in India are freer to consider such options while reality constrains its likelihood of occurrence.

Most of the people either wanted to find their mates on their own or were open to a semiarranged method of selection. They wanted a choice in the matter and had definite ideas of what characteristics they wanted and did not want in a mate. In 80% of the cases, the individuals were less constrained with respect to the prospective mates' community, religion, and nationality. The typical individual in either group preferred someone who was of Indian origin and of their own religion, but the individual's caste did not matter.

With respect to the economic background of the mate, most preferred those at or about the same level. Some individuals were worried that too much of a discrepancy in levels would create problems in social compatibility. For example, Rani stated,

I don't want someone who is dirt poor. Someone who has a job, who is going to be able to pay the bills along with me and will have a little left over to insure that we are comfortable, have a nice place to live. But I don't want someone who is too rich either, because of the Indian families I have seen here who have a lot of money. I see something lacking in their personal lives, I don't know what it is, I just think that they have, their priorities are just a little bit different than mine.

Jay, raised in America, said that he would prefer someone from his own economic strata because "somehow I think we are alike." He also thought that differences might affect the relationship "like mannerisms, you know, if it's something you couldn't get used to." The two groups did not differ significantly with respect to what they desired in their mate in terms of economic status. Social status of their prospective spouse was not stated to be of any importance.

The education of the prospective mate, or at least the intelligence of the mate, seemed to be an important part of these individuals' choice. All of the subjects were college educated, many in graduate school. Most of them also came from highly educated families. Every individual preferred a mate who had a college degree. All the women in the sample preferred someone who was intellectually compatible if not more intelligent than they were. Some men stated they wanted an intelligent individual although intellect should not be equated with a college degree. For example, Vinay, a 28-year-old man raised in America said,

> I don't think intelligence is measured by having a PhD in physics. It could be the person could be smart in other ways and they are happy doing what they are doing, that's a big important part and I don't need somebody with a PhD in chemistry and hates her job. I think I measure education much more differently than the conventional wisdom.

Most of the individuals did not care what field the mate would be in except that he or she be happy in it. Only a 30-year-old man raised in India wanted someone in the sciences to be able to understand and support him in his career.

In summary, members of both groups wanted a mate who was approximately at the same economic level as they were and someone who had at least one college degree. The women specifically wanted someone who would be at least intellectually compatible with them. Only a few of the men expressly stated that they would prefer someone who would be able to stimulate them intellectually.

The first thing that attracted men of either group to any particular woman was physical attributes, such as a pretty face and a nice body. For example, Banshi, a 20-year-old man raised in America states,

> The first thing that attracts me is the body. If I pass her and I turned around and nobody was around and that was good, then I'd slow down and I'd make sure she would remember me, that there is nobody on campus like me. And if I really liked her, by the way how she dresses and how she carries herself, whatever, you know, it will put a smile on her face and will make her remember me. So when she sees me again, she'll think, hey, this guy said this. That might be smooth talk to you, but it's me to me.

Most of the men stated that looks were the first thing that attracted them but that they would make their choice on personality and not just looks. Although the women also said that they would respond to looks, that was not on top of their list. Some women responded to education first and others to personality characteristics, such as wit, humor, or presence.

For men, the top five attributes preferred in a woman were physical attraction, open-mindedness, social compatibility, sensitivity (understanding and interest in the other person), and values. For example, Sarma, a 27-year-old man raised in India, stated that he wanted somebody compatible.

> Compatibility means, basically, being honest about your true feelings, how you feel about the other person, being open about the things that you like, the things that you

don't like, and being very optimistic about a relationship working out, not being always pessimistic or trying to find fault with the other person. That is, saying okay, I have my own weaknesses too, problems and weaknesses too, I think we can cope up with all these things.

The top five attributes that the women preferred in a man were intellectual compatibility, sense of humor, ambitiousness (aggressive), respect (manners, etiquette, not chauvinistic), and values.

Although several people stated that they would date, very few said that they have or definitely would engage in premarital sex or that it would enter into their decision in the choice of a mate. Less than half of either group said they would consider premarital sex or that it would influence their decision of mates. In both groups, the women consistently did not accept premarital sex or its influence. The question arises, how much do family cultural prohibitions affect the behaviors and attitudes of these women and men differently, or do the prohibitions differ by gender?

Given all the data on the different factors that affect mate choice and the manner in which the subjects responded in the interviews, for a majority of women, the family played a mild to strong influence on the choice of mate and for the men, a mild to no influence. Of course, age again confounds the results here as it does in many of the other areas. In general, women looked for intellectual compatibility and personality and men wanted physical attractiveness. Both found that values are important in the mate. The women tended to be more strongly influenced by parents and culture relative to the method of choosing the mate and premarital sex than did the men.

Conclusions

More similarities than differences were found among the two groups compared in this study. Both groups tended to prefer semiarranged methods or complete freedom of choice in mate selection. Both groups valued education and, in general, culture and religion to the extent that the majority wanted someone within the same religion and nationality. However, both tended to disregard caste as being an important factor in the choice of a mate. More of the locally raised Indians accepted dating than the Indians from India.

Differences were apparent between the sexes with respect to women desiring intellectual compatibility, being more strongly influenced by the parents and culture, indulging less in premarital sex, allowing sex less influence in mate choice, and looking for a sense of humor in the mate. The men definitely focused more on the physical attractiveness and then personality; they were less influence by family, although both extremes were found in the group. The men would, in general, allow sex to influence their decision of mate choice.

A few of the findings of this study were similar to Buss and Barnes' findings[6] of what men and women want in a mate. For instance, the idea that men would consider physical attractiveness highly important coincided with those findings. Also, the finding that women wanted ambitiousness in a mate occurs in both studies.

Mate selection is a complicated process that takes a long time and great effort in an individual's life. For the first generation of immigrants from a very traditional culture like India, adapting to the culture and keeping only certain values and rejecting others is a difficult process. In the process of choosing a mate, one may indicate how much tradition he or she wants to keep or throw out. This paper is a beginning to understanding the dynamics of what is involved in assimilating cultures and traditions and what is important in one major life occupation, the selection of a life partner.

Discussion Questions

1. Do you agree with Krishnagiri that mate selection is an occupation?
2. As suggested by Krishnagiri's paper, how might studies of occupation reveal the influence of culture on daily choices for action?

References

1. Kenrick, DT, and Trost, MR: A reproductive exchange model of heterosexual relationships: Putting proximate economics in ultimate perspective. In Kenrick, C (ed): Close Relationships. Sage, Newbury Park, CA, 1989, p 92.
2. Saran, P: The Asian Indian Experience in the United States. Schenkman Publishing Co., Inc., Cambridge, 1985.
3. Darwin, C: The Descent of Man and Selection in Relation to Sex. Murray, London, 1971.
4. Eckland, BK: Theories of mate selection. Eugenics Quar 15:71–84, 1968.
5. Buss, DM: Marital assortment for personality dispositions: Assessments with three difference data sources. Behav Genet 14:111–123, 1984.
6. Buss, DM, and Barnes ML: Preferences in human mate selection. J Pers Soc Psychol 50:599–570, 1986.
7. Kenrick, DT, Sadalla, EK, Groth, G, and Trost, MR: Evolution, traits, and the stages of human courtship: Qualifying the parental investment model. J Pers 58:97–116, 1990.
8. Winch, RF: Mate-selection: A Study of Complementary Needs. Harper & Brothers, Publishers, New York, 1958.
9. Murstein, BI: Who Will Marry Whom? Theories and Research in Marital Choice. Springer Publishing Co., New York, 1976.
10. Buss, DM: Sex differences in human mate preferences: Evolutionary hypotheses tested in 37 cultures. Behav Brain Sciences 12:1–49, 1989.
11. Buss, DM, and Angleitner, A: Mate selection preferences in Germany and the United States. Personal Indivi Dif 10:1269–1280, 1989.
12. Siddiqi, MU, and Reeves, EV: A comparative study of mate selection criteria among Indians in India and the United States. Internat J Compar Sociol 27:226–233, 1986.

by Wendy Wood, PhD, OTR

20

Biological Sex, Gender, and the Work of Nonhuman Primates

Two stories raise the central questions of this paper. I am personally acquainted with the first story, which took place within a psychiatric teaching hospital that was affiliated with a major medical school. In the 1970s, a large department of occupational therapy existed at this hospital that was composed of 20 to 30 therapists. For reasons that remain unclear, the department was abruptly disbanded by the hospital's administration. All occupational therapists were laid off, while music, drama, and art therapists were hired to take their places. It was not until the early 1980s that an occupational therapist was once again hired, partly in response to Medicare requirements.

Question #1: Why is it that occupational therapy, a predominantly female profession devoted to caregiving, has often failed to defend its professional turf against the encroachment of others?

Question #2: Could women phylogenetically be "locked into" a nurturing mode of behavior that renders them relatively ineffective, in contrast to men, in territorial defense?

The second question captured considerable media attention in California in 1993. It had to do with the decision of a tenured professor of neurosurgery at Stanford University's School of Medicine, Dr. Frances Conley, to resign from her position. Dr. Conley wrote in the *Los Angeles Times* that she submitted her resignation because:

> I was tired of being treated as less than an equal person. I was tired of being condescendingly called "hon" by my peers, of having honest differences of opinion put down as a manifestation of premenstrual syndrome, of having my ideas treated less seriously than those of the men with whom I work. I wanted my dignity back. . . . Those who now administer my work environment have never been able to accept me as a peer, not because I lack professional competence, but because I use a different bathroom. I lack the appropriate gender identification that permits full membership in the club.[1]

My next question concerns why Dr. Conley experienced a sexual division of work such that she, as a woman, could not be fully admitted to the male club of neurosurgeons.

Question #3: Was it because Dr. Conley chose to work in a territory that sociocultural forces have essentially limited to men only?

My fourth question summarizes the first three and is the central question that I am exploring in this paper.

Question #4: Does the sexual division of work among humans persist, in part, because of innate biological differences that women and men have phylogenetically inherited through millions of years of evolutionary engineering?

The purpose of this paper is to look at the sexual division of work among nonhuman primates to provide a perspective on the last question. Given that occupational scientists are concerned with the phylogenetic history of human occupation and in particular with why people pursue some occupations and not others,[2,3] this is an important question to investigate. A primary reason for using primate research for this investigation lies in the observation that nonhuman primates do not transmit gendered norms and values guiding who should do what kinds of work to one another.[4-6] In other words, whereas nonhuman primates have cultural traditions of tool use and even food preparation, only human primates explicitly, for example, shame women for being "unlady-like" or men for being "wimps." Nonhuman primates do, however, demonstrate a range of patterns with respect to the sexual division of work. Primatological research thus offers an important perspective concerning how biological sex alone does or does not influence division of work among the sexes when unconstrained by a sociocultural construction of gender.

Biological sex is genetically determined and refers to the different primary and secondary reproductive characteristics with which females and males are either born or that they develop at puberty.[7] Gender, in contrast, is socioculturally constructed and refers to the psychological, social, and cultural meanings associated with genetically determined sex differences between women and men.[8] Discussion of the work of nonhuman primates is delimited to two activities: care of offspring and territorial defense. These activities were chosen for discussion because they reflect the greatest variation in the sexual division of work across the primate order. They also reflect a highly polarized sexual division in American society as indicated by the observations that women still perform the bulk of child care,[9,10] while men, as witnessed in the Persian Gulf war, are the only sex currently allowed by United States law to engage in direct combat during territorial defense. Whereas the various species discussed herein do not provide an exhaustive overview of nonhuman primates with respect to these two activities, they do represent the most prevalent ways in which work is sexually divided among monkeys and apes.

Care of Offspring

Female involvement in care of offspring ranges from those females who only birth and nurse their infants to females who provide all vital offspring care for extended periods of time. In a parallel fashion, male involvement in the care of offspring ranges from males who are primary care providers of infants to males who tolerate infants but rarely interact with them.[11] There are many gradations between these extremes that, when taken together, represent points on a continuum rather than distinct patterns. For our purposes, however, three essential patterns of offspring care are briefly described.

Male Primates as Primary Care Providers to Infants

The species in which males are the primary providers of care to their offspring include marmosets, tamarins, owl monkeys, and titi monkeys. These are New World species of monkeys, that is, monkeys who live in South America. Significantly, all of these species are monogamous. Mothers' involvements with their infants is limited primarily to nursing, whereas monogamous New World fathers assume all parental duties, with the exception of nursing, soon after the infant's birth.[11,12] Fathers remain the primary care providers of their offspring until infants become capable of independent locomotion. After this developmental point, fathers and offspring continue friendly associations as noted by the frequency with which they travel, groom, sit, and rest together.[11]

Female Primates as Primary Care Providers to Offspring: Male Involvement Typically Affinitive

Gorillas represent species in which mothers primarily care for infants through provision of food, bodily contact and care, and protection against danger. Nonetheless, fathers often develop strong and lasting relationships with their offspring.[11] Infants frequently seek close proximity to a dominant silverback male and turn to him when they are distressed. Quite significantly, Dian Fossey, the occupational therapist turned primatologist, observed silverbacks who took over full mothering duties of orphans whose mothers had been killed.[11] These males not only held, comforted, and protected the infants from danger, they also carried them and allowed them into their sleeping nests at night.

Female Primates as the Only Care Providers to Offspring: Significant Male Involvement With Offspring Atypical

Chimpanzees are characteristic of species in which males may have only occasional, short-term affiliations with some infants. Mothers in these species are the only care providers of infants and usually develop enduring bonds with their offspring. Jane Goodall[5] has documented how important these bonds are to the development of later social competence in chimpanzees. However, Goodall's[13] research also has revealed that male chimpanzees, like male gorillas, sometimes adopt unrelated juveniles or younger siblings who have lost their mothers. Although such adoptions are rare, when they have occurred, males have carried their adopted orphans, shared food and nests with them, and sometimes maintained emotional bonds that persevere over years. In two instances, Goodall[13] credited male adoption with saving an orphan's life.

Territorial Defense

Not surprisingly nonhuman primates defend their territory for two main reasons: food and sex. Several patterns emerge among males and females with respect to which sex defends territories for which reason. Comparable to the sexual division of care of offspring, these patterns represent points on a continuum. Once again, however, for the purpose of facilitating discussion, three basic patterns are described.

Female and Male Primates Defend Territories for Food and Access to Mates

Among tamarins, marmosets, titi monkeys, and owl monkeys, that is, the monogamous New World monkeys previously discussed, both sexes cooperate to defend their territories against neighboring monogamous pairs. Territorial defense is accomplished through vocal duets followed by occasional fighting.[12,14–15] Generally, although there are exceptions, females aggressively fight females, while males aggressively fight males. Individuals thus actively limit the possibility of cuckoldry, or what we call adultery, on the part of the mate. Joint territorial defense simultaneously enables a monogamous pair to reinforce its boundaries and to ensure adequate nutritional resources for themselves and their offspring.

Female Primates Defend Territories for Food: Males Defend Territories for Access to Mates

Various species of macaques, baboons, langurs, and vervet monkeys demonstrate a pattern whereby females defend territories primarily for food and males defend territories primarily for access to mates. These are all Old World monkeys, that is, monkeys who live in Africa and Asia. All are characterized by male dispersal, meaning that when the male reaches maturity, he leaves his natal group to join another group where he will be able to find mates. Needless to say, when an immigrant male attempts to join a new group, the resident males are not particularly welcoming. Fighting often ensues and can be quite fierce. Conversely, females in these species stay in their natal groups and form very close and enduring ties with kin. Because many of these species live in relatively high population densities, fighting with neighboring groups in a competition for resources frequently occurs and much more commonly involves females than males. Females advantageously use their kin-based political alliances with one another in these encounters.[16]

Female Primates Do not Defend Territories at all: Males Defend Territories for Access to Mates

Female gorillas and chimpanzees typically do not defend territories at all, whereas males are often aggressively involved in defending their access to mates (Fig. 20–1).[16] It is not fully understood why neither sex in these species defends a territory for the purpose of protecting food resources. It has been hypothesized that because gorillas live in a veritable salad bowl, territorial defense of food is unnecessary. In contrast, the patchy distribution of food in time and space in the habitats in which chimpanzees live may preclude its effective defense.[5,17]

Males of these species are involved in fighting other males for access to breeding opportunities. A male gorilla needs to challenge the resident silverback male if he is to have a chance at propagating his genes. In contrast to the typical one-male groups of gorillas, chimpanzees have multimale social groups. Chimpanzee males thus often engage in intense hostility between neighboring communities of males. Goodall has used the term "war" to describe these intergroup battles that account for significant mortality rates among wild chimpanzees.[13,16] Young females are not attacked, so it is generally theorized that these hostilities ultimately relate to competition between males for mates.[16] However, a sterile female by the name of "Gigi" has been observed to join males in gang attacks of neighboring individuals.[13] The question is why.

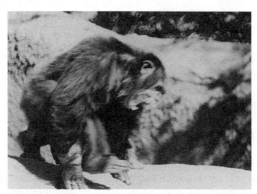

Figure 20–1. Male chimpanzee assuming an aggressive posture as he patrols his territory. (Photo by Paula Schoenwether.)

Implications for Occupational Science

What implications for occupational science might we derive from these snapshots of primate life? Only females are capable of bearing and nursing infants, and only males are capable of inseminating females. What is less obvious is that phylogenetic inheritance as a destiny for what kind of work each sex will perform largely appears to end at this juncture. The primate record instead suggests that the female capacity for gestation and lactation is an insufficient condition to have "hard wired" all primate females into nurturing types of mothering work. Similarly, the male capacity for insemination is an insufficient condition to have "hard wired" all primate males into the work of defending territories. Rather, interspecific variation across the primate order reveals that females of certain species are typically fierce warriors in territorial disputes, whereas males of certain species are typically attentive and highly capable primary care providers to offspring. Moreover, as illustrated by the choices that some gorillas and chimpanzees make that run counter to the typical division of work in their respective species, the work of nonhuman primates, perhaps particularly that of the higher primates, does not appear to be genetically determined in a rigid kind of way. The primate record suggests that the sexual division of work among humans is far more socioculturally constructed than it is phylogenetically determined. If so, the implications for occupational science are considerable. Rather than viewing our primate biological inheritance as mostly constraining the kinds of work that male and female humans have been phylogenetically predestined to pursue, this inheritance might more accurately be viewed as offering biological potentiality for behavioral flexibility and innovation. Such potential is obviously of enormous adaptive advantage to individuals as they construct and orchestrate, through their work, strategies for adapting to ever-changing environmental conditions. Thus, at the level of ultimate causation, which is concerned with the ways in which behavior influences the survival or success of individuals over evolutionary time,[18] our primate inheritance has provided us with the biological means for vitally important behavioral flexibility with respect to what work we do or do not choose to pursue.

However, this is not to deny that biology also may constrain the sexual division of work at a more proximal level of causation, that is, at the level of what underlies or prompts behavior at any specified moment. For example, the actions of Gigi, the sterile female who accompanies males on their war patrols raises questions concerning interactions between hormonal states and social contexts. Does Gigi defend the group's territory because, as a sterile female, she is hormonally more prone to do so than are fertile females? Is Gigi simply free to choose to travel with the males, whereas females with offspring are not due to the demands of motherhood? The example of Gigi thus raises further questions concerning relationships among her inherited biological potential for action as a representative of a sophisticated primate species and her immediate biological impetus for engagement in some kinds of work and not others.

It is beyond the scope of this paper to investigate these questions, but the larger point is that primate research can potentially contribute to occupational science by elucidating relevant phylogenetic, biological, social, ecological, and personal variables that influence specific occupations, such as work, across the primate order. For instance, social variables that have been identified by primatologists as influencing the work of nonhuman primates include population density, alliance formation with peers, and rank within the dominance hierarchy.[16] Ecological variables that influence the work of nonhuman primates include the respective constraints and plentifulness of one's habitat and the degree of control that one may have over defending that habitat.[19] Goodall's[5,13] work also has revealed how personal variables affect the life of an individual, for instance, how vagaries in ontogenetic development differentially influence competence as an adult or how key events in an individual's life history may affect the actions undertaken later in life. Primatological research points out not only the importance of these variables, but how they might play out within the context of the full diversity of occupational patterns of behavior that are phylogenetically accessible to humans. Therefore, if occupational scientists can cultivate a deep understanding of this diversity among our closest evolutionary relatives, we will gain great insight into the nature of ourselves as occupational beings.

Discussion Questions

1. How is (or is not) an understanding of humankind's primate heritage of value to occupational therapists and scientists?
2. What emerging views of biology are suggested by Zemke's (paper 15), Chamove's (paper 17), and Wood's papers?

References

1. Conley, FK: Why I am leaving Stanford: I wanted my dignity back; a brain surgeon gives up her teaching job in protest over a system that reinforces men's ideas that they are superior beings (column). *Los Angeles Times* 110:M1, June 9, 1991.
2. Clark, F, Parham, D, Carlson, M, Frank, G, Jackson, J, Pierce, D, Wolfe, R, and Zemke, R: Occupational science: Academic innovation in the service of occupational therapy's future. Am J Occup Ther 45:300, 1991.
3. Yerxa, E, Clark, F, Frank, G, Jackson, J, Parham, D, Pierce, D, Stein, C, and Zemke, R: An introduction to occupational science, a foundation for occupational therapy in the 21st century. Occup Ther Health Care 6:1–17, 1989.
4. Bonner, J: The Evolution of Culture in Animals. Princeton University Press, Princeton, NJ, 1980.
5. Goodall, J: The Chimpanzees of Gombe: Patterns of Behavior. The Belknap Press of Harvard University Press, Cambridge, MA, 1986.
6. Fouts, D: Signing interactions between mother and infant chimpanzees. In Heltne, P, and Marquardt, L (eds): Understanding Chimpanzees. Harvard University Press, Cambridge, MA, 1989, pp 242–251.
7. Fausto-Sterling, A: Myths of Gender. Basic Books, New York, 1985.
8. Williams, C: Gender Differences at Work: Women and Men in Nontraditional Occupations. University of California Press, Berkeley, CA, 1989.
9. Berk, R, and Berk, S: Labor and Leisure at Home: Content and Organization of Household Day. Sage Publications, Beverly Hills, 1979.
10. Robinson, J: How Americans Use Time: A Social-Psychological Analysis of Everyday Behavior. Praeger Publishers, New York, 1977.
11. Whiten, P: Infants and adult males. In Smuts, B, Cheney, D, Seyfarth, R, Wrangham, R, and Struhsaker, T (eds): Primate Societies. University of Chicago Press, Chicago, 1987, pp 343–357.
12. Hrdy, S: The Woman That Never Evolved. Harvard University Press, Cambridge, MA, 1981.

13. Goodall, J: Through a Window: My Thirty Years with the Chimpanzees of Gombe. Houghton Mifflin Co., Boston, 1986.
14. Leighton, D: Gibbons: Territoriality and monogamy. In Smuts, B, Cheney, D, Seyfarth, R, Wrangham, R, and Struhsaker, T (eds): Primate Societies. University of Chicago Press, Chicago, 1987, pp 135–145.
15. Robinson, J, Wright, P, and Kinzey, W: Monogamous cebids and their relatives: Intergroup calls and spacing. In Smuts, B, Cheney, D, Seyfarth, R, Wrangham, R, and Struhsaker, T (eds): Primate Societies. University of Chicago Press, Chicago, 1987, pp 44–58.
16. Cheney, D: Interactions and relationships between groups. In Smuts, B, Cheney, D, Seyfarth, R, Wrangham, R, and Struhsaker, T (eds): Primate Societies. University of Chicago Press, Chicago, 1987, pp 267–281.
17. Stewart, K, and Harcourt, A: Gorillas: Variation in female relationships. In Smuts, B, Cheney, D, Seyfarth, R, Wrangham, R, and Struhsaker, T (eds): Primate Societies. University of Chicago Press, Chicago, 1987, pp 343–357.

Co-occupations of Mothers and Children

We most frequently think of occupations in terms of the activity of one individual and its meaning to him or her. However, as social beings, much of our time is spent in occupations carried out in the presence of others. Much of this activity occurs through parallel occupations, in which participants are individually involved in their own occupation while others nearby are carrying out similar or related ones. Browsing shoppers, commuters, and assembly line workers are in parallel occupations.

At a deeper social level of involvement, shared occupations could be carried out individually but instead are enriched by give-and-take between people. Communities are built, physically and socially, from shared occupations, such as barn-raising, harvesting, quilting bees, and volunteer fire fighting.

The most deeply social occupations, by definition, are activities that can be considered co-occupations, which by their very nature, require more than one person's involvement. Of these, caregiving occupations are easily dismissed as active occupation on the part of the giver, while the other person involved is seen as a passive recipient of care. In the nature of occupation, the active agency of the participant is requisite; that is, both people must be seen as actors to define their activity as co-occupation. Thus, our view, as occupational scientists, of caregiving activities must explore, recognize, and celebrate the active agency of both participants. We must acknowledge and reframe the data available today that identify, even in the newborn infant-mother occupations of feeding, diapering, dressing, and playing, the elements of the nature of the human infant, which make them active agents in co-occupation with their primary caregiver.

In the first paper of this section, Zemke and Hunt present the results of a study of mother and infant co-occupation that compares the interaction of 4-month-old infants born full-term to that of infants prematurely born when both groups are at the same gestational age of 4 months after a normally expected birth date, that is,

56 weeks since conception. Supposedly universal mother-child games, such as "so big," "peek-a-boo," and "pat-a-cake" were observed in both groups but were less frequent and of significantly shorter duration in the premature infant-mother play. Field[1] has suggested that difficult temperament in high-risk infants may affect play patterns such as these, as a mother-infant pair adapts to the style of the infant. The developmental and maturational differences in these infants suggest the possibility of a developmental spectrum of play in which the complexity of the co-occupation increases with time, in which earlier, simpler forms provide a basis for later, more complex interactions.

Anne Dunlea notes that the primary co-occupations of mothers and infants involve visual contact and access to visual information, which is lacking in infants born blind. She suggests that if much of the interactive repertoire of mothers and infants is universal and essential to development, then infants born blind and their mothers will, through a process that might be considered co-adaptation, find alternative strategies for the basis of their interactions. She reports on a longitudinal study of the development of mother-infant interaction. This collaborative process requires a temporal synchronicity, a co-timing that is not solely under the mother's control but is built by infant and mother together out of their joint experiences. In the early weeks and months, visual responding is one part, but not necessarily an essential condition, for mother-child interaction. As Knox describes in her paper, other sensory systems, such as smell, touch, and sound, play a more vital role. The development of alternative interactive strategies seems to include combined use of vocalization and tactile or kinesthetic stimulation to produce smiles and laughter and maintain the turn-taking routines of social interaction. Similar to the games mothers and their sighted premature infants play (according to Hunt and Zemke), the game-like activities that were most successful with the infants who were blind were nursery rhymes that involved mutual vocalization. In contrast to this adaptation of familiar interactions, Dunlea points out that children who are blind demonstrate a lack of offering and showing objects, which is based on visual information. It would appear that for the infant without vision, action rather than vision provides the base for the development of interactive occupation.

In the second year, the children who were blind used only simple manipulation of objects for play, while children who were sighted began to develop a much more symbolic level of object play. However, the use of routine maternal language patterns as a possible route into pretend play is suggested as an alternative strategy for caregivers and therapists in support of the child's development.

It would be interesting to study infants who are blind who have been raised in other cultures, especially those where body contact is more constant, and mother's touch is a frequent and major form of interaction. Perhaps occupational scientists can explore further how actions can be used to promote developmental adaptation by providing alternatives to visual offering or showing and to encourage reaching and pointing. Is the intrinsic exploratory drive of the infant satisfied with manipulation activity and aural information from the environment?

Thus, the co-occupations of mothers and infants are seen not as universals to be imposed on every situation, but as opportunities for alternative strategies of co-adaptation for development, using the existing abilities of the infants rather than focusing on disabilities. Can therapists creatively assist mothers in using the tactile, action, and language-based routes into pretend play that have been described not as inadequate or abnormal, but as successful co-adaptation? Martin Krieger, a single-parent, primary caregiver to his infant approached his role (father? mother?) with all the social science information at his fingertips. He quickly saw that much of the science literature bore little resemblance to the reality that he was experiencing. Engagement in an enthralling, and at times, overwhelming, interaction with an infant caused him to rethink the focus of science, its jargon, and its traditional rules.

Perhaps we listen first because of the incongruity of this "Mommy" with a male voice, but his story is that of mother and infant, joined in an intimacy that defines both and draws us deep into a recognition of the genderless reality of that narrative. Traditional social science, he suggests, has attempted to abstract away the intimacies of the moment and by doing so, has lost reality from its knowledge base. Perhaps, to be useful to mothers in their co-occupational interaction with their infants, occupational scientists must learn to listen more carefully to the story of mothering and respect more highly the validity of the individual experience. As occupational therapists, we can learn, in the same way, to listen with respect to the experience of the parents of children in our care. Although we may have a resource of treatment knowledge, parents have a depth of knowledge of their lives as it is entwined with that of their child. They must make realistic decisions about the home programs developed and given to them by occupational therapists and the techniques recommended that they apply. As Bernheimer, Gallimore, and Weisner suggest,[2] strategies must be meaningful and sustainable to become part of the routine of family life and are most sustainable when they fit the family activity pattern. They can do that only when they become a part of the family's valued routine occupations.

Valerie O'Brien focuses on the social development of early childhood. She acknowledges that the basis of that development is simple infant-mother game-like interactions. Awareness of self and others arises from the developing mastery of social exchange. Through participation in the culture within the home and family, children learn the social meaning of their actions. This meaning is internalized through narrative and provides a basis for the further development of social skills. The importance of the child's daily activity patterns in the development of social competency is noted. She reminds us that as occupational therapists, we need to evaluate social competencies as much as motor or cognitive skills. This is best facilitated through home visits and visits to day care, classroom, or playground settings to observe children in the fullness of the sociocultural environment of their occupational routines.

References

1. Field, TM: Games parents play with normal and high-risk infants. Child Psychol Human Devel 10(1):41, 1981.
2. Bernheimer, LP, Gallimore, R, and Weisner, TS: Ecocultural theory as a context for the individual family service plan. J Early Intervention 14(3):219, 1990.

*by Doreen Fraits-Hunt, MA, OTR
and Ruth Zemke, PhD, OTR, FAOTA*

21

Games Mothers Play With Their Full-term and Pre-term Infants

Method

Data Analysis

Results

Discussion

Replication of Results

New Results

Game Choice

Relationship of Games and Development

Challenges in Mother-Infant Play

Conclusion

Game playing during early infant-parent interactions helps to lay a crucial foundation for normal, healthy development. Research has suggested that early interactions of pre-term and high-risk infants and their parents differ significantly when compared with parents with full-term infants.[1-3] The purpose of this study was to provide partial replication of a 1979 study by Field,[4] investigating game playing in samples of white, middle-class, full-term and premature infant-mother dyads; it described some of the supposedly universal games that comprise playful interactions between mothers and their babies. Additional purposes of this study were to determine if there were significant differences in game playing between this sample of full-term and premature infant-mother pairs and to provide descriptive data on previously unidentified games occurring during early mother-infant interactions.

An infant's temperament may have an effect on the mother-infant relationship and quality of interaction.[1] Infants born prematurely are more irritable and generally more "difficult" temperamentally than healthy full-term infants.[4-5] Mothers of pre-term infants and other sick infants rate their infants' behavior as somewhat difficult during the 1st year of life.[6-7] Moreover, parents of pre-term infants often have to work harder to "read" their infant's cues. This is because pre-term babies, due to their immaturity and high risk for sickness, do not show the same ability to enter into dialogue-like exchanges as full-term babies.[2]

Game playing during early infant-parent interactions provides a vital foundation of physical, sensory, cognitive, and social skills that is important for normal, healthy development.[8-9] In playful co-occupation with a caretaker, infants are supported and encouraged to process information from the environment about their location in time, space, and personal relationships. Piaget suggested that in the first 3 or 4 months of life, reflexes provided the means by which infants achieve sensorimotor interaction with the world.[10] Meltzoff[11] challenged the view that "primitive reflexes are the newborn's only way of 'knowing' the world." His research demonstrated that infants have innate capacities to recognize certain similarities between themselves and other humans, to act on abstract intermodal representations of things and people in the world, and to organize and control their behavior. A study by Meltzoff and Moore[12] of infants ranging from 12 to 21 days old showed that infants could imitate four different adult gestures: lip and tongue protrusion, mouth opening, and finger movement. Even newborns younger than 72 hours imitated adult mouth opening and tongue protrusion.[13]

Field et al.[14] reported that recognition of the mother by her newborn appears to occur within hours after birth and that pre-term and full-term infants are capable of discriminating between their mother's and a stranger's face. Field[15] also found that average looking times were generally shorter for pre-term infants than full-term, and fewer of the pre-term infants showed an initial preference for their mother's face or face and voice. She suggested that neonates who can discriminate the mother's face may elicit more nurturant behavior; that is, the infant's response to the mother encourages playful, interactive co-occupation, even within the limited common caregiving occupations, such as feeding and diapering.

There is increasing evidence that full-term and pre-term neonates can discriminate and imitate facial expressions, such as happy, sad, or surprised, shortly after birth.[16] These abilities provide one means by which mother-infant interactions are temporally synchronized. Thus, Brazelton and his colleagues'[8] study of 12 mother-infant pairs in the first 5 months of the infants' lives found a cyclical pattern of attention and action on the part of infant and mother.

In her study of 3-month-old infants, Field[17] found that when mothers of pre-term and post-term infants did not give their babies enough time to respond to them, the infants turned away from the interaction. When mothers gave infants more time to respond, infants looked at their mothers more and had more positive expressions on their faces.

Patterns of caregiving and play emerge between the infant and mother that are, at least in part, a response to the characteristics of the baby. A mother's sensitivity toward her infant and ability to read her infant's cues will accordingly affect the quality of their interaction. A sensitive mother will adapt her behaviors to encourage responsive interaction with her infant.[18]

Infant games are highly repetitive, with simple and stereotyped roles for the parent and child. Infant games provide and facilitate a positive affect, building trust between the infant and the parent. Greenberg[3] and Field[4] found that early interactions of high-risk or developmentally delayed, atypical infants and their mothers featured very few games. Field[4] suggested that difficulties experienced by premature infants affect the mothers' playfulness and result in significantly less interactive game playing between mothers and pre-term infants in contrast to mothers and full-term infants. Does this difference suggest that the kinds of interactions that occur between mothers and their pre-term infants are somehow deficient, or do they suggest simply a different form of interaction than might typically occur between mothers and their full-term infants?

Method

This two-sample study compared the interactions of full-term infant-mother dyads with those of premature infant-mother dyads. Each group was composed of 10 infant-mother pairs with five male and five female infants in each group. Mothers of the infants were married, white, middle-class high school graduates living in the Reno (Nevada) area.

Infants, both full-term and pre-term, participated in the study when they were 4 months beyond the normally expected birth date (40 weeks gestation). Thus, full-term infants were chronologically 4 months old (after full-term birth), while pre-term infants ranged in chronological age from 5 months to 7 months (after premature birth). Full-term infants had been born between 38 and 41 weeks gestation, weighing more than 2500 g. Premature infants were born between 26 and 36 weeks gestation with birth weights between 1000 and 1800 g.

Subjects in this study were similar to those in Field's[4] study in gestational age and birthweight, differing only in the length of time the premature infants spent in the intensive care nursery (Table 21-1). However, the mean intensive care time is affected by two subjects who spent 155 and 157 days, respectively, in intensive care. Without these two subjects, mean days in intensive care for the other eight premature infants would be 37.5 days, similar to that of Field's subjects.

Mothers were videotaped in their homes, playing with their infants for 10 minutes. The videotaping was scheduled for the infant's approximate feeding time so that the infants' behavioral state was likely to be similar and active. The baby was placed in its upright infant seat on the table, and the mother was seated opposite, facing the infant, about 18 inches away. The mothers were instructed to "play with your infant just as you would without using any toys."

Six games were previously identified by Field[4] in more than 50% of infant dyads studied: "tell me a story," "I'm gonna get you," "walking fingers," "so big," "pat-a-cake," and "peek-a-boo." Frequency and duration of these games were observed and measured. Other games that mothers and infants played were identified and measured. Interaction was considered a game when the mother moved a part

Table 21–1 Comparison of Premature and Full-term Infants Participating in Field's[4] and This Study

	Field	This Study
Full-term Infants		
Number participating	20	10
Mean gestational age (at birth)	40 wk	40 wk
Mean birth weight	3300 g	3376 g
Premature Infants		
Number participating	20	10
Mean gestational age (at birth)	32 wk	31 wk
Mean birth weight	1600 g	1583 g
Mean days in intensive care	32 d	61 d*

*Without two infants' extreme length of stay, the mean was 37.5 days.

of the infant's body or moved her body in some relationship to affect the infant and spoke words pertaining to the action in a high-pitched, playful voice.

Interrater reliability was established with a second researcher rating six of the 20 videotapes (three of pre-term pairs and three of full-term). Observations were considered reliable with an agreement of 88% for frequency and 84% agreement for duration across all games.

Data Analysis

Because the frequencies of game playing were discrete variables and were not normally distributed, a nonparametric test (chi-square) was used to test the presence of an association between groups (premature and full-term infants) and frequency of game playing. Because numerous cells would have a frequency of less than five, the "other" games that were identified were grouped together for analysis as a seventh game. The total and average durations of games approached normal distributions of continuous ratio level data; thus, parametric two-sample nondirectional t tests were used for analysis.

Results

Statistically significantly less game playing of the six universal games occurred in the preterm infant-mother dyads than in full-term pairs. Frequency of universal game playing was significantly associated with group (pre-term $M = 2.7$, full-term $M = 8.3$, $x^2_5 = 16.225$, $P < .01$). Using two-sampled, two-tailed t tests, total duration of universal game playing also was significantly less in the pre-term group ($M = 29.3$ seconds) than in full-term pairs ($M = 110$ seconds) across the six games ($t_{18} = 3.53$, $P < .005$). Average universal game duration also was significantly less in the pre-term pairs ($M = 5.9$ seconds) than in the full-term pairs ($M = 8.6$) ($t_{18} = 2.17$, $P = .05$).

When the other games were included in the calculation (combined as a seventh game to keep frequencies in each cell above 5), a significant association with group occurred again for game frequency (pre-term $M = 7.3$, full-term $M = 11.9$,

x^2_6 27.655, $P < .001$). Results of two-sample, one-tailed t tests found significant differences in total duration of all games played (pre-term $M = 88.9$ seconds, full-term $M = 177.7$ seconds, $t = 2.58$, $P < .05$) and in average duration (pre-term $M = 7.2$, full-term $M = 10.5$ seconds, $t_{18} = 2.28$, $P = .05$).

Among questions answered descriptively by the data were "How many mother-infant dyads played games?" and "How many games did they play?" All of the subjects in both groups played at least one game during the 10 minutes of videotaping. One hundred percent of the full-term group and 80% of the premature group played at least one of the six "universal" games. One playful dyad engaged in each of the six universal games at least once.

The total number of different games played was the same, 15, for both groups; however, the combination of universal and other games differed. The full-term group played all six universal and nine other games, while the pre-term group played five of the universal and 10 of the other games. The number of different games played by an infant-mother dyad ranged from one to nine, with a mean of 4.8 games for the full-term and 3.1 games for the pre-term group.

The next question answered descriptively by the data was "What games did the mothers and infants play?" Table 21-2 lists the percentage of each group that played the games observed by the researchers. Five of the six universal games were played by both groups, as were two of the other games. The rest of the games (16) were played only by a pair or pairs in one or the other group but not by members of both groups.

"I'm gonna get you" was the most popular with both groups, although more so with the full-term infant-mother pairs. "Tell me a story" and "so big" also were played by 70% of the full-term pairs but were played infrequently by the pre-term pairs (20% and 10%, respectively). Field[4] defined her term "universal" games based on participation by 50% or more of the subjects in her sample. For this sample, "walking fingers" and "peek-a-boo" would not have met the criterion for the full-term group, and none of the universal games would have reached criterion level of participation in the pre-term group.

Of the 17 other games observed in this study, only two were played by both groups. "Tickle" was played by 50% of the pairs in each group, second in popularity across groups only to the universal game "I'm gonna get you." The other game observed in both groups' play was "where's your nose—where's mommy's nose?" played by one pair in each group. Another game, "get your feet," met the 50% criterion for the pre-term group only. All of the other games were played by less than 50% of the pairs of one group and none of the other group.

Discussion

Replication of Results

Field[4] described six familiar infant-mother games and found differences in game playing between pre-term and full-term infant-mother pairs. This finding was supported by this study, with significant differences found in frequency and playing Field's six games, duration of game playing, and average game duration. These differences may reflect differences in the amount of mother-infant interaction between the two groups with possibly negative implications for the development of prematurely born infants. These differences, however, may reflect differences in

Table 21–2   Percent of Mother-Infant Pairs Observed Playing Each Game

Game	Full-term* (%)	Preterm† (%)
"Universal" Games		
1. Tell me a story	70	20
2. I'm gonna get you	70	40
3. Walking fingers	30	10
4. So big	70	0
5. Pat-a-cake	50	20
6. Peek-a-boo	30	20
"Other" Games		
1. Tickle	50	50
2. Running	30	0
3. This little piggy	20	0
4. Where's your nose—where's mommy's nose?	10	10
5. Slap me five	10	0
6. Do Indian	10	0
7. ABC song	10	0
8. Animal sounds	10	0
9. Can I see your teeth?	10	0
10. Get your feet	0	50
11. Blowing bubbles	0	30
12. Hands together-clapping	0	10
13. Riding a horse	0	10
14. Itsy bitsy spider	0	10
15. Stick your tongue out	0	10
16. What's that sound?	0	10
17. Where did it go?	0	10

*$n = 10$.
†$n = 10$.

the quality of the interaction of the pairs and as such, implications may be negative, but they also may be positive, reflecting a better match between infant abilities and maternal behavior (Fig. 21-1).

New Results

In addition to the six games described by Field,[4] 17 other games were observed during the videotaped 10 minutes of play. Play was classified as a game if the mother moved any part(s) of the infant's body or the mother's body in some relationship to affect the infant and words pertaining to the actions were spoken in a high-pitched, playful voice. When these games were considered in the statistical analysis, significant differences between groups were again present. However, the preterm infant-mother pairs played more of the other games than the games that had been described by Field, while the full-term infants played more of Field's supposedly universal games. One interpretation of these differences is that mothers are choosing games that match their infants' needs and desires. In other words,

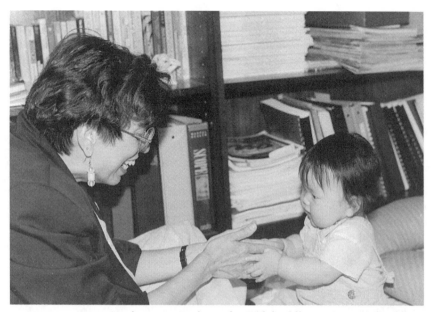

Figure 21–1. Occupational scientists need to understand the differences in mother–infant co-occupations. Here a mother is engaged in a game with her infant. (Photo by John Wolcott.)

mothers may be responding to cues from their babies by choosing optimally appropriate kinds of interactions. If so, then the mother's choice is being influenced, to a major degree, by her infant. Reviewing the games themselves and how subjects participate in them may assist us in understanding these transactions.

Game Choice

Field[4] found the most popular games were "tell me a story," "I'm gonna get you," and "pat-a-cake." The first two of these games also were among the most popular in this study, along with the game "tickle" from the "other" games. The popular games of "I'm gonna get you" and "tickle" are effective elicitors of smiles and laughter in infants younger than 4 months of age.[3] The mothers' selection of these games is probably reinforced by the full-term and preterm infants' frequent smiling, cooing, and laughing responses.

"I'm gonna get you" and "tickle" were popular games with both groups, but "tell me a story" was considerably less popular with mothers of pre-term infants. This game is often started when the infant coos and the parent treats the infant's vocalizations as words. The mother responds to the infant first by assuming the infant's role and "translating" the infant's cooing into a story and then by responding as the parent, acting as if the infant fully understands the words of the game.[19] The infant responds to the mother's vocalization, and the game continues. However, premature infants vocalize less than do full-term infants.[20] This game may therefore be initiated less and may be less satisfying as a synchronous activity in preterm infant-mother pairs.

"So big," while highly popular with full-term pairs, was not played at all by the mothers of pre-term infants. Perhaps awareness of the infant's small size makes this game less appealing psychologically, or stretching the infant's arms above the head is too bold a game to be played with babies whose extremities often appear frail. Similarly, the game "pat-a-cake" includes a variety of strong upper extremity movements that may not seem as appropriate to mothers of at-risk infants as it does to the mothers of full-term infants. "Peek-a-boo" was not played frequently by either group. Perhaps the appeal of this game comes later as the infants begin to struggle cognitively with issues of object permanence.

Except for the popular "tickle" (and one pair from each group who played "where's your nose—where's mommy's nose?"), the games in the "other" group were played by either full-term or pre-term pairs but not both. Because a large number of these games (11 of the 17 games) were played by only one subject pair, it is hard to draw general conclusions. However, many of the other games preferred by a preterm pair only, such as "get your feet," "hands together-clapping," and "stick your tongue out," involved simple movement of the infant's body rather than the more active involvement of complex games; in fact, some games played only by pre-term pairs, such as "get your feet," may be developmentally earlier versions of later games played only by full-term pairs, such as "running."

Relationship of Games and Development

The basic skills nurtured by these game-like, playful interactions have implications for later social and cognitive development. The games described provide socially and personally meaningful input to multiple sensory systems: the tactile sense in response to touch; the vestibular/proprioceptive response to movement; and the visual and auditory response to mother's face and voice. Meaningful multisensory play with an infant is critical for healthy physical, socioemotional, and cognitive development. Play provides an integrating mechanism, linking developmental progress of components.[21] Mother-infant games also provide and facilitate positive affect, building on basic trust between infant and parent. Successful play experiences are important to the maintenance and further development of the mother-infant relationship.

Challenges in Mother-Infant Play

Field,[4] using a temperament scale, found all of the pre-term infants in her study to be difficult, presenting additional challenges for mothers attempting to establish interactions. Although such a scale was not used in this study, mothers' comments indicated that the pre-term infants had poorer schedules for sleeping, eating, and alertness. It was more difficult for mothers' of the pre-term infants to predict a good time for the researcher to come to their homes to videotape. These mothers found it more difficult to set a time after the baby's nap and prior to a feeding. Additionally, three of the 10 pre-term pairs had to be rescheduled due to infant illness. Further, the psychosocial characteristics of the tiny, thin pre-term infant may psychologically affect the mother's desire to engage the child playfully. The concept of sickness permeates the early interactions, and the risk of error may seem great to these mothers. All of these factors might affect the mother-infant interaction. However, the result, although different from that of mother-infant co-occupational play with full-term infants, is not necessarily poorer. It may, instead, reflect the adaptation of the duo to the needs of the baby and may be a successful coadaptation.

Conclusion

Our data suggest that not only is there significantly less game playing and shorter duration of game playing in pre-term infant-mother pairs than in mothers with full-term infants, but there are qualitative differences in playful co-occupation as well. One could point to the physical and temperamental differences of pre-term infants as a causative factor in what could be considered poor co-occupation within the dyads. However, these authors suggest that it is a co-adaptation of game play in infants and mothers, in which the nature of the mother-infant play is guided successfully by the temperamental and developmental characteristics of the infant. Some of the games played by mothers with their pre-term infants appear to be forerunners to the universal games described previously. Further research is needed to determine whether the games seen in the pre-term infant-mother play gradually develop into these universal games and in contrast, whether the "other" games are seen in the co-occupations of full-term infants and their mothers.

Occupational scientists need to understand better qualitative differences in mother-infant play so that occupational therapists can have a stronger knowledge base for assisting parents in their daily occupations as mothers of at-risk infants. Further research, including longitudinal qualitative study of mother-infant games, may provide the needed knowledge and allow us to better assist mothers in the co-occupation of play with their infants.

Discussion Questions

1. How can the study be used to justify the therapeutic benefits of family-centered therapy?
2. What are the main insights that this study offers with respect to how the co-adaptation of mothers and infants influences the development of co-occupation?
3. What are the implications of this study for viewing pre-term infants as following a course of development in which they are primary agents of their own adaptation?

References

1. Crockenburg, SB, and Smith, P: Antecedents of mother-infant interaction and infant irritability in the first three months of life. Infant Behav and Dev 5:105–119.
2. Goldberg, S: Premature birth: Consequences for the parent-infant relationship. Am Sc 67:214, 1979.
3. Greenberg, NH: A comparison of infant-mother interactional behavior in infants with atypical behavior and normal infants. Except Infant 2:68, 1971.
4. Field, TM: Games parents play with normal and high-risk infants. Child Psych and Human Dev 10(1):41, 1979.
5. Schwartzberg, NS: Born too soon. Parents April:114, 1988.

6. Field, T, Hallock, N, Ting, G, Dempsey, J, Dabiri, C, and Shuman, H: A first year follow-up of high-risk infants: Forming a cumulative index. Child Dev 49:119, 1978.
7. Torgersen, AM, and Kringlen, E: Genetic aspects of temperamental differences in infants. J Am Acad Child Psych 17:433, 1978.
8. Brazelton, T, Tronick, E, Adamson, L, Als, H, and Wise, S: Early mother-infant reciprocity. Parent Infant Interaction. Ciba Foundation Symposium 33, Amsterdam, 1975.
9. Medvescek, C: Eight silly little games (and why they're so important). Parents June:92, 1987.
10. Flavell, JH: The Developmental Psychology of Jean Piaget. D. Van Nostrand Co., Inc., New Jersey, 1963.
11. Meltzoff, AN: The roots of social and cognitive development: Models of man's original nature. In Field, TM, and Fox, NA (eds): Social Perception in Infants. Ablex Publishing Corp, Norwood, NJ, 1985, p 2.
12. Meltzoff, AN, and Moore, MK: Newborn infants imitate adult facial gestures. Science 198:75, 1977.
13. Meltzoff, AN, and Moore, MK: Newborn infants imitate adult facial gestures. Child Dev 54:702, 1983.
14. Field, TM, Cohen, D, Garcia, R, and Greenberg, F: Mother-stranger face discrimination by the newborn. Infant Behav and Dev 7:19, 1984.
15. Field, TM: High risk infants "have less fun" during early interactions. Topics in Early Child Sp Ed 3:77, 1983.
16. Meltzoff, 1985.
17. Field, TM: Effects of early separation, interactive deficits and experimental manipulations on infant-mother face-to-face interaction. Child Dev 48:763, 1977.
18. Lozoff, B, Brittenham, GM, Trause, MA, Kennell, JH, and Klaus, MH: The mother-newborn relationship: Limits of adaptability. J Pediat 91(1):1, 1977.
19. Stern, D: The goal and structure of mother-infant play. J Am Acad Child Psych 13:402, 1974.
20. Crawford, W: Mother-infant interaction in premature and fullterm infants. Child Dev 53:957, 1982.
21. Holt, K: Movement and child development. Clinics in Developmental Medicine 55, JB Lippincott, Philadelphia, 1965.

by Anne Dunlea, PhD

22

An Opportunity for Co-adaptation: The Experience of Mothers and Their Infants Who Are Blind

Social Interactions and Co-occupation

Many of the principal occupations of mothers and infants center on the repertoire of social interactive routines that evolve within the mother-infant dyad. Indeed, the introduction of the human infant into the social world is based on the pattern of parent-infant interaction beginning in the neonatal period. The infant's first exposure to the world is largely composed of his or her mother's activities, especially her "infant-elicited behaviors."[1-3] These consist of exaggerated facial expressions accompanied by vocalization and mutual gazing. The infant has a strong propensity to observe and even imitate these facial expressions and engagement behaviors[4,5] with the result that they form the basis of episodic play interactions.[6] Recent experimental evidence[7] corroborates the suggestion from naturalistic observations that early interaction does not merely involve the caregiver tuning into the infant, but also requires the infant to engage, attend to, and react to its interactive partner.[8-10] The contemporary view of the infant increasingly emphasizes competence. Thus, these basic interactive routines constitute an important occupation in the daily lives of *both* parents and infants; they are in effect "co-occupations."

These rudimentary exchanges are structured along the same lines as the adult discourse system and are characterized by turn-taking episodes, a quality first observed by Bateson[11,12] and widely reported since. Such exchanges quickly develop into a communicative framework that increasingly encourages vocal interchanges, establishment of shared topics, the emergence of social routines, and eventually, verbal interactions. The infant's interactive competence increases through a growing ability to adhere to social and linguistic conventions and through the activation of cognitive, social, and motor mechanisms that support the development of interaction. Thus, during the second half of the first year, children typically exploit pointing and reaching gestures to establish reference or to request things.[13] They also use routines,[14,15] practice making sounds, and eventually begin to use language as the primary means of interaction.

Parents and infants thus collaborate to configure their time so that it includes frequent chunks of joint attention characterized by various sorts of interactive routines ranging from simple engagement to highly conventionalized games or verbal exchanges. The ramifications of this enterprise are presumably many and include a warmth of sharing, the introduction of the infant into the social routines of his or her culture, an exchange of information, and the strengthening of bonds between parent and child. They also are critical for the development of language and for providing opportunities for the infant to observe, explore, and imitate the behaviors and activities of others. In short, these co-occupations provide the stage for much of the infant's experience with the world.

Universal Behaviors and Their Developmental Significance: The Special Case of Children Who Are Blind

As is evident from two papers presented at Occupational Science Symposium II,[16,17] which are presented in this book, parent-infant routines have commonalities that span cultures and species. To at least some extent, there are universals in the co-occupations of mothers and infants, and at least some of these are shared by several species of primates. The observation that there are universals in mother-infant interactions does not necessarily mean that these are derived from some inherent or prewired system. Although it *could* mean that, it is also plausible that what is regarded as "universals of behavior" result from independent factors or from functional solutions to common problems. In the case of adults and infants, for example, the problems may be those of ensuring that an adult cares for a highly dependent offspring and of ensuring that the infant becomes equipped to participate appropriately in its social and physical universe.

Given the presence of apparent "universals of behavior," it is seductively easy in science to assume that what we observe as "normally occurring" is in fact developmentally necessary. This is especially true in developmental studies where the typical sequence of events is generally assumed to be the necessary one. Whenever something appears to be universally observed or species typical, it needs to be probed carefully. In particular, it is important to consider whether there are alternative routes that can lead to a similar end and to evaluate how plastic and adaptable the mechanisms are that prescribe the apparently universal occurrences.

In an effort to explore some of the potential for plasticity or flexibility in behavioral development, much of my recent research has focused on the interplay between language, social, and cognitive development in a special population of children: those who are born blind but who have no additional impairments. The rationale for this is that children who have no exposure to visual information will necessarily construct a somewhat different concept of the social and material world than their sighted peers. Moreover, they must rely on different strategies to gain access to that world.[18]

The primary co-occupations of mothers and infants, as previously outlined, crucially involve visual contact and access to visual information. The many social cues for engagement depend on mutual eye contact: Visual information is critical for activities involving smiling, imitating, pointing, gesturing, and most of the other behaviors in the interactive repertoire of mothers and infants. If this apparently universal repertoire is, in fact, an essential co-occupation of mothers and infants, then mother-blind child dyads will be compelled to find alternatives for these normally visually based strategies. Scholars are presented with the possibility to observe alternative strategies of co-adaptation between mothers and infants.

Several previous studies have considered various aspects of interaction between parent and a child who is blind and describe a decreased pattern of responsiveness on the part of the children. Fraiberg,[19] in particular, reported that infants who are blind are often "unresponsive" to their parent's bids for interaction and have a restricted range of facial expressions (Fig. 22-1). She suggested that smile and hand "language" substitute for "eye language." However, it is unclear from her reports whether these behaviors were actually directed toward others, or were even intentional interactive signals, or whether they were simply produced in response to stimulating sounds or caresses.

Rowland[20] focused specifically on three mother-infant pairs and used temporal contingencies to identify the maternal behaviors that most frequently elicited responsive behavior in the infant who was blind and infant behaviors that most strongly elicited maternal responses. Rowland analyzed films of interaction at 2-second intervals to code mother and infant behaviors and then used a fairly sophisticated statistical technique for her probabilistic analysis (Sackett's lagged conditional probability program).[21] Rowland's results indicated that infants between 11 and 18

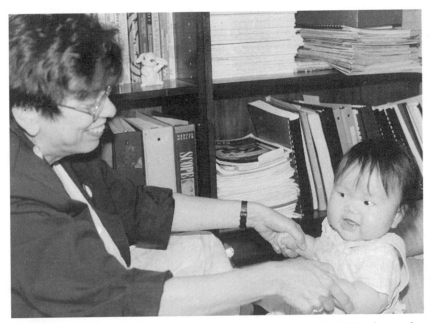

Figure 22–1. Infants with vision imitate the expressions of their mothers while infants without vision develop a restricted range of facial expressions. (Photo by John Wolcott.)

months who were blind affected their mother's behavior far more strongly and systematically than the mothers affected their infants' behavior. The mothers she studied were especially responsive to their infants' smiles and curiously, also were most likely to smile in response to their infant's vocalizations—a behavior that is imperceptible to the infant who cannot see it! One of Rowland's most striking findings was a lack of mutual responsiveness involving vocal behavior, which contrasted vividly with the conversational quality of interactions reported for dyads of a mother and an infant with vision. This stunning finding seems counterintuitive, because listening and responding to auditory information is the chief basis for the child who is blind to glean information about the environment beyond arm's length. However, Rowland proposed that her subjects, infants without vision, may have maintained silence to avoid cluttering the environment with their own vocalizations: An infant's silence when and after its mother vocalizes may, in fact, indicate attention and may be a "safe" response that keeps the auditory channel clear.

Overall, the picture portrayed by the Fraiberg and Rowland studies suggests that the parent-child dyads have difficulty in adapting to the constraints imposed by the child's congenital blindness. However, both researchers considered heterogeneous samples of children who were blind where other disabilities and prematurity were not factored out. Rowland's results, in particular, must be viewed with caution because all three of her subjects were severely developmentally delayed (although they had no concomitant sensory disabilities).

A more positive picture is presented by Urwin,[22,23] whose pioneering study of early language in two children who were blind found that nursery rhymes involving such gross motor routines as clapping or rocking were unusually frequent and that imitation, maintenance, and control of these rhymes provided an important means for parents to gain and maintain the attention of their infant. Urwin suggested that representational play and language were rooted in nursery routines for the children she studied. However, a consistent finding across research projects[18,19,22–26] also has been that there is a tendency for children who are blind to engage in a considerable amount of sound and motor play that is not directed toward others.

The present report is an opportunistic one in which data gathered for a longitudinal investigation of language and related development in children provided films and other records suitable for at least an anecdotal discussion of the co-occupations of mothers and infants who are blind. Thus, this chapter draws together some recent data and findings in a preliminary effort to examine this unusual opportunity for co-adaptation. In particular, I want to consider the kinds of activities observed in the mother-infant dyads with respect to two general issues. First, are there alternative routes to the visually based interaction strategies of mothers and infants that can lead to similar ends or serve similar needs in mother-infant dyads in which the infant is blind? Second, how plastic and adaptive are the mechanisms that prescribe seemingly universal observations about the nature of mother-infant co-occupations? These are rather ambitious questions, and at best, only a few rather global answers to them will be offered.

Method

The findings reported here are drawn from an extensive longitudinal study of communicative competence and related cognitive and social development in eight children representing a range of visual function. (For a broader perspective of the research, see Andersen, Dunlea, and Kekelis;[25,26] Dunlea;[18] Dunlea and Andersen;[27] Kekelis and Andersen[28]). As presented in Table 22-1, two children are totally blind from birth, three have severe relative blindness from birth but have some shadow or motion sense in a portion of one eye, and three children are fully sighted. The children who are blind have no additional impairments.

Table 22–1 Subjects and Their Level of Visual Functioning*

Subject†	Level of Visual Function‡
Teddy	Absolute blindness
Lisa	Blind, possible light sensation
Julie	Shadow perception for items within a few inches of inner periphery of one eye
Lydia	Shadow and some form perception, periphery of one eye
Ruth	Shadow and form perception
Bonnie	Fully sighted
Brett	Fully sighted
Nickie	Fully sighted

*Complete subject descriptions are available in Dunlea.[18]
†Names are pseudonyms.
‡All of the visually impaired subjects have absolute or relative blindness; that is, none of them has vision sufficient to measure by the familiar Snellen Scale of Visual Acuity.

All eight children come from intact (two-parent), monolingual, English-speaking families from middle and upper middle socioeconomic groups, and all score significantly above average on the Maxfield-Buchholz,[29] the Vineland Scale of Social Maturity,[30] and the Bayley Scales of Infant Development.[31] (Full details of subject characteristics and assessments are presented in Dunlea.[18]) The subjects were followed from the preverbal period, beginning between 5 and 11 months, through the preschool years. This report concerns only the period of infancy through 24 months.

Data are drawn from films and transcripts of audio and video recorded interactions between the subjects and their caregivers that occurred spontaneously during monthly home visits. These are supplemented by parental diaries and interviews. Home visits generally lasted more than 2 hours and included experimental and naturalistic probes; approximately 30 to 45 minutes of unrestricted interaction were recorded per visit. Information about the earliest periods is drawn exclusively from parent and physician interviews.

Description of the Developmental Co-occupations Between Mothers and Their Infants Who Are Blind

The First Months

The mutual orientation that is so strongly characteristic of early parent-infant interaction, one of the first co-occupations of parents and children, is inevitably disrupted by infant blindness. The intriguing question is when and how does this disruption manifest? Surprisingly, retrospective reports from the parents in our studies* indicate that the early weeks of mother-infant interaction progress in the usual way, especially when the visual deficit is not physically obvious. Among our subjects, only Julie, born with microthalmia, showed physical signs of visual impairment, but Julie does have some motion sense in one eye.

Why should the early weeks have appeared so "normal?" Abundant research indicates that young infants orient to smell and sound by turning their faces toward the stimulus source.[32,33] Thus, otherwise intact infants who are blind should quite reliably turn toward their parents as they attend to a variety of sensory cues. It seems to me that mothers may be seeking facial orientation as much as visual attention. This is especially feasible, given that infants attend to the periphery of objects, seeking points of contrast, rather than centering on objects in their visual field, and therefore do not necessarily lock into mutual gazing. Moreover, the parent must fine tune the face-to-face engagement with their motorically immature neonate. (See Atkinson and Braddick[34] and Bower[35] for detailed reviews of neonatal perception.) Perhaps the mothers richly interpreted their infant's orienting behavior, imposing the meaning "mutual visual engagement" when the infants, although blind, turned their faces toward their mothers.

---

*In this paper, use of the first person plural refers to the larger collaborative research project[18,24–27] from which the present data are drawn or refers to subjects shared in this larger project (hence, "our subjects"), and use of the first person refers to material unique to the study presented here or to work that is uniquely my own.

As Stern and Gibbon[36] and others have amply documented, mothers typically reward an infant's gaze with exaggerated facial expressions of greeting or mock surprise, thereby encouraging face-to-face engagement. During the early weeks, however, mothers have a back-up reward—they vocalize to elicit a response. At this age, the response is typically a flailing of limbs or smiling. The strongest evidence we have that vision is not crucial to mother-infant interaction during the first few months is that parents of the children who were blind did not suspect something was wrong for 3 to 6 months. (This is further corroborated in similar findings reported by Lairy and Harrison-Covello[37]). We consequently have no films of the first few months because children are not yet identified as blind. Thus, visual responding between parent and infant is one piece of the pattern of social coordination, but it is not an essential condition for caregiver responsiveness during the earliest weeks of an infant's life.

From 3 to 8 Months

Parents of infants who are blind begin to notice oddities during the 3- to 6-month period, which is precisely when an infant's interest in face-to-face interaction normally peaks.[38] Two particularly robust findings have been that engagement and disengagement are predictable on the basis of the infant's visual attention to its parent[2,3] and the infant's smile is a highly reliable response to interaction.[38] Infantile blindness means not only that this trigger for engagement is absent, but that its absence has significant consequences. Moreover, like Fraiberg,[19] this study found smiling to be a curiously unreliable response from infants who are blind. This implies that smiles are a signal for others at least as much as they are an indication of internal state and gives further credence to the view that the social aspect of smiling is primary.

Without visual attention to trigger engagement and smiling to sustain interaction, mother-infant dyads must find alternative means to coordinate activity. Several researchers, including Fraiberg,[39] have reported that infants who are blind may actually begin to avoid social encounters. This was not the case in the children I observed, but compensatory strategies on the part of the mothers, particularly extensive tickling and gross body stimulation, such as moving the infant's arms or legs, were clearly evidence of such avoidance. Both of these strategies were reported by Fraiberg.[39] This kind of stimulation regularly produced smiles, laughter, and vocalizations in the infants in this study and thus appeared to be the first adaptation to the infants' blindness that the mothers made.

Interestingly, the mothers' vocalizations alone did not elicit an adequate response from the infants to sustain the interaction. Like Rowland,[20] our video records clearly indicated that the infants reliably "stilled" when hearing their mothers speaking to them, but this clue indicating their interest or attention was missed or dismissed by all the mothers of the subjects who were blind. (This response was clearly evident throughout the children's first 2 years.) As a result, in lieu of the turn-taking routines of visual attention and vocalizing reported in mother-infant dyads and observed extensively in our subjects with vision, the mothers and their infants who were blind evolved routines that combined physical stimulation with vocalization.

This contrast may be quite strong. The videotapes from Teddy (who is absolutely blind) between 5 and 8 month of age indicated that if mother and infant were specifically involved with each other, that is, the mother was not simply vocalizing while attending to other tasks, the mother simultaneously touched Teddy and vocalized 79% of the time. In contrast, records of a mother-sighted infant dyad recorded at this same age range indicated that the mother incorporated physical contact into the interactions only 35% of the time. These findings must be regarded as highly tentative because data were not available for all subjects. They do, however, match my subjective impressions.

From 8 to 12 Months

The pattern of physical stimulation seems to lead to the discovery that nursery rhymes that incorporate body activities, such as clapping and rocking, are an extremely effective means of gaining and maintaining attention of an infant who is blind. This was first observed by Urwin[22,23] and strongly supported in the present study.

During the second half of the first year, mother-infant dyads in which the infant has vision typically engaged in the following co-occupations: shared involvement with independent objects (toys); vocalized conversations; gestures, especially pointing and reaching; games of offering and showing; and nursery rhymes, such as pat-a-cake. Mothers of the children who were blind attempted to engage their infants in all five of these activities but were mainly successful only with the last item, nursery rhymes. From as early as 7 months, each of the children who were blind vocalized to nursery routines and began to coordinate hand movements to accompany them. (Some of this information is based on parental interviews and retrospective reports from parents and the children's physicians.) These routines became the first vehicle, aside from fussing or crying, that empowered the infants to engage their mothers deliberately. They appeared to be the first unequivocally interactive behaviors produced by the those infants.

Thus, at 10 months, Julie was observed clapping and rolling her hands repetitively until her mother began singing pat-a-cake. Also at 10 months, Teddy was recorded moving his fingers mysteriously through the air, a signal his mother interpreted as a request to sing "the itsy bitsy spider." Notice that if one is not specifically attending to the infant's activities, these bids for interaction are missed. Perhaps as a consequence of this, by the time they were 12 months old, the infants who were blind began to vocalize a (very) rough approximation of the tune associated with a nursery rhyme and its accompanying hand gesture, thereby using a far more reliable method for them to garner attention.

The Second Year

While the exploitation of nursery rhymes points to an effective adaptation strategy evolved by mothers and their infants who are blind, other aspects of the usual interactive repertoire may show deviance or may not be observed at all. This is especially true of gesturing.

Offering and showing are seemingly ubiquitous rituals, at least in western cultures. Indeed, all of the mothers in our studies used these routines, but these were of little interest to the children who were blind. Lisa and Teddy, the two infants who were totally blind, were never observed to hold out an object to another person as a way of offering it. Further, they never displayed an object in any way to draw attention to it. Julie, who has a minute amount of sensation for movement in the periphery of one eye, did not offer or show objects, but did elicit attention by saying "this" while holding an object. Moreover, she fussed and manipulated the object if no one responded to her bid for attention. In contrast, both Lydia and Ruth, who have a small amount of shadow perception in one eye, offered objects if asked, that is, in response to utterances, such as "Can I see your truck?" and both extended their arms in an attempt to get an object returned to them.

The importance and universality of offering and showing as a shared act between parents and infants is evident in Goodall's research with chimpanzees. As she discussed in her keynote presentation at Occupational Science Symposium II[16] (see also paper 5), infant chimpanzees have been observed showing their mothers sticks and other items. In one more elaborate display of showing, Goodall described an infant chimpanzee who showed her mother termites that she had just retrieved on a stick.

It is not a trivial point that this kind of sharing through offering and showing items is missing in the repertoires of children who are blind. We can infer that this is an instance of cross-cultural and cross-species behavior. However, it is not in itself "prewired," or it would be in evidence with these children. Rather, offering and showing are effective strategies for sharing the immediate context and are probably induced by access to visual information and the coordination of *visual* attention. I would suggest that there is a biologically prescribed potential for these kinds of social gestures but that these rely on social needs and the coordination of perceptual and motor processes for their manifestation (see paper 5).

The gestures that have been most posited as universal because they have been observed throughout the world's cultures are pointing and reaching. Both are conspicuously absent in all of the subjects who were blind, including those with some residual visual sensation. During the second year, the children were certainly able to explore their immediate environment, and they regularly reached to grasp an object they encountered while moving about. (All of the children walked independently by this time.) However, none of the children were observed spontaneously extending their arm toward an object, even when sound clues informed the child of its existence. These kinds of gestural routines, both the offer/show and the point/reach activities, have been assumed to provide a vital link for interactions between mothers and older infants, a link that scaffolds development from gazing and vocalizing to interactive communication involving objects and events removed from the infant. Actions also seem to initiate the child who is blind into cooperative interactive occupations. The gestures of nursery routines appear to serve a similar function for children who are blind as the more prototypical gestures appear to serve children who can see. Both allow the child to engage others in a specific shared routine, to control the nature and duration of the routine, and to pace and terminate an interaction. It is possible then that communication founded in action enables the older infant to evolve into a competent social partner.

Thus far, the discussion of shared occupations has primarily focused on the infant, yet it also is important to consider how infants who are blind and their mothers share attention and activities relating to independent objects. One of the ways I examined this was by introducing a set of toys to each of the subjects at regular intervals during the longitudinal study. During infancy, these were presented at 12, 18, and 24 months. The set consisted of a doll and some doll props, such as a full-size baby bottle, and doll-size baby bottle, and a blanket; a variety of common household objects, such as cup, glass, spoon, and hairbrush; items for personal adornment, such as glasses and necklace; and a realistic telephone and toy cars, stuffed animals, and the like. (See Dunlea[40,41] for detailed discussion of object manipulation and play.)

Playing with objects is one of the hallmarks of early childhood and emerges during the second year of infancy. In play, the child builds knowledge and skills about how items can be used and through imitation, explores the culturally valued use of objects and the various roles of individuals. (See Bretherton,[42] Sutton-Smith,[43] and Yawkey and Pellegrini[44] for reviews of the functions of play in development.) Indeed, this kind of play activity is characteristics not just of human culture, but also of other primates (see paper 5). The ability to engage in activities with objects, other than simply manipulating them, requires the child to decenter, that is, to recognize and explore perspectives other than his or her own. Simply, the child observes how others use objects and imitates or pretends at these possibilities. Early on, mothers are a prime source for this kind of information with the consequence that play is a common co-occupation of mother-infant dyads during the baby's second year. The early interactions with objects of the subjects who were blind became the first clue in this study that the challenge to explore the properties and roles of people and objects would be an enormous one for them.

The following examples illustrate the enormous contrast in mother-infant interaction of the dyads with infants who were blind versus sighted. Example A involves Julie, who is blind but has some movement sensation in the periphery of one eye. Example B involves Brett, who is fully sighted, and his mother. Both children have just been given the opportunity to play with the toy box provided by the researcher.

A. Julie (blind, 22 months). Julie's mother picks up a stuffed animal and makes it dance up Julie's arm; Julie reaches for the toy and holds it, saying:

Julie	Mother
dai:i/*	
	What do you have?/
doggie/	
	Is it a puppy?/
puppy/	
	How's the puppy go?/
woof/	
	What do you do when the puppy barks?/
woof/	
	What do you say?/

---

*The first utterance is nonconforming and is therefore presented in the international phonetic alphabet; all other utterances are presented in standard orthography. Throughout the research project, children's utterances were initially transcribed phonetically and then analyzed for lexical and grammatic content so that both phonetic and interpreted representations are available in the data.

woof/

> What do we say to Goldie?/ (family dog)

woof/

> We say hush./Hush Goldie./

woof/

> Do we give Goldie cookies?/

woof/

> Shall we take puppy for a walk?/

walk/

Julie throws the stuffed animal aside. She then touches several other toys and names them, then walks away.

B. Brett (sighted, 23 months). Brett has a doll and a plastic camel. He is sitting on the floor, holding the doll.

Brett	**Mother**
	What's that?/
baby/	
(doll drops)	
fall down/baby/	
(puts camel next to doll, then pulls it away)	
no/my sheep/	
	Did the baby take your sheep?/
my sheep/	
	Are you sure it's a sheep?/
sheep/	
	Maybe it's something else./
huh?/	
	It's a camel./
my camel/	
(pauses, then picks up doll)	
go sleep now?/	
	Shall we put the baby to sleep?/
go sleep/	
bath?/	
	No/I don't think we need to give the baby a bath now./

In example B, the child with vision spontaneously begins to play with the toys. The complete script of this episode clearly indicates that he is first representing himself by the doll, re-enacting a scene from several days earlier in which he was fighting with a cousin for possession of a toy (this is the probable meaning of the "no/my sheep" scene). He then begins to enact the roles of a caregiver with a baby. (The scene continues with an elaboration of feeding, sleeping, and bathing in a delightfully illogical sequence that is rich in detail.) This contrasts rather vividly with the episode involving Julie, the infant who is blind. Notice first that the mother, rather than the child, initiates object play. In fact, Julie's mother goes to considerable effort to engage her. An overall theme seems to be that she is attempting to help Julie become aware of the symbolic relationship between a stuffed animal and a family pet, in effect instructing her in the possibilities for pretend play. She is working hard to draw Julie into a normally expected childhood occupation, adapting her contributions so that she leads rather than responds to her child's play.

Notice also that she doesn't talk about how dogs run and play, something that Julie would not readily apprehend; rather, she mentions familiar routines in which Julie could reasonably participate—hushing, walking, or feeding the dog.

Perhaps these seem like unfair or nonequivalent examples because Julie's persistent repetition of a few words (especially "woof") seems vastly less sophisticated than Brett's more varied utterances. The children's language as measured by vocabulary size, the expression of semantic roles, and illocutionary force is comparable. However, there are important linguistic differences that point to a relative lack of creativity in the children who are blind and a striking absence of decentration in language that parallel the impoverished object play scenes. (See Dunlea[18] for detailed analysis of these linguistic measures and Dunlea[40,41] for parallels between the development of language and play.) The striking difference in the two excerpts is largely related to the observations that while infants who can see and their mothers develop a repertoire of play schemes, children of comparable ages who are blind do not engage in any object activity spontaneously other than very elementary manipulation, and their mothers seem unable to elicit more sophisticated kinds of object play.

There is, however, one way in which children who are blind *may* begin to engage in play: they seem to recreate typical maternal language associated with familiar situations. Example C below is illustrative:

C. Teddy (blind, 21 months). Teddy is jumping in his crib after taking a nap:

jump/
jumping/
stop that jumping/

The language Teddy uses in example C reproduces what his mother typically says when she finds him jumping on the bed, "Stop that jumping." He also identifies his own activity ("jump/jumping"), evidencing a close relationship between producing an activity and encoding that activity verbally. Linguists regard utterances of this sort as language routines or language formulas. Such routines are reminiscent of the nursery rhymes that are so pervasive in the interactions of children who are blind because in both cases, chunks of routinized, or formulaic, language accompany physical activities. These pairings of language and action routines constitute a focus of occupation for the blind children.

My colleagues and I have argued elsewhere[26] that the repetition of language that is typical of other speakers by children who are blind contributes to certain language problems. For example, it seems to extend the period of time in which the blind children show pronominal confusion (e.g., using "you" to refer to oneself as in saying "pick you up" rather than "pick me up"). It also may contribute to a delay in their recognition that words are symbolic rather than isomorphic, that is, a word and its referent are distinct.[18] Nevertheless, I think such language routines provide a route into pretend play for mother-infant dyads when the infant is blind. By tuning into this language and participating with the child, mothers of infants who are blind have an opportunity to establish mutually satisfying routines that initiate the child into the culturally valued activities and roles of various individuals.

Conclusion

We return to the central questions posed in the introductory remarks: Are there alternative routes that can lead to similar ends in development? How plastic and adaptive are the mechanisms that prescribe apparently universal developmental occurrences in the co-occupations of mothers and infants?

Many of the crucial early signals that normally draw mother and infant together are absent when vision is not available to coordinate and facilitate interaction; infants who are born blind lack the means generally thought most effective in initiating contact with their mothers in nonstressful situations. Although they may fuss when distressed, they cannot gaze at their caregiver to attract and monitor attention. However, in the earliest weeks, the impact of this may be negligible, suggesting that vision is only one of several factors that induces mother-infant interaction. However, in the ensuing months, the mother-infant dyads with infants who are blind are confronted with a series of challenges that force co-adaptation. For example, the use of tactile stimulation in conjunction with vocalization emerges in place of the usual coordination of vocalization and eye gaze. This later leads to the discovery that nursery routines that incorporate formulaic physical actions are unusually interesting to infants who are blind. Through these, such infants are able to initiate and control interactions with their caregivers by substituting physical activities for visually based attention-getting devices. These nursery routines may parallel such physical gestures as pointing, reaching, offering, and showing, which are observed throughout the world's human cultures extending to nonhuman primates as well. This suggests that the use of conventionalized physical actions is an intermediate stage in coordinating interaction between infants and older interactional partners and is possibly a necessary scaffold for mature interactional competence. Finally, we see some suggestion that the use of imitation and pretend play with objects to transmit culturally valued roles and activities, again something that is apparent in chimpanzees and humans, may be an alternative route in conventionalized verbal routines.

The research my colleagues and I have been doing for the past several years has revealed numerous areas of linguistic, conceptual, and social development that are negatively impacted by congenital blindness. The initiation of the infant into the social world through adapting the usual repertoire of mother-infant co-occupations, however, need not be one of them. The presumed imperative to establish a mutually rewarding and binding pattern of interactive occupations between mother and infant seems to trigger a series of co-adaptions that enable mothers and their infants who are blind to discover alternative mechanisms for the visually based strategies that are so widely reported in the literature.

Acknowledgments

This research was supported by grants from the National Science Foundation and the Spencer Foundation.

Discussion Questions

1. What are the ways in which this research views disability, in this case, blindness, as an opportunity or impetus for developing adaptive strategies that, while different from those of children with sight, are nevertheless largely effective?

2. How does this study underscore occupational science's and therapy's view of human beings as agents?

References

1. Stern, DN: Mother and infant at play: Dyadic interaction involving facial, vocal, and gaze behavior. In Lewis, M, and Rosenblum, L (eds): The Effect of the Infant on Its Caregiver. Wiley & Sons, New York, 1974, p 187.
2. Stern, DN: The First Relationship: Infant and Mother. Harvard University Press, Cambridge, MA, 1977.
3. Stern, DN: The Interpersonal World of the Infant: A View from Psychoanalysis and Developmental Psychology. Basic Books, New York, 1985.
4. Meltzoff, AN, and Moore, MK: Imitation of facial and manual gestures by human neonates. Science 198:75, 1977.
5. Meltzoff, AN, and Moore, MK: Newborn infants imitate adult facial gestures. Child Dev 54:702, 1983.
6. Schaffer, HR: Studies in Mother-infant Interaction. Academic Press, New York, 1977.
7. Murray, L, and Trevarthan, C: The infant's role in mother-infant communication. J Child Lang 13:15, 1986.
8. Kaye, K: Toward the origin of dialogue. In Schaffer, HR (ed): Studies in Mother-infant Interaction. Academic Press, New York, 1977, p 89.
9. Trevarthan, C: Communication and cooperation in early infancy: A description of primary intersubjectivity. In Bullowa, M (ed): Before Speech: The Beginnings of Interpersonal Communication. Cambridge University Press, Cambridge, 1979, p 321.
10. Trevarthan, C: Sharing makes sense: Intersubjectivity and the making of an infant's meaning. In Steele, R, and Threadgold, T (eds): Language Topics: Essays in Honour of Michael Halliday, vol 1. John Benjamins, Philadelphia, 1987, p 177.
11. Bateson, MC: The interpersonal context of infant vocalization. Quar Report Res Lab Electr 100:170, 1971.
12. Bateson, MC: Mother-infant exchanges: The epigenesis of conversational interactions. Ann NY Acad Sci 263:101, 1975.
13. Bates, E, Camaioni, L, and Volterra, V: The acquisition of performatives prior to speech. Merrill-Palmer Quarterly 21:205, 1975.
14. Carter, A: Prespeech meaning relations: An outline of one infant's sensorimotor morpheme development. In Fletcher, P, and Garmen, M (eds): Language Acquisition. Cambridge University Press, Cambridge, 1979, p 93.
15. Peters, A: The Units of Language Acquisition. Cambridge University Press, Cambridge, 1983.
16. Goodall, J: The independent and interdependent occupations of chimpanzee infants and mothers. Keynote address, Occupational Science Symposium II, Los Angeles, CA, 1989.
17. Fraits-Hunt, D, and Zemke, R: Games mothers play. Paper presented at the Occupational Science Symposium II, Los Angeles, CA, 1989.
18. Dunlea, A: Vision and the Emergence of Meaning: Blind and Sighted Children's Earlier Language. Cambridge University Press, Cambridge, 1989.
19. Fraiberg, S: Insights from the Blind: Comparative Studies of Blind and Sighted Infants. Basic Books, New York, 1977.
20. Rowland, C: Patterns of interaction between three blind infants and their mothers. In Mills, A (ed): Language Acquisition and the Blind Child. Croom-Helm, London, 1983, p 114.

21. Sackett, GF: Lag sequential analysis as a data reduction technique in social interaction research. In Sawin, DB, Hawkins, RC, Walker, LO, and Penticuff, JH (eds): Exceptional Infant. Vol. 4: Psychosocial Risks in Infant-Environment Transactions. Brunner-Mazel, NY, 1980, p 300.

22. Urwin, C: The Development of Communication Between Blind Infants and Their Parents. Unpublished doctoral dissertation, Cambridge University, 1978.

23. Urwin, C: The development of communication between blind infants and their parents. In Lock, A (ed): Action, Gesture and Symbol: The Emergence of Language. Academic Press, London, 1979, p 79.

24. Wilson, B: The Emergence of Semantics of Tense and Aspect in the Language of a Visually Impaired Child. Unpublished doctoral dissertation, University of Hawaii, 1985.

25. Andersen, E, Dunlea, A, and Kekelis, L: Blind children's language: Resolving some differences. J Child Lang 11:645, 1984.

26. Andersen, E, Dunlea, A, and Kekelis, L: The impact of input: Language acquisition in the visually impaired. First Lang 13:23, 1993.

27. Dunlea, A, and Andersen, E. (1992). The emergence process: Conceptual and linguistic influences on morphological development. First Lang 12:95, 1992.

28. Kekelis, L, and Andersen, E: Family communication styles and language development. J Vis Impair Blind 78:54, 1984.

29. Maxfield, KE, and Buchholz, S: A Social Maturity Scale for Blind Preschool Children: A Guide to Its Use. American Foundation for the Blind, New York, n.d.

30. Vineland Scale of Social Maturity, rev ed. The Training School, Vineland NJ, 1979.

31. Bayley, N: Bayley Scales of Infant Development. Psychological Corporation, New York, 1969.

32. Muir, D, Abraham, W, Forbes, B, and Harris, L: The ontogenesis of an auditory localization response from birth through four months of age. Can J Psychol 33:320, 1979.

33. Rieser, J, Yonas, A, and Wikner, K: Radial localization of odours by human newborns. Child Dev 47:856, 1976.

34. Atkinson, J, and Braddick, O: Sensory and perceptual capacities of the neonate. In Stratton, P (ed): Psychobiology of the Newborn. John Wiley & Sons, Chichester, 1982, p 191.

35. Bower, TGR: Development in Infancy. Freeman, San Francisco, 1974.

36. Stern, DN, and Gibbon, J: Temporal expectancies of social behavior in mother-infant play. In Thoman, EB (ed): Origins of the Infant's Social Responsiveness. Erlbaum, Hillsdale, NJ, 1979.

37. Lairy, GC, and Harrison-Covello, A: The blind child and his parents: Congenital visual defect and the repercussion of family attitudes on the early development of the child. Reprinted as the American Foundation for the Blind, Research Bulletin 25, 1973.

38. Bullowa, M: Before Speech: The Beginning of Interpersonal Communication. Cambridge University Press, Cambridge, 1979.

39. Fraiberg, S: Blind infants and their mothers: An examination of the sign system. In Lewis, M, and Rosenbaum, A (eds): The Effects of the Infant on Its Caregiver. Wiley & Sons, New York, 1977, p 215.

40. Dunlea, A: Parallels in the development of object play and lexical semantics: Evidence from blind and sighted children. Paper presented at the Biennial Meeting of the Society for Research in Child Development, Seattle, WA, 1991.

41. Dunlea, A. Parallels between lexical development, object exploration behavior, and representational play, Forthcoming.

42. Bretherton, I: Symbolic Play. Academic Press, New York, 1984.

43. Sutton-Smith, B: Play and Learning. Gardner Press, New York, 1979.

44. Yawkey, TD, and Pellegrini, AD: Child's Play: Developmental and Applied. Erlbaum, Hillsdale, NJ, 1984.

by Martin H. Krieger, PhD

23

A Phenomenology of Motherhood

If social science has developed under the influence of a managerial and hermeneutic ethos, it now might take seriously the experience of mothers—those who bear a primary responsibility for their children—in formulating its models and concepts. I want to draw some lessons from a descriptive phenomenology of my work of being a mother (as a single-parent father), lessons for the practice of theorizing about society and human nature.

As Winnicott[1] points out, your baby knows what he or she wants, what is good for him or her, and how to train you to be a good mother. You are seduced into being a good mother; and if you are failing, baby will take you to task and further train you. Correspondingly, you know your baby; you give meaning to what he or she does, and how you respond constitutes what he or she is up to. You know your baby intimately. Your baby's needs are not expressed as demands but as necessities that define who you both are. If you try to avoid that intimate knowledge, there will be disaster, that is, a moral failure to acknowledge a relationship both of you are given the moment you are together the first time.[2] This is not all about a mechanism such as bonding, but rather about a situation that demands our response if we are to define ourselves as human beings.

Most mothers recognize the truth in the previous paragraph, but in the matter of course, the description denies the usual social science categories of demand, choice, and knowledge as decoding. Necessity, devotion, and intimate knowledge are fundamental to the experience of mothers. For a conventional social science, it is always assumed that the intimacies of the moment can be abstracted away, which then becomes the moment of disaster in bringing up your baby.

Whatever else mothers are doing with their crying babies, they are not "solving" problems. Advice about how to solve child-care problems is useful before one has a baby, because it calms anxiety. Later on, however, advice mostly induces guilt, unless it is of the sort that recommends trying something else (without claiming much for that option other than it is the next one). The real value of advice, in any case, is that it provides a line of action that then can be abandoned for another. You discover that nothing matters and everything does. In other words, either nothing will work, or just about anything will make a difference when your baby is hysterical. The situation feels both decentered and at the same time robust and overdetermined. If the last thing you do works and focuses your child and brings him or her out of hysteria, that last thing won't work as the first thing next time. History matters here: The history of failed attempts and successful comfortings sets the stage for what finally does work. In your best moments you know that it will not go on forever. Whether diaper rash, loose bowels, or crying occurs, there will be a resolution, but doing nothing, a null hypothesis, is not morally acceptable. Situations of motherhood are not only complex, they are so overdetermined that the attempt to isolate factors or causes is likely to make action seem either hopeless or arbitrary.

Mothers know that gender matters enormously. At least, you do not know how to treat a baby who is without a gender. This is not a matter of gender stereotyping, but rather that people come with genders no matter how problematic they are for getting to know those people.

Your major task as a mother is to bring your infant into the world so that he or she can be a member. Your child becomes disciplined, fitting into your life. He or she comes to recognize your authority through the joys of participating in a much larger life than when he or she is first born.[3] Through this acquired discipline, your infant learns to be effective and have his or her own authority. Incentives rarely work in these circumstances because what is desired by both mother and child is membership, not compliance.

The constitution of society is here a matter of authority and membership, in contrast to the economic viewpoint of incentives and markets.[4] Your life with your baby is perhaps highly scheduled and predictable but not at all managerial and bureaucratic. It is all of a piece and not at all modular and interchangeable. The flexibility you surely have with your child, and he or she with you, is a matter of constant conversation rather than negotiation and bargaining.

According to Winnicott,[1] the good-enough mother is devoted to the child. Diapering-time counts at least as much as any other times. "Quality time" makes no sense when mothering means to be fully present to your child. We are unavoidably bound up in "everydayness." Mommy-and-me class is a luxury. What really counts is mommy and me (Fig. 23-1).

The usual story of time in social science is about a commensurable linear unit, but mother-infant time is defined by necessity and emergency and development.

In such a context, time does not come in nice units to be allocated and used efficiently. Rather, there is never much breathing room, there is always more to do, and what counts in the end is the responsiveness the mother exhibits. Necessity gets you through what you must do, so you discover what does not have to be done. (Cole and Zuckerman[5] show how scientists who become mothers do not show it in their scientific productivity; other formerly necessary tasks get dropped.) Moreover, emergencies and overloads are not statistical fluctuations, subject to queuing theory regimens. The events here are not at all independent or mildly correlated variables. The world falls apart totally and together. Emergencies and overloads are occasions for extraordinary and heroic effort.

Developmental time is not at all linear. Development comes in stages (because a large number of subtasks need to be potentiated for a single task, such as

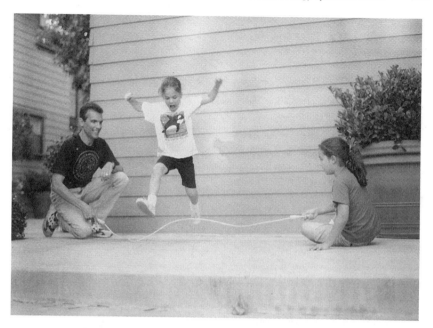

Figure 23–1. This single father takes delight in the accomplishments of his daughter as he assumes "mothering" responsibilities. (Photo by John Wolcott.)

walking, to take place). Stages of development are real, and markers of development are socially transformational. When your baby walks, he or she becomes a new kind of person within the family.

Motherhood is the existential truth of the present, a matter of concreteness and immediacy. Moreover, every mother is a single mother, or so most mothers report of their experience. The trick, as the airline emergency procedures tell us, is to "put on your oxygen mask first," and then you can take care of your baby. Be there in the present (rather than "losing it"), and if you can, "stay on the same side as your baby."[6] Babies, even your own, are not always so interesting, and sometimes they are downright boring, but it has to be done, and what counts is doing it, whatever it is that needs to be done. No wonder there is a romanticizing of motherhood, when the appropriate response, in retrospect, is perhaps one of anger, ambivalence, devotion, and wonder. The murderous feelings you sometimes have toward your beloved children when they insist on themselves *just* when you have a moment to yourself and the ambivalence you feel when you avoid their need to have that moment alone versus when you meet their need but ignore your own—these are on what motherhood insists and for which social science finds it difficult to account.[7,8] That is why the operative categories must be ones of necessity, need, devotion, intimate unavoidable knowledge, emergency, and individual experience. Someone has to bring up the children, and, it seems, it has to be mothers.

Discussion Questions

1. Both Krieger and Seward Johnson emphasize being in the moment. In what ways does or does not being in the moment reinforce occupational scientists' contention that to engage in occupation is to seize control?
2. How might Krieger's operative categories of motherhood (necessity, needs, devotion, intimate unavoidable knowledge, emergency, and individual experience) be applied to other occupations?

References

1. Winnicott, D: The Child, the Family, and the Outside World. Penguin Books, Baltimore, MD, 1964.
2. Cavell, S: The avoidance of love: A reading of *King Lear*. Reprinted in Disowning Knowledge. Cambridge University Press, Cambridge, 1987.
3. Hearne, V: Adam's Task. Knopf, New York, 1986.
4. Buchanan, J: The constitution of economic policy. Science 236:1433, 1987.
5. Cole, J, and Zuckerman, H: Marriage, motherhood and research performance in science. Sci Am 256:119, 1987.
6. Leach, P: Your Baby and Child. Knopf, New York, 1979.
7. Ignatieff, M: The Needs of Strangers. Viking, New York, 1985.
8. Rich, A: Of Woman Born: Motherhood as Experience and Institution. Norton, New York, 1986.

by Valerie O'Brien, MS, OTR

24

Early Childhood: The Social Domain

Social Interaction: Theorists Revisited

Who Influences the Child in the Early Years?

Implications for Occupational Therapy

Many occupational therapists are keenly interested in the development of children. Traditionally, we evaluate motor skills, sensory-integrative abilities, visual-perceptual skills, or reflexive development and base our treatment goals on standardized assessment results. While we characterize the child's behavior during evaluation and treatment sessions, the child's interactive skills and social maneuverability may be most important for a child's perceived success within the treatment session, in the home,[1] and within the classroom.[2] As we evaluate a child's performance, it would greatly enrich our knowledge to examine the child's daily interactions including the who, what, where, how long, and the quality of interaction, that is, whether or not it is successful, unresponsive, or directive. This paper accordingly explores the theoretical development of early childhood social interactions and the importance of examining children's social maneuverability to gain a richer insight into their competence.

Social Interaction: Theorists Revisited

Children are social beings and are born within a social group. No surviving child has been without a social context throughout human history.[3] Born with a specific genotype, with human predisposing tendencies to learn about sounds and images in a symbolic sense,[4,5] children grow and develop within the context of the family, neighborhood, and community, which are influenced by county, state, and country values.

Mother-infant dyads are clearly noted as the earliest sources of social interaction. Eibl-Eibesfeldt[6] described individual bonding from an evolutionary perspective with a parent, especially mother, and child actively seeking proximity and reciprocity. Occurring in birds and mammals, individualized bonding, or parental care, could be conceived as the impetus for developing higher and more differentiated social systems. Bowlby[7] and Ainsworth[8] are renowned for providing ample literature into the study of mother-infant attachment and the impact that appropriate bonding may have on future development. Research has generally revealed the significance of the initial attachment as it affects future behavior, in positive and negative contexts.[9,10]

The early cues to sociability and appropriate learning of rules is evident in infancy. Bruner and Sherwood explored the acquisition of the "rules of the game" of peekaboo in infants from 7 to 17 months old.[11] They noted that within the interaction, there "rapidly develops a set of reciprocal anticipations in mother and child that begin to modify it and, more importantly, to conventionalize it."[12] The child knows the rules of the game and acts as initiator and agent as he or she matures. However, if the rules provided by the mother are initially too varied and prematurely cued, the game does not develop. Interaction ceases to occur in the playful manipulation. Understanding and social meaning are a reciprocal process, and if miscalculation or miscuing are evident, then meaning may be lost or misconstrued and interaction stymied.

This is further supported in a study by Harris and associates of language development in children younger than 24 months.[1] When mothers failed to provide appropriate nonverbal context, language development was slower. Additionally, failure to cue the child's attention and lack of appropriate object references also related to slower language development. A young child's environment affects his or her level of social understanding and expression.

The very young child is able to produce and respond to social interactive cues, but it is not until the child is able to interpret symbolically these cues that we may understand his or her perception. Jean Piaget's theory of intellectual development notes that a child begins a stage of representational thinking within the second year and attempts symbolic and preconceptual development through environmental interaction up until the fourth year.[13] Once the child becomes somewhat adept at symbolic expression and interpretation, an intuitive phase can develop from about 4 to 7 years. At this level, the child enters an area of self-perception through intuitive thought.

While Piaget[14] did not explicitly delineate social intelligence, he did underscore that a child develops cognitively only through interaction with the external environment. Piaget characterized the young child between 2 and 4 years as especially egocentric in his or her concept of the world.[13] He or she progresses into a stage of somewhat diminished egocentricism based on a maturation of cognitive abilities and notes that all children follow a specific, sequential course to formal logical thought. Piaget, however, leaves one only to infer the importance of social interaction to intellectual development and diminished egocentrism.

Dunn explores the appreciation of self and others when she links self-awareness to awareness of others and to emotional experience.[4] She suggests that the developmental psychologist's view of self-awareness (i.e., self-awareness parallels an increase in the awareness of others) and the sociologist's view of self-awareness based on Mead (i.e., the self is seen as the product of the individual's social exchange with others) should be combined to elicit the sense of self arising from a cognitive and cultural inception. She arrived at this after examining young children in varied cultures and noting, "A sense of self-efficacy comes from managing a particular cultural world; all gain pleasure from their own mastery of the difficulties—social and psychological—that face them, and their own powers within that world."[15] In Dunn's view then, social interaction is pivotal in a child's sense of self-awareness.

Dunn further explores the emotional component to the development of self-awareness. Rather than reiterating the support for the role of cognition in emotional development, that is, change in emotional development depends on cognitive change or growth, she explores the possibility that emotional experiences themselves may contribute to cognitive change. Based largely on observation of children in discord with mother and siblings, growth in understanding seemed highly linked with instances that involve expression or experience of intense emotions.[4] Dunn also described a study by Arsenio and Ford that demonstrated that the emotion experienced by first and third grade children in response to particular events was highly related to their memory, coding, and differentiation of those events. She further postulated that "situations of conflict and threatened self-interest are encounters in which the child's growing understanding of the social world is not only revealed but fostered."[16]

Bruner has explored the understanding of the sociocultural development of the child through the narrative.[5] Based on his extensive history and research into language acquisition, he postulated that as the child becomes more symbolically adept, internalization of the "system of signs"[17] allows that child to be able to interpret his or her world. Bruner theorized that there "are certain classes of meaning to which human beings are innately tuned and for which they actively search."[18] Through participation within the culture, we thereby learn the significance and meaning of our actions that become internalized through the use of narrative. The importance of interaction and interpretation is accordingly pivotal in the child's development.

Bruner was influenced by Vygotsky's theory that stressed the necessity of appropriate social interaction to push cognitive development.[19] Unlike Piaget, who realized the necessity of environmental interaction, according to Wertsch,[20] Vygotsky stressed that internalization is a "process wherein an internal plane of consciousness is formed" based on an external reality that is socially interactional. The mastery, or correct interpretation, of external signs results in the internal consciousness plane being based on a "quasi-social nature because of its origins."[21] Wertsch further notes that Vygotsky described the child's advancing development as occurring only through an interactive process within the zone of proximal development. The zone of proximal development can be defined as:

> the distance between a child's actual developmental level as determined by independent problem solving and the higher level of potential development as determined through problem solving under adult guidance or in collaboration with capable peers.[22]

Many theorists are concerned with child cognitive development. Although it is clear that a child matures only within a social-interactive environment, Vygotsky, Bruner, and Dunn are focused on the importance of the sociocultural influence in social understanding and cognitive growth, especially through the preschool years. Born into a social world, only through interactions does a child gain self-awareness, perception, and meaning in his or her world (Fig. 24-1).

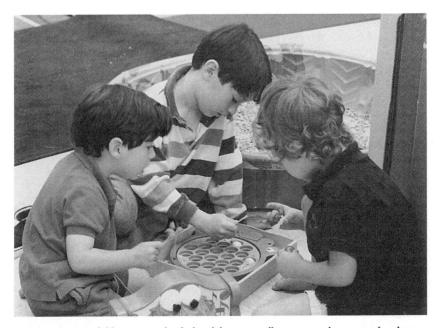

Figure 24–1. As children enter school, the ability to socially maneuver becomes related to peer acceptance and social status. (Photo by Shay McAtee.)

Who Influences the Child in the Early Years?

As previously noted, the first interactions occur within the mother-infant dyad, with the quality of attachment purported to have developmental effects.[10] Intentions and cues between caregiver and infant would seem to begin the first interactive processes, and cognitive growth could be presumed to occur as caregivers enlist the infant within Vygotsky's zone of proximal development.[9] As the child enters its second year and symbolic interpretation and expression gain prominence, interactions with siblings, peers, and parents provide an increasingly complex environment in which the child learns to maneuver in social and cognitive contexts.

Dunn eloquently explored the influence of siblings in the social interactions of the young child. In her study of children within the home, she noted the interactive and cooperative effects on the development of symbolic play of a younger child when engaged by an older sibling. The beginnings of joint pretend play were evidenced in children as young as 18 months. However, it was previously believed that this ability was not evidenced until well into the third year.[4]

As the interactive ability becomes more sophisticated in a young child, peers take on increasing significance in the process of invoking and learning to interpret social encounters. Brownell[23] noted that toddlers in mixed-age dyads were able to adjust their social behavior and complexity of the social interaction to the age of their partners, supporting the notion by Dunn that by 2 years, children possess the ability to accommodate their play, an accomplishment not considered attainable until the third year.[4]

Krasnor and Rubin explored the ability of preschoolers to achieve goals through social interaction and noted their social maneuvering strategies.[24] Persistence, flexibility, and cost were examined in success of goal attainment. They noted that often the more socially acceptable strategy was less effective, but they supported that a balance between social acceptability *and* effectiveness may be a basic component to social competence.

As children enter school, this ability to socially maneuver becomes related to peer acceptance and social status. Dodge and associates studied the ability of kindergarten, second-, and fourth-grade children to detect intention cues, that is, to interpret accurately the intention of another's behavior.[25] This intention-cue skill increased as the child's age increased, and popular and average children scored more highly in their ability to detect intention cues accurately than did socially neglected or socially rejected children. The socially inept children tended to interpret positive social intentions as hostile. Dodge and colleagues noted that "certainly one must first be able to discriminate and identify the intention of an act before one can make sophisticated moral judgment decisions about the act"[26] and supported the concept of a developmental lag in the acquisition of some social-interactive skills. This would seem to imply that the child perhaps had an incomplete narrative, or interpretation, of the social interaction.

It is hardly surprising, then, that Guralnick and Weinhouse[27] noted unusually noticeable deficits in peer interactions of developmentally delayed toddlers and preschool-age children. Considering their presumed cognitive delay, Guralnick and Weinhouse[28] conceived that the "disruptive effects on the socialization process may alter the entire course and outcome of the development of peer interaction." They offered some intervention strategies to increase the frequency of social interaction of developmentally delayed children with normally developing children.

That social competence is correlated with age and peer status and is influenced by disability is not surprising. It becomes increasingly clear that social interaction and interpretation are primary components of a child's ability to function successfully within his or her sociocultural environment. Initial interactions between infant and caregiver form a beginning of cue interpretation that expands and internalizes as a child grows and interacts with siblings, peers, and parents. However, as Bornstein and Bruner[29] aptly state, "The child does not get something simply from interacting with peers and parents. The nature of the interaction, its timing, and its reciprocity must all be taken into account."[30]

Implications for Occupational Therapy

In addition to the motor, sensory-integrative, or reflexive functions of a child, it would behoove therapists to explore a child's social competencies. Through home visits, day care, classroom, and more importantly, playground observations, a view of the child as social learner would appear to have great impact on social acceptance, skill, and ultimately, functional abilities. To consider a child only within the context of the therapy room or treatment session would be akin to interpreting a movie after viewing only 5 minutes of it. Understanding where and how the child maneuvers within his or her sociocultural sphere and the importance of that system with his or her everyday activity is surely of vital interest to every occupational therapist involved in the treatment of children.

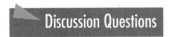
Discussion Questions

1. What kinds of evaluation tools might occupational therapists use or create that would be sensitive to the importance of the social domain with respect to developing occupational competence?
2. Do you think attention to the social domain has been lacking in our field? If so, why?

References

1. Harris, M, Jones, D, Brookes, S, and Grant, J: Relations between the non-verbal context of maternal speech and rate of language development. Brit J Develop Psychol 4:261–268, 1986.
2. Ladd, GW, and Price, JM: Predicting children's social and school adjustment following the transition from preschool to kindergarten. Child Dev 58:1168–1189, 1987.
3. Scarr, S, and Kidd, KK: Developmental behavior genetics. In Mussen, PH (ed): Handbook of Child Psychology (Vol 2). Wiley, New York, 1983.
4. Dunn, J: The Beginnings of Social Understanding. Harvard Press, Cambridge, MA, 1988.
5. Bruner, J: Entry Into Meaning. Harvard Press, Cambridge, MA, 1990.
6. Eibl-Eibesfeldt, I: Human Ethology. Aldine de Gruyter, Hawthorne, NY, 1989, pp 167–238.
7. Bowlby, J: Attachment and Loss (Vol 1) Attachment. Basic Books, New York, 1969.
8. Ainsworth, MD: Patterns of Attachment: A Psychological Study of the Strange Situation. Halstead Press Division of Wiley, New York, 1978.
9. Jacobson, JL, and Wills, DE: The influence of attachment pattern on developmental changes in peer interaction from toddler to the preschool period. Child Dev 57:338–347, 1986.
10. Matas, L, Arend, RA, and Sroufe, LA: Continuity of adaptation in the second year. The relationships between quality of attachment and later competence. Child Dev 49:547–556, 1978.
11. Bruner, JS, and Sherwood, V: Peekaboo and the learning of rule structures. In Bruner, JS, Jolly, A, and Sylva, K (eds): Play—Its Role in Development and Evolution. Basic Books, New York, 1976, pp 277–285.
12. Bruner & Sherwood, p 283.
13. Piaget, J: Play, Dream and Imitation. Norton, New York, 1962.
14. Piaget, J. The Origins of Intelligence in Children. Norton, New York, 1952.
15. Dunn, p 80.
16. Dunn, p 82.
17. Bruner, p 69.
18. Bruner, p 72.
19. Wertsch, JV: Vygotsky and the Social Formation of the Mind. Harvard Press, Cambridge, MA, 1985.
20. Wertsch, p 66.
21. Wertsch, p 67.
22. Wertsch, p 67–68.
23. Brownell, CA: Peer social skills in toddlers: Competencies and constraints illustrated by same-age and mixed-age interaction. Child Dev 61:838, 1990.
24. Krasnor, LR, and Rubin, KH: Preschool social problem solving: Attempts and outcomes in naturalistic interaction. Child Dev 54:1545–1559, 1983.
25. Dodge, KA, Murphy, RR, and Buchsbaum, K: The assessment of intention-cure detection skills in children: Implications for developmental psychopathology. Child Dev 55:163–173, 1984.
26. Dodge et al., p 170.
27. Guralnick, JJ, and Weinhouse, E: Peer-related social interactions of developmentally delayed young children. Development and characteristics. Dev Psych 20:815–827, 1984.

28. Guralnick & Weinhouse, p 816.
29. Bornstein, MH, and Bruner, JA: On interaction. In Bornstein, MH, and Bruner, JS (eds): *Interaction in Human Development.* Lawrence Erlbaum Associates, Hillsdale, NJ, 1989.
30. Bornstein and Bruner, p 12.

Perspectives on Occupation

Occupation is complex and multidimensional. There are many ways of approaching an understanding of occupation. Part of the process of the developing occupational science is the exploration of these different ways of understanding. Perhaps as a result of this exploration, the unique perspective of occupational science will be further developed. The papers in this section reflect a wide variety of perspectives for the understanding of occupation. Each of them brings a light to focus on certain elements, and together, they increase our awe at the complexity of what we have chosen to study, occupation.

The first paper in this section addresses how emotions, narrative interpretation, and even neural selection (consistent with the ideas put forth by Zemke in Section IV) guide choices of occupation and the meaning with which it is imbued. In this paper, White uses three theoretical perspectives to interpret the meaning of occupation in the life of the famous jazz musician Miles Davis: narrative meaning as described by Jerome Bruner[1]; action psychology as described by Harre, Clark, and de Carlo[2]; and Edelman's theory of neural selection.[3]

Essentially, White's paper addresses the general question of why Miles Davis chose to be consumed by music and by the other occupations in which he periodically or recurrently engaged. Thus, a key question posed by occupational science is this: Why do certain occupations achieve preeminence in people's lives, while others are not engaged in at all or are engaged in but are not meaningful enough to be recalled in a personal narrative? With respect to this question, the theoretical frameworks discussed by White may help therapists extract their patients' personal and cultural narratives. By doing so, therapist and patient might gain a sense of emotions that unconsciously influence patients' readiness to re-enter the world of occupation. Moreover, they might better comprehend the social and cultural patterns that are influencing patients' process of making meaning. The three perspectives used by White to examine occupation may turn out to have potent therapeutic application, bolstering therapists' ability to motivate their patients to engage in occupations that will enhance their recovery.

In her paper on running, Primeau approaches this occupation from several perspectives. First, the history of running as a competitive and fitness-related occupation is presented, reminding us how the cultural environment affects meaning of occupations in different historical times.[3] In addition to the meaning ascribed by a particular culture, a society's class structure promotes different meanings for occupation to different groups. While the high culture in European and American society was based on valuing the predominantly intellectual artifacts arising from a wealthy leisure class (such as arts and philosophy), sport and physical leisure occupations tended to be identified as lower class, for whom physical labor was necessitated for survival. Only with the industrial and technological changes of this century, along with increased focus on health and fitness, has running become an acceptable leisure occupation throughout society. Thus, not only has the sociocultural meaning of running changed, but running has become an element of contemporary attempts to effect more healthy adaptation to the dominant sedentary life-style.

This cultural adaptation, which has accepted running as a leisure occupation, is not the only adaptive aspect of this occupation reviewed by Primeau. Occupational scientists at the University of Southern California developed a model with potential use in organizing information about the human as an occupational being.[4,5] Primeau's use of those subsystems provides another perspective for examining occupation. That perspective explores the knowledge we have about running that is related to adaptation at the physical, biological, information processing, sociocultural, symbolic-evaluative, and transcendental subsystem levels. Each of these approaches contributes to our understanding of the complexity of an occupation such as running.

In contrast to the large physical motions and traditionally male participation in running, the last paper in this section explores an occupation using more fine movement that has been traditionally associated with female participants. Pendleton, in her paper on the occupation of needlework (sewing with a hand-held needle) also begins with a historic perspective that once again reminds us of the changing cultural meaning of occupation. That meaning has related to historically changing views of appropriate men's and women's occupations. It is interesting to note the changes in valuing the occupation that accompanied meaning changes. For example, when needlework was considered artwork, women were only allowed to fill in the detail of male artists' designs, and craft guilds were used to control entry into practice. The sewing that produced clothing was highly valued in a preindustrial society but became a symbol of leisure activity later. It reminds us, as occupational therapists, to look again at occupations that might be useful in therapy and to attempt to recast their meaning for today's society.

As Primeau noted, occupations include adaptive skills. Pendleton's paper on the occupation of needlework also reflects on the adaptive skills required to participate. She focused on the ontogenetic development of motor skills inherent in the occupation. From this perspective, current theories of motor learning and motor planning may offer concepts useful to our patients' learning and relearning occupations. In conclusion, Pendleton shares a delightful personal narrative that incorporated information about her own history with needlework, including her developing skills. Particularly interesting is focusing on the meaning that the occupation has had for her at different times. Most therapists could share that internal exploration of the meaning of a particular occupation in their lives and through doing so, refresh their approach to patients beyond the simple so-called activities of daily living, to assist in the patient's return to occupations of much greater personal meaning in many cases.

McLaughlin Gray, Kennedy, and Zemke present two papers that explore potential application of concepts from dynamic systems theory to aid in our study of an understanding of occupation. Occupational therapy has used the concepts of general systems theory for a number of years, but increasing familiarity has raised a number of questions about some of the concepts, especially hierarchy as a control mechanism in the human open system. The idea of heterarchy, with no predetermined control element, reflects much of what we see happening in human function. The concepts of this approach are examined, and in the second paper, an example of application of some of them is considered. Whether this theory will be used metaphorically or explicitly in the development of occupational science remains to be seen.

References

1. Bruner, JS: Acts of Meaning. Harvard University Press, Cambridge, MA, 1990.
2. Harre, R, Clarke, D, and de Carlo, N: Motives and Mechanisms: An Introduction to the Psychology of Action. Methuen, London, 1985.
3. Edelman, GM: Neural Darwinism: The Theory of Neuronal Group Selection. Basic Books, New York, 1987.
4. Edelman, GM: The Remembered Present: A Biological Theory of Consciousness. Basic Books, New York, 1989.
5. Reed, KL: Tools of practice: Heritage or baggage? 1986 Eleanor Clarke Slagle Lecture. Am J Occup Ther 40(9):597, 1986.
6. Clark, F, Parham, D, Carlson, M, Frank, G, Jackson, J, Pierce, D, Wolfe, R, and Zemke, R: Occupational science: Academic innovation in the service of occupational therapy's future. Am J Occup Ther 45(4):300, 1991.
7. Clark, F, and Larson, E: Developing an academic discipline: The science of occupation. In Hopkins, H, and Smith, H (eds): Willard and Spackman's Occupational Therapy. J.B. Lippincott, Philadelphia, 1993, pp 44–57.

by John A. White, Jr., MA, OTR

25

Miles Davis:
Occupations in the Extreme

Life History

Theoretical Perspectives on the Life of Miles Davis

Bruner

Harré, Clark, and De Carlo

Edelman

Conclusion

The narrative of the life of musician Miles Davis is truly remarkable. It could be likened to the wave form of a musical note in the way it traces into the depths of despair and self-destruction and moves to the heights of achievement and acclaim. It spans more than 60 years, and in it, one can find little that most would consider ordinary. His life was unique from the way he played music to the way he dressed to the political views he held. To apply a term used by Jerome Bruner, the narrative of Davis's life was "noncanonical," that is, unusual and totally varying from the standard.[1] Bruner suggests that such exceptional or noncanonical stories are the ones most retold as people attempt to construct their sense of reality.[1] The ordinary events of life need little explanation and share common interpretations. However, the noncanonical stories enable us to define the boundaries of reality as we try to make sense of life. Because Miles Davis's life was so unusual, it offers an excellent opportunity to investigate a number of issues surrounding human occupation (Fig. 25-1). The compelling occupation of music framed and suffused his life in a unique way, for few lives are so dominated by a single activity. The intention of this paper, therefore, is first to present an account of Miles Davis's life story largely

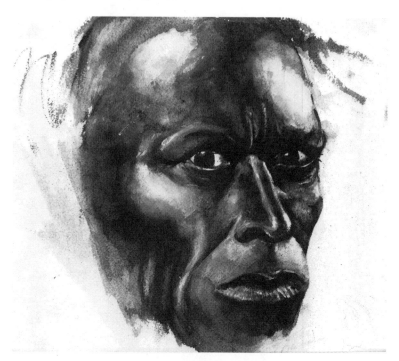

Figure 25–1. Miles Davis' life provides a model for understanding how a life trajectory can be influenced by total commitment to a single occupation. (Illustration by Steven R. Morrone, Philadelphia, PA.)

drawn from his autobiography in collaboration with Quincy Troupe.[2] Secondly, this paper strives to explicate salient aspects of his life that relate to various theoretical perspectives as they apply to occupational science and occupational therapy. Specifically, the story presented in the next section will be the basis of analysis using Bruner's[2] narrative perspective; Harré, Clark, and De Carlo's[3] action theory; and Edelman's[4,5] theory of neuronal group selection.

Life History

There is much in the Davis autobiography to suggest that his life trajectory was propelled by a need to recover the intense feeling he had when he first heard two exceptional jazz musicians play in his hometown of St. Louis, Missouri. Dizzy Gillespie played trumpet and Charlie "Yardbird" Parker was on saxophone in Billy Eckstein's band in 1944, the year Davis graduated from high school. Davis opens his book with the following: "Listen. The greatest feeling I ever had in my life—with my clothes on—was when I first heard Diz and Bird play together . . . [the] music was all up in my body, and that was *all* I wanted to hear."[6]

Davis was already an accomplished trumpeter in 1944 and, by chance, got to play with his musical heroes. This exposure led him to move to New York City so that he could be close to the source of the music and the people who were playing it. Within 5 years, Davis had gained equal status to his musical idols and had become a noted band leader with several records to his credit.[2] They played a new form of jazz called bebop, which derived from classical and swing and was the first true modern jazz style.[4] Davis was immersed in the sounds of the new improvisational music. In spite of responsibilities to his girlfriend and their two children, he was playing for low wages in clubs until midnight and then moving to after-hours clubs and jamming until dawn. The fast life-style led him into many of the vices prevalent in the music scene of that time: alcohol, cocaine, and in 1949, heroin.[2]

Miles eventually developed a more unique sound as his confidence grew and by 1949, had recorded "Birth of the Cool" with a nine-piece band he had put together. That album clearly defined Davis as a leading musician in his own right and laid the foundation for a new sound in jazz that would last through the 1950s. The new style would be called "cool" jazz because of its lighter and easier to listen to, although no less complex, sound.[7]

A tour of France brought even more acclaim to the young musician, and while in Paris, he fell in love again in spite of being in a relationship with the mother of his children. Despite his successful tour and a new love, Miles felt compelled to return to New York where the jazz scene was most active. A deep depression ensued, and his casual drug usage became a self-destructive habit. Music jobs were harder to find, he had encounters with the police, and he neglected his girlfriend and their two children. He sent them back home to St. Louis and continued on a downward spiral until he was finally able to kick his heroin habit in 1954.[2]

To improve his musical performance and help him put his life back together, Davis took up boxing and started a disciplined training regimen.[2] He brought together a new quintet, which, in a short time, became the second truly great band Davis had assembled and led. With John Coltrane on saxophone and a dynamic rhythm section, this group became one of the greatest in jazz history, a musical legend.[7]

Cannonball Adderley joined the band in 1958 to make it a sextet. Adderley's blues sound would take the group into a style that would totally redirect jazz going into the 1960s. When Davis described the process of improvisation among the players of this band, he used words like "chemistry,"[8] "synchrony,"[9] and playing off each other's "voices."[10] Miles knew what sound he wanted for this group, but he had to find a way to bring it out in the members:

> See, if you put a musician in a place where he has to do something different from what he does all the time, then he can do that—but he's got to think differently in order to do it. He has to use his imagination, be more creative, more innovative; he's got to take more risks. He's got to play above himself. . . . So then he'll be freer, will expect things differently, will anticipate and know something is coming down. I've always told the musicians in my band to play what they *know* and then play *above that*. Because then anything can happen, and that's where great art and music happens.[10]

Two great and very different albums came out of this period, "Kind of Blue" and "Sketches of Spain." Each incorporated totally new and different musical concepts that cemented Davis's reputation as a composer, arranger, and performer.[7] Despite his success, in only a few years, Miles was getting bored with his life and turning more to alcohol and cocaine. His drug use was further promoted by hip pain and the death of his father in 1962.[2]

Once again, his music gave Davis a reason to cut back on his drug use. A fiery drummer named Tony Williams set off a new creative streak for Davis and a need to play: "He [Williams] made me play so much I forgot about the pain in my joints. . . . he was something else, man."[11] The new band formed around this drummer enabled Davis to use the influence of rock music to create yet another wave of change in jazz. This time the music was called "fusion," capturing or fusing jazz and rock.[2] "Bitches' Brew" was the album that premiered this sound and brought together a new, younger audience with Miles' jazz fans and led to his title, "avatar of jazz-rock fusion."[12]

Experimenting with electronic instruments and exposure to pop music greats like Jimi Hendrix, Sly Stone, and "soul" singer James Brown again inspired a new musical direction. The resulting music was a "funk" styled jazz with lots of electronic music and as many as three pianos backing up the lead horns.

In spite of the continuing stream of creativity that Davis was producing, he continued to abuse drugs. With a second major depression, he essentially became a recluse from 1975 to 1981, not picking up his trumpet even once in those five years. In that time, "sex and drugs took the place that music had occupied in my life until then and I did both of them around the clock."[15] As a testament to Davis's influence on his musical genre, critic Francis Davis[14] commented that "jazz took a nearly fatal commercial dive during the 6-year period that Davis withdrew from recording and live performance."[15]

Propelled by gentle prodding of friends and the sudden awareness of his rapidly failing health, Davis returned to music, putting together another band and successfully touring Europe. Davis also began sketching and drawing at this time, and he viewed these activities as therapeutic, "now that I wasn't smoking, drinking, or snorting. I had to keep myself occupied so that I wouldn't start thinking about doing those kinds of things again."[15] Davis continued to paint until his death, often working at the easel for several hours a day. He found it soothing and a positive outlet for his creative energy. He felt that it balanced his sometimes demonic drive to play music and allowed him to keep his life more relaxed and in control.

Near the end of his life, as he brought his self-destructive habits under control, Davis looked back on a number of aspects of his life with regret. He realized how his children and the women in his life had suffered because of his obsessive experimentation with music and drugs. In his book, he speaks frankly of his neglect and even physical abuse of his wives and girlfriends and how he had used women to help support his heroin addiction in the 1950s.[2] In his professional life and for his personal interactive style, however, Miles made no apologies. He treated friends and peers with respect, but if he sensed any pretension or insincerity, he was quick to call it for what it was and had therefore made many enemies.

Part of what made Davis so reactive to insincerity were his feelings about the state of race relations in the United States. He learned from his father and other relatives that it was possible to achieve status and power as a black but that life for blacks in America was definitely a struggle.[2] This was borne out in Miles' career experiences watching less talented white musicians gain greater recognition than he and his fellow black players, even though the white artists were actually copying the style the black musicians had created.[7] His outspoken views were not always accepted by those who wished to believe all was well between races in the United States.

Davis also was consistently outspoken regarding fashion. In high school, he copied the styles of Fred Astaire and Billy Eckstein. By the 1950s, he was creating his own fashion statements, and the 1960s allowed him the stylistic freedom of bright colors and outlandish accessories. An example of his iconoclastic styling occurred at a 1987 Presidential dinner honoring Ray Charles. Davis wore tails embroidered with a sequined serpent, a bright red vest, and black leather trousers. The only times in his life when he failed to maintain his appearance occurred during his depressions. In the midst of his "darkest period," Davis remembered, his house was trashed, because he had ceased to care about keeping himself or his house clean.[2]

Just before his death in the summer of 1991, Miles Davis was still performing in concerts and searching for new sounds in music. He had been responsible for at least four major shifts in the course of jazz. Dozens of great names in jazz emerged from Davis's tutelage, leading their own bands and setting new musical trends. Davis had won every major award in the jazz field and had received some of the annual awards several times. Although technically not the most skillful trumpeter of his era, his great creativity and completely unique style of playing overwhelmed any technical deficits.[14]

Theoretical Perspectives on the Life of Miles Davis

Bruner

Bruner holds that an autobiography is not a veridical account of what has transpired in a life; rather, it is a constructed story of the narrator's life as a longitudinal sequence of events and actions.[1] The sequence leads to the present in a way that is justified by exceptional occurrences as those occurrences are interpreted in light of the teller's current circumstances, beliefs, and social "situatedness." In Bruner's view, the creation of meaning through narrative involves two levels of discourse: the personal story that helps one interpret the outstanding or noncanonical events and the collective one that offers a cultural framework with which the individual can compare and refine his or her personal narrative. These two levels are used to interpret Davis's life story.

It seems reasonable to speculate that as Miles Davis reached his sixth decade, he felt a need to review his life and place that story in perspective. The resulting autobiography was frank and open about Davis's accomplishments and his failings and was written in a style that revealed much about the character of the man. It was uncensored in his use of street jargon, filled with profanity and blunt honesty in the style he used in everyday speech. The critic Francis Davis believed that "his profanity gives his speech its rhythmic thrust" and would not reflect the true nature of the man if it were bowdlerized.[15]

Davis's personal narrative begins as he recounts his first memory. It is that of a "whoosh of blue flame" jumping off a gas stove:

> And that stove flame is as clear as music is in my mind. I was 3 years old. I saw that flame and felt that hotness of it close to my face. I felt fear, real fear, for the first time in my life. But I remember it also like some kind of adventure, some kind of weird joy, too. I guess that experience took me someplace in my head I hadn't been before. To some frontier, the edge, maybe, of everything possible. I don't know; I never tried

to analyze it before. The fear I had was almost like an invitation, a challenge to go forward into something I knew nothing about. That's where I think my personal philosophy of life and my commitment to everything I believe in started, with that moment. . . . In my mind I have always believed and thought since then that my motion had to be forward, away from the heat of that flame.[16]

Miles then described a bad tornado in St. Louis the year after he was born and speculated that it may have left him some of its violent creativity and a strong wind with which to play the trumpet. These retrospective omens certainly portended the tumultuous and creative life that Davis lived, or perhaps, as Bruner might suggest, they were simply good matches with the story that Miles has created from the place where he arrived 60 years later.[1]

As already suggested, Bruner goes beyond the narrative of the individual and proposes that a collective narrative exists that represents the experience of cultures.[1] Collective narratives influence the development of individual narratives through the situatedness of the individual within the culture. This leads to a recursive process of feedback that has the sum of individual narratives shaping a collective narrative that emerges to influence the individual's story again.

Two of the collective narratives in circulation during Davis life reflect that complex interaction between the individual and group narrative. Black Americans were considered second class citizens. Black patrons were often not allowed admission to many of the clubs in which Davis played. African Americans frequently received harsh treatment by police (e.g., Davis was beaten for standing outside a club just after he escorted a white friend to her car). Second, black musicians were expected to use illegal drugs as members of the jazz scene. Many contemporaries of Charlie Parker took heroin in hopes that it would free them to play like he did.[2]

These collective narratives seemed to shape the way Davis interacted with his audiences, music critics, record companies, and politicians. He felt compelled not to be treated in a certain way simply because of his skin color. However, much of his behavior confirmed stereotypes of a "drug-addicted musician pushing back against the social currents" that were created by the collective narratives. These narratives shaped Davis's life, the way he acted and interacted with people, and the stories he created about himself even if he didn't specifically articulate those stories until years later.

Bruner uses the terms "praxis" and "logos" in his discussion about how early childhood language arises out of the need to understand the environment.[1] Praxis refers to what people actually do, while logos refers to how they explain what they have done in words. He contends that praxis and logos are culturally inseparable. "The cultural setting of one's own actions forces one to be a narrator."[17] Much of our action occurs in the context of occupation, and narrative constitutes one way in which meaning arises out of our occupations.

An understanding of the link between meaning and occupation can be deepened by considering the social context of many occupations. The occupation of dressing was influenced by the story Davis had created for himself and the message he wanted to impart to others. "Slick, clean, hip, and sharp" are just some of the adjectives Miles used to describe his clothing styles and those of others he admired. The individuality he expressed through this occupation told the world that he was his own man and in control of his destiny. Leonard[18] considers this part of the "rituals of appearance" that were an important part of the "religion" of jazz.[19]

These rituals helped sweep Miles into the music scene as he admired and mimicked the "styles" of the greats he first saw and took those to new sartorial heights of his own.

Davis' occupation of music was even more socially connected. Throughout his book, he tells of the importance of sharing his music with others. He felt most content when he was communicating through music. The times in his life when he felt his best were when he was either listening to great musicians or improvising with other great musicians.[2] He felt compelled to share his music with the widest possible audiences, so he toured extensively and recorded well over 200 albums. Although he eventually became wealthy through his music, many years went by before money could be seen as a primary motivator for him to play such grueling schedules. He simply loved the feeling of sharing music: "All I ever wanted to do was blow my horn and create music and art, communicate what I felt through music."[20] Late in his career, Davis used his talent to try to influence social conditions. Such an attempt can be seen in his 1986 record "Tutu" named after South African activist Desmond Tutu. He also played many benefit concerns, especially if the proceeds went to improve the conditions of African people anywhere in the world.[2]

Harré, Clark, and De Carlo

The social aspects of Bruner's narrative formation[1] fit into a theory of action psychology proposed by Harré, Clark, and De Carlo.[3] Application of the theory of Harré et al. additionally allows exploration of the impact that emotion played in Davis' life and occupations. In their theory of action psychology, Harré et al. have proposed that meaning, emotion, and activity engagement must be considered in the context of one's relationships to others. Emotion, meaning, and subsequent activity are primarily shaped and mediated for the individual through conversation with others. Harré et al. maintain that by studying conversations, one can learn the most significant lessons for understanding human behavior and thought.[3] They make a distinction between actions, which a person uses to communicate to others or to affect their environment, and acts, the social meanings that are attributed to such actions.[3]

Harré's group integrates the act/action concept into a three-level hierarchy that has both regulative (top down) and constitutive (bottom up) features. According to their model, our choices of occupation will be governed by "deep structures of the mind" (including emotions, social orders, and cultural values) that are unconscious. These structures are depicted as a "supraconscious" contained at the top of what they describe as a constitutive hierarchy that controls one's decisions to act in particular ways. The middle level of this hierarchy, labeled conscious awareness, is where one perceives consciousness, and therefore it includes our perceptions and thoughts. Finally, our wishes and intentions are carried out at the lowest level consisting of behavioral routines.

Harré et al. argue that the deep structures of the mind (the supraconscious) are constantly, but unconsciously, exerting a substantive influence over our conscious decisions. This "superconscious" level is an integration of individual and social dimensions and shapes thought, emotion, and action in a top-down manner. The individual component is the person's emotional makeup, whereas the social dimension is a summation of the social relationships and institutional structures within which a person must interact and function.[3] They believe that "there is an elusive pattern to emotional life which structures everything we do."[21]

Davis said that his music, a reflection of his emotions, was influenced by the immediate environment within which he played: "When I'm out of the country I play different because of the way people treat me with a lot of respect."[22] Sometimes the music could be strongly impacted by the emotional situation:

> When we came out to play, everybody [in the band] was madder than a motherfucker with each other and so I think that anger created a fire, a tension that got into everybody's playing and maybe that's one of the reasons everybody played with such intensity.[23]

Returning to the hierarchy proposed by Harré et al., the middle level is where we perceive consciousness and are aware of the actions and thoughts we experience. This is "where we live" and is open to observation and recording. Behavioral psychologists have typically studied this tier. It is described as depending on the smooth functioning of the lowest level, which controls the unconscious maintenance of the physical self and allows us to act on and move within the environment.

This bottom level provides the means with which we carry out the wishes and intentions of the higher levels. As the goals and purposes of the individual are executed by the two lower systems, they are controlled by the highest level, the superconscious influence of emotion and social order. Hence, the top level has a regulatory, top-down control function in the system. In turn, the two higher levels are constrained in what they can do and how they direct the person's actions by the lowest level. The organism is limited by its physical capabilities, and this is what the Harré group considered to be a constitutive role of the bottom or physical system.[3]

Harré et al.[3] proposed that "our behavior toward other people, and their reactions to us, are some of the most powerful triggers to emotional change; it is for the most part by systematic employment of social life that we engineer our emotional life."[24] If we accept this notion and apply it to Davis' life, we can better understand some of the choices and actions Davis made in his life. He reflected on that transforming experience of hearing Eckstein's band:

> I've come close to matching the feeling of that night in 1944 in music, when I first heard Diz and Bird, but I've never quite got there. I've gotten close, but not all the way there. I'm always looking for it, listening and feeling for it, though, trying to always feel it in and through the music I play every day.[25]

From an opportunity to play as an equal in a big band composed of most of the jazz giants of the late 1940s, Miles recalled:

> That music was all over the place, up in everyone's body, all up in the air. . . . It was one of the most exciting spiritual times I have ever had, next to that first time I played with B's [Billy Eckstein] band in St. Louis. . . . It was electric, magical. I felt so good being in that band. I felt that I had arrived, that I was in a band of musical gods, and that I was one of them. . . . We were all there to do it for the music. And that's a beautiful feeling.[26]

Bob Brockmeyer observed this spiritual phenomenon within jazz music. "Jazz is the most ecstatic form of creativity. No form of music is as intense emotionally for the men making it as jazz. It is an immediate, sensate emotion that does not last."[27] In contrast to painting or sculpting, which is slow to build, "In jazz when you're playing with the right people, you can hit that pitch frequently in a night, and when you do, it's a thrill exceeded only by making love."[28]

It seems that this emotional drive also fueled Davis' craving for drugs and his highly active sexual life. After first snorting cocaine in 1946, Miles reported, "All I know is that all of a sudden everything seemed to brighten up and I felt this sudden burst of energy."[29] Davis felt that cocaine increased his abilities as a musician as well: "It was especially good when you were creating and going to be in the studio for a long time. . . . My mouth would get numb but I sure wouldn't run out of creative ideas; they'd be jumping out of my head."[30]

A recurrent theme in Davis' autobiography is the similar satisfaction he derived from music, drugs, and sex. The following example connects the ecstasy of drugs and sex:

> When I see it [that sex thing] I get a feeling in my stomach. It's like I get a rush, like from a snort of cocaine—a big one. It's the anticipation of being with someone like that makes me feel so good. That feeling is so great that it is almost better than any orgasm. Nothing can match that.[31]

Especially after his first depression, Davis engineered his social life to protect his emotions at almost any cost, as seen in this description of the reunion with his former French lover:

> I had gone inside myself to protect me from what I thought was a hostile world. And sometimes, like in the case of Juliette, I didn't know who was my enemy or my friend and many times I didn't stop to find out. I was just cold to mostly everyone. That was the way I protected myself, by not letting hardly anyone inside of my feelings and emotions. And for a long time it worked for me.[32]

In summarizing this section on the Harré group theory, the facts of Davis' life support the notion that people structure their lives and behaviors in ways that satisfy their emotional needs. These needs are determined by multiple influences. From the top, there is the regulative and guiding control of the affective state in interaction with collective social influences. A case has been made to illustrate how emotions, social order, and culture at the supraconscious level governed the kind of occupational being into which Miles Davis evolved.

Edelman

Edelman's original theory[4] (see Zemke's paper) allows us to take a more detailed look at the workings of the lower tier physical subsystem as described by Harré et al.[3] Edelman's work, *The Remembered Present*, addresses the middle- and top-level system[5] in relation to how neural mechanisms ultimately affect consciousness and supraconsciousness. In general, Edelman's work provides an explanation of how a biological substrate may impact the meaningfulness and attractiveness that particular occupations will have for individuals. It also sheds light on how individuals develop the skills and capacities that enable them to excel in occupations. This analysis focuses on the latter. Edelman, a neuroscientist, contends that the development of mental structures and even consciousness can be understood by applying selection principles, such as those seen in evolutionary natural selection to neuron populations within the brain.[5] In his theory of neuronal group selection (TNGS), he posits that nervous system function is shaped by experiences of the organism.[4] This shaping occurs at the synaptic and neuron population group level by selection from variant groups of neurons. That is, different groups of neurons have varying characteristics of transmission and selectivity. These characteristics can make one particular group more "fit" to carry certain signals.

Once a perceptual signal has been transmitted over a pathway within a specific neuron group, the chances are increased that the triggering stimulus will follow that path in future perceptions. This selective process occurs through neurophysiological mechanisms and structures too detailed to pursue here. The more a particular stimulus or signal is encountered, the more it is likely to be processed for awareness or automatic response by that specific neuron group. The signals under consideration here arise out of the environment and are relayed to the brain by way of a multitude of sensory receptors, such as visual, pressure, auditory, and kinesthetic.[4]

A premise on which Edelman bases much of his work is that categories of objects or events do not exist in the world; they are created through a process he calls perceptual categorization.[4] This view runs counter to a common understanding of perception based on the Piagetian model, which suggests that the developing child must discover the categories of objects and events that already exist in the world. Edelman's perceptual categorization, on the other hand, emerges as the brain develops the ability to process and then categorize the incoming perceptions. This ability develops in individuals through a process of selection of variant neuronal groups.

Neuron populations exist throughout the central nervous system (CNS). The CNS structure is based on a design set by the genotype. Through embryologic development of the individual, a primary repertoire of neuron groups unfolds. These primary groups have been designated by the genotype and offer certain constraints to the individual's categorization process. For example, the human visual system is equipped to handle only specific range wavelengths of the light spectrum. Therefore, categorization of light beyond that spectrum was limited until instruments allowed improved perception. There are many other examples of human perceptual limits set by the genetic blueprint on physiology. These constraints are most evident early in individual development.

However, as maturation proceeds, populations of neurons in the structure of the brain are continuously being selected and in the process, develop increasingly complex interconnectivity. These neuron groups are not the circumscribed nuclei depicted by classic neuroanatomy, although a nucleus or nuclei can and do make up parts of them. Edelman's concept is that a group is actually composed of thousands of dendritic and axonal interconnections *distributed* throughout various anatomic levels of the brain. These groups he also calls neural maps. Neural maps consist of large numbers of neurons that have ordered arrangements and activity in their interconnections between and among functionally related areas of the brain. These should be thought of as ensembles of connections related to specific functions. There are literally hundreds of thousands of these maps in the brain, perhaps even millions.[4] An analogy of a telephone system in a large multistory corporate building may be helpful. The connections can run in any direction, up, down, and across the physical and departmental boundaries, and all of the connections should be considered reciprocal. This analogy will be applied to the concept of maps in Edelman's TNGS.

Selection of neural groups or maps occurs through the simultaneous processes of degeneracy and re-entry and results in formation of secondary repertoires. Degeneracy means that while multiple neuron populations exist that can be used to record experiences in the brain, only some populations are used or selected over others. Once a group is selected, it is more likely to mediate that perception in the future, through such mechanisms as synaptic reinforcement. This mapping of neurons becomes the basis for a perceptual category. As mapping and selection proceed, the groups not selected actually lose their ability to mediate future signals (degenerate) and hence the process is termed degeneracy. Edelman states that these processes are ongoing through life; therefore, the secondary repertoire is a dynamic and constantly evolving neural feature. Applying the phone analogy, the connections between departments that are never used are eventually taken out of the system; overused lines will be multiplied to optimize efficient communication. Recall that all the connections building in the telephone system analogy are reciprocal; the same also is true for many of the connections in neural groups, and Edelman calls this reciprocity "re-entry."

Re-entry is a phenomenon that results from parallel or reciprocal neural connections between maps. This promotes instantaneous comparison between several maps and increases the flexibility of the nervous system to deal with novelty. The reciprocal connections allow novel events in the environment to be categorized based on the preexisting categories. Through re-entry, existing categories can be compared instantaneously to see if any fit the incoming stimuli. If there is no immediate fit, a new group will be created, or an old one modified. This could be considered an example of learning. Applying the telephone analogy again, if a novel event impacts the corporation, several departments will set up "conference calls" to compare findings and opinions to make a decision. First they will categorize the event in some way and then develop a plan of response.

The categorization process is assumed to continue to develop as the secondary repertoires become increasingly complex. This adds to the ability of the brain to form intricate associations among increasing numbers of categories. Therefore, the individual has the potential to deal with more and more novelty and complexity. This becomes the foundation for, and eventually the process of, learning. As these maps and neuron groups become more complex and their inter-relationships become more intricate, the individual is capable of higher mental operations expanding in a multiplicative fashion. As selection proceeds, other nonused groups degenerate.[4] This aspect of degeneracy helps explain why adults have difficulty reproducing the way they thought and solved problems as children. For example, once a person learns how to perceive the three-dimensional structure of a drawing, it is difficult to recapture the two-dimensional perspective. That way of categorizing has been lost to the increasing complexity of the neural group interconnectivity.

The significance of Edelman's work to Miles Davis' story can be understood in the way Davis was able to shift continuously his thinking about music.[4] Every musical era has an individual who puts his or her mark on the sound and style of music played, but with Davis, at least four distinct periods of jazz and popular music bore his unique signature.[7,14,33] Davis appeared to be able to grow in this way because he possessed certain capacities that relate to TNGS.[4] Davis' primary neural group repertoire must have been richly endowed. This would have involved such elements as a strong sense of rhythm, including perhaps a cerebellar time keeper,[34] musical or sound memory, and an ability to shift thinking "sets." All of these elements are explained in Edelman's elaboration of the theory. As for the rhythm aspect, Miles himself was amazed by his ability to stay in time. "It's always been a gift with me hearing music the way I do. I don't know where it comes from, it's just there and I don't question it. . . . I can start my tempo off and go to sleep and come back and be at the same tempo I was in before I went to sleep."[35] This was confirmed by the jazz historian Gridley: "Much of his work is characterized by unusually skillful timing and dramatic construction of melodic figures."[36]

Davis' musical memory was both a blessing and a bane in his performances as he recounted in a recorded interview. "People ask me to play an old tune. When I do it, it's different than the way they're used to hearing it and they get mad. Man, I can't even remember what I played yesterday! My mind's too busy thinking about what I want to play tomorrow."[37] Such a phenomenon could be attributed to Edelman's concept of degeneracy.[4] As Davis was hearing new sounds, either in his imagination or from other musicians, previously used neuron groups would degenerate due to lack of selection or use. The old tunes would remain in memory, but the rapidly evolving new repertoires would impose new styles on the old music.

An acute musical memory was needed for playing bebop at the demanding level that Dizzy Gillespie and Charlie Parker required. Miles was able to memorize thousands of chord progressions, recognize them, and fit them appropriately into the improvisation of the moment.[34] The process of improvisation, especially when played in the lightning-fast style of bebop, would require a phenomenon like re-entry to allow for the split-second comparison of incoming sound sensations with the production of outgoing music. Considering all the synapses that must be traversed and the physiologic constraints of reaction time, it is difficult to explain a rapid-fire communication process like jazz improvisation in any other way. The instantaneous comparison of incoming information and resulting decisions would allow for the synchronous way the music changed so rapidly.[4]

In summarizing the relationship of Edelman's work to Davis' story, we see how the neuronal group selection theory can account for the radical shifts in musical style the musician pioneered. The TNGS also offers a rationale for several of the technical skills that Davis perfected in his trumpet playing, composing, and band leading. The TNGS explains how Davis developed the neurobiologic substrate that undergirded his musical capacities. In turn, that Davis possessed these capacities was a crucial factor in how he developed as an occupational being.

Conclusion

As stated in the introduction to this paper, there was little in the life of Miles Davis that could be construed as normal. His life was full of extremes, from the way he pursued music to the lack of balance in his occupational routine. Through that pursuit, he also experienced the extremes of emotion, from the depths of despair to heights of accomplishment and hedonistic indulgence. By viewing these extremes through the lenses of three contemporary theorists, we can gain a deeper understanding of the multiple dimensions of occupation. In the process, we can take this noncanonical narrative and use it to foster our creation of meaning for ourselves and hence promote the same in our patients.

The life story of Miles Davis offers interesting lessons about the importance of occupational balance in life. In each period in which Davis recovered from severe depression or drug addiction, he broadened his occupational routine to help him redirect his energy and bring his addictive urges under control. His boxing provided a physical outlet for the rage and tension that built up over his frustrations with American society. It also provided discipline that he could apply to music and to control his drug usage. Painting during his last decade seemed to fulfill the remaining need to express himself creatively and to balance the demands he had always struggled to meet through music.

Narratives in general are defined as "a discourse form in which events and happenings are configured by means of a plot into a temporal unity."[38] They capture the purposefulness of involvement in activity within the framework of a life. Through the process of narrative configuration, Polkinghorne claims a variety of episodes, acts, and things that happen are synthesized into a whole with temporal organization. They are given coherence through their relationship to a plot. Bruner[1] described the function of the narrative as finding intentions that render understandable the departures in individual lives from the ordinary. Davis' interpretation of his life history, his personal narrative, gives us a profound understanding of why he dedicated his life to his music and participated in the other occupations that consumed him.

This paper also has illustrated how the collective narrative of American culture during the time in which Miles Davis lived influenced him. According to Bruner, the cultural narratives provide frameworks for apprehending norms and interpreting experiences according to cultural patterns and beliefs. The American cultural narrative that delineated what the lives of African Americans were apt to be like was highly influential in how Davis eventually lived out his life. Davis' acts were situated within the American culture, and its symbolic structure shaped how he would interpret his encounters in the world of activity.

The significance of the three theories I have used in my analysis for occupational therapy is in how we interpret the stories of our patients and recognize that we enter the treating relationship with a narrative of our own. Our narrative will influence the way in which we treat and interact with the patient. Continuing in the spiraling feedback process, this relationship impacts how the patients are able to reshape their lives as they adapt to the circumstances of chronic disability. This perspective is from Bruner's contribution.[1]

Perhaps even more important to consider is how the collective narrative of our health care culture and our specific treatment settings impact the configuration of the patient's narrative and that of our own. This demonstrates ideas from Bruner and Harré et al. Concerning how the individual interacts with the social order. If we go a step further with the work of Harré et al., we are led to consider how our emotional needs are shaping our therapeutic relationships.

Looking finally at Edelman's TNGS, I find it promising that such a process of selection may account for much of the brain's activity. It offers further evidence of the plasticity of the nervous system and may unshackle practitioners from their limiting prognostic traditions. Edelman's theory suggests that how we emerge as occupational beings may begin with how the neural architecture of our brains develops. The architecture of one's brain to some extent shapes one's capacities. Together, these theories provide a multidimensional view of Miles Davis as an occupational being and elaborate the complex factors that interact in the construction of the self as an agent in the world of activity with distinct interests and talents.

Discussion Questions

1. White has offered three theoretical perspectives by which he has interpreted the unusual and highly creative life of Miles Davis. How might each of these perspectives be used to substantiate occupational therapy's foundational belief that engagement in occupation has the potential to serve as a medium for adaptation and health?
2. A related but more open-ended question is this: How does a noncanonical life, such as that of Miles Davis, inform the practice of occupational therapy and enrich our understanding of humans as occupational beings?
3. What insights might be gained from Miles Davis' life story with respect to how the narrative of a clinician might optimally interact with that of a patient?

References

1. Bruner, JS: Acts of Meaning. Harvard University Press, Cambridge, MA, 1990.
2. Davis, M, and Troupe, Q: Miles: The Autobiography. Simon and Schuster, New York, 1989.
3. Harré, R, Clarke, D, and De Carlo, N: Motives and Mechanisms: An Introduction to the Psychology of Action. Methuen, London, 1985.
4. Edelman, GM: Neural Darwinism: The Theory of Neuronal Group Selection. Basic Books, New York, 1987.
5. Edelman, GM: The Remembered Present: A Biological Theory of Consciousness. Basic Books, New York, 1989.
6. Davis and Troupe, p 7.
7. Gridley, MC: Jazz styles: History and Analysis (3rd ed). Prentice-Hall, Englewood Cliffs, NJ, 1988.
8. Davis and Troupe, p 222.
9. Davis and Troupe, p 198.
10. Davis and Troupe, p 220.
11. Davis and Troupe, p 264.
12. Davis and Troupe, p 91.
13. Davis and Troupe, p 336.
14. Davis, F: Outcasts: Jazz Composers, Instrumentalists, and Singers. Oxford University, New York, 1990.
15. Davis, p 90.
16. Davis and Troupe, p 11.
17. Bruner, p 81.
18. Leonard, N: Jazz: Myth and Religion. Oxford University, New York, 1987.
19. Leonard, p 88.
20. Davis and Troupe, p 206.
21. Harré et al., p 36.
22. Davis and Troupe, p 398.
23. Davis and Troupe, p 206.
24. Leonard, p 33.
25. Davis and Troupe, p 10.
26. Davis and Troupe, p 100.

27. Leonard, p 56.
28. Davis and Troupe, p 56.
29. Davis and Troupe, p 96.
30. Davis and Troupe, p 179.
31. Davis and Troupe, p 403.
32. Davis and Troupe, p 186.
33. Roland, S, Troupe, Q, Abrams, L, and Allison, J: Sound Recording "The Miles Davis Radio Project" (Audio Recording). Corporation for Public Broadcasting, Zoot Productions, Minneapolis, MN, 1990.
34. Ivry, RB, Keele, SW, and Diener, HC: Dissociation of the lateral and medical cerebellum in movement timing and movement execution. Exp Brain Res 73:167–180.
35. Davis and Troupe, p 397.
36. Gridley, p 209.
37. Roland et al., Part 5.
38. Polkinghorne, D: Narrative Knowing and the Human Sciences. State University of New York Press, Albany, NY, 1988, p 2.

by Loree A. Primeau, PhD, OTR

26

Running as an Occupation: Multiple Meanings and Purposes

Running has been described as a "way of life."[1] To millions of people, running is more than keeping in shape; it is "a mental and spiritual experience" and "an exquisitely physical pastime."[2] To quote one runner:

Running is extremely personal to each runner; its importance shapes the lives of many people who enjoy running long distances. I can really never see myself quitting unless an accident should occur. It has been an integral part of my life for a number of years and I am quite happy with myself and my life and I wouldn't trade places with anyone.[3]

It is estimated that today in the United States alone, 20 to 30 million people regularly incorporate running into their daily lives.[4,5] Several different reasons may be advanced to explain the participation of the general public in the occupation of running. Technological developments occurring throughout the world's industrial and postindustrial nations have resulted in a decrease in physical labor with a concomitant increase in devastating medical consequences of a sedentary life-style.[6] Equally important, technology has expanded leisure time but just as frequently has created a psychologically stressful and alienating life-style. Running, with its physical, psychological, and social benefits, has become a popular occupation in a daily balance of work, play, and rest.

This paper addresses running as a leisure occupation of choice among the general population of industrialized nations. Running is a physically active occupation in which people engage, generally as a form of nonwork. Running can be a vocation, as in the case of professional athletes or racers. The meaning and purposes of running may vary within the individual and across individuals. Different frames of reference are used to view running as an occupation. First, a history as an occupation is provided. Second, the concept of running as a cultural adaptation of the individual to the modern environment is advanced. Finally, the physical, psychological, and social adaptive skills developed through participation in the occupation of running and their relationships to subsystems of the human as an occupational being are discussed.

History of Running

The first Olympic Games were held in Greece around 776 BC. In the classic Olympics, the longest footrace was the dolichos, which was 24 lengths of the Olympic stadium, a distance of 2.618 miles.[1] Although there were trained long-distance runners, or couriers, who ran messages between city-states, there was not a marathon race event in the classic Olympics.

The classic Olympics were held for political reasons, those of democracy and political harmony. Unfortunately, as the city-states began to compete for championships, some cities began to hire the best athletes, and training for the Games became a full-time profession. Olympic champions were given valuable gifts, stipends, and other rewards. Although they were supposed to receive only a crown of wild olive leaves, the long-standing symbol of amateurism, athletes were able to make a substantial living from their winnings.[1] The Games were halted in AD 393 due to the growth of athletic professionalism and elitism.

Professionalism continued through the 1840s to the 1920s in the form of pedestrianism. Pedestrian was the term used in England and America for a professional runner who was paid to travel great distances on foot. Commonly called "go-as-you-please," pedestrians could hop, skip, run, walk, or crawl, stopping to rest and eat as they pleased.[1] Both men and women made a living from participation in 24-hour, 48-hour, 72-hour, and 6-day races. The 1870s and 1880s were a time when the popularity of distance walking and running was at its height.[7] Interest in the sport has gone unequaled, although the current sport of ultramarathoning does come close. Compare Mary Marshall's 1877 achievement of 50 miles in 12 hours with Amy Trason's historic milestone in 1989 of a record-setting 143 nonstop miles in 24 hours, winning her a national championship against top-ranked men.[7,8] During the 1880s, the general public tired of being spectators and began to participate in the "professional" sprint and distance races. Because there were no public athletic facilities, running soon became a form of public recreation, similar to today's "fun runs" and road races.[1]

The birth of the modern Olympics was in April 1896 in Athens. It was here that the first marathon was run in honor of Pheidippides. There were 25 official entrants and one unofficial female entrant who completed the course in 4.5 hours.[1] The Boston marathon, the country's oldest road race, was run for the first time in April 1897 and continues to be a prestigious event.

In the 1928 Olympic Games, there were three running events for women. It was after the 800-meter event that the International Olympic Committee (IOC) ruled that long distance running was unhealthy for women and removed that event from the program, restricting female racing to distances of 100 meters or less.[1] The event was not reintroduced to the Olympics until 1960. Similar reasoning prevented women from officially participating in amateur marathons until 1971. The Amateur Athletic Union (AAU) ruled that women could not withstand the stress of long distance running and therefore forbade their entry into any AAU-sanctioned races. It was not until 1981 that elite women runners were able to convince the IOC that women could run long distances without damaging themselves. In that year, the IOC announced that the first women's Olympic marathon would be held at the 1984 Los Angeles Olympic Games.[9]

During the 1960s and 1970s, several milestone events occurred that affected the history of running as an occupation. In 1961, the President's Council on Physical Fitness and Sport published a report on the decline of the physical fitness of the American public. On the basis of that report, President John F. Kennedy restored the tradition of 50-mile training hikes for armed forces personnel and encouraged civilians to exercise.[1,4] President Kennedy's fitness-minded administration had an influential effect on Americans, who began to take an interest in active sports and in having a healthy body. In 1966, Dr. Warren Guild published the results of an experimental program with cardiac patients that suggested that the prescription of physical exercise, instead of rest, speeded recovery from heart attacks and that consistent aerobic activity might prevent heart disease.[1] Dr. Kenneth Cooper, already conducting research on improving the physical fitness of Air Force recruits and astronauts, used Guild's study in the development of his book *Aerobics*, which had a profound effect on distance running. At the time of its publication in 1968, there were approximately 100,000 runners or joggers in the United States.[1] Also in 1968, the American Medical Joggers Association was founded. This was a group of medical practitioners who were runners and could provide medical services and research-based information to the general public. A Gallup poll in 1970 reported that approximately 2 million Americans said they ran or jogged at least three times a week.[1]

Media exposure of the Olympic distance running events in the 1970s, particularly Frank Shorter's victory in the 1972 Olympic marathon before millions of worldwide television watchers, led to a new consumerism in the sport of road running.[1,4] Top amateur athletes were sponsored by running gear companies and lured to road race events by generous "expense" money. Placement of the top athletes in the public eye in such a manner encouraged large numbers of runners to participate in racing events and to buy running gear.[1] Media exposure also is credited for the "running boom" that occurred in the 1970s, specifically late 1977 and 1978.[4,10,11] In the United States alone, 80,000 runners were estimated to have completed a marathon in 1979.[12] By 1980, between 20 and 30 million Americans had made running a part of their daily lives.[5]

Early 1980 studies suggested that the running boom was over.[11] Circulations of popular running magazines and sales of running shoes plateaued. The number of people participating in road races, especially the marathon, declined.[10] The death of Jim Fixx, a best-selling author and runner, had a negative effect on people's perception of the occupation of running. The most recent statistics indicate that the running boom may have peaked, with one interesting exception. The number of women runners increased steadily throughout the early 1980s; women now comprise 20% and 32% of the marathon and 10-kilometer race populations, respectively.[10] Comparison of 1975 and 1985 data on gender differences in participation in jogging demonstrates that although men are still more likely to jog than women, the gap between the genders is closing. In two age groups, the ratios of number of men to women joggers decreased from three men to every woman in 1975 to less than two men to every woman in 1985.[13]

Although it appears as if participation in organized races and fun runs has declined, the literature indicates that people are increasingly incorporating running into their daily routines.[10] As one race organizer stated, "We're just beginning to see a second generation of runners. Parents who have become fit are interested in seeing their kids do the same. Running and fitness are no longer just a rage, but a life-style. In some ways, the movement is just beginning."[14]

Running as a Cultural Adaptation

It has been only in the last few decades that sport in general, and running in particular, has become a popular leisure occupation. To understand this phenomenon, it is necessary to know that until recently, the general public did not have time for leisure. The worker when not working was resting to recover from and to prepare to return to work.[15] Although most human societies throughout the ages have supported a leisure class, leisure was available to a privileged few made possible by the labor of several. Through the millennium up to the industrial revolution, hard labor was required for human subsistence. However, with the advent of modern technique and technology, it was hypothesized that leisure no longer would be a privilege, but a right for all humankind.[16] In the past, a small leisure class created the arts, the philosophies, and the sciences. The high socioeconomic few represented the model for a high culture that was representative of the total culture. It is to this narrow view of culture that this paper refers in the following discussion. Russell[16] believed that the wise use of leisure required education and an introduction to such culture. Sport occupations, however, were not included as cultural pursuits.

Although sport and culture were both founded on the use of leisure time, there are few connections today between sport and what are considered to be cultured activities.[15] In today's societies, traditional high culture continues to lie beyond the interest of the masses, while sport is firmly embedded in the lives of the general public.[15] Current intellectual thought, as evidenced by the high culture of our society, values the heart, mind, and soul above the body. The lack of respect for the body present in today's intellectual and cultural climate separates sport from culture.[15]

The industrial revolution in the late 1800s and the technologic revolution in the late 1900s transformed humans from Homo faber into Homo sedentarius. Transportation became mechanized, production became automatized within the home and places of employment, and workers became bureaucratized.[15] The physical form of labor is no longer predominant in industrial societies, and with its decline, many humans lost their sense of movement and their natural relationship with their bodies. Rapid cultural changes resulted in a sedentary life-style and an inability of the body to biologically adapt to this life-style. Modern degenerative diseases, such as heart disease, cardiovascular accidents, and cancer, are thought to be directly related to physical inactivity, along with poor diet, stress, and cigarette smoking.[17,18] Heart disease in the early 1800s was a rarity, but by the 1970s, 14 million people were being treated for this disease, while another 600,000 died from heart attacks each year.[17] To adapt to these changes, people began to respond to the need for activity, and the awareness of running as a healthy activity became valued by the same middle class that aspired to higher culture. In summary, the occupation of running, as one form of sport, may be viewed as an adaptation to cultural changes occurring in modern industrial and postindustrial societies.

Demography of Runners

What is known about the 20 to 30 million runners in the United States? The average runner is in his or her early 30s.[19,20] The majority of runners are men, comprising 82% to 85% of the total numbers given in various studies, with the percentage of female runners ranging from 15% to 18%.[19,20,21] Sixty-five percent of this group is married,[19] yet the divorce rate among runners is three times that of the national average.[22] A breakdown of the running population by vocation indicates that the majority are professionals or are in business; 56% and 75% were cited in two different studies.[20,21] Sales-related vocations account for another 14%.[20,21] Full-time students and other vocations each comprise 16% of the remaining population.[20] Only one study provided information on ethnicity, and it was conducted in the American Southwest.[23] Regional differences must be considered when looking at these data. The population consisted of White Americans (68%), Hispanic Americans (18%), Native Americans (9%), Black Americans (2%), and others (2%). Most often cited motivations for reasons for running are physical fitness, psychological benefits (i.e., mood elevation, feeling good after running), weight control, and enhanced self-concept and identity.[8,24–29] Now that the characteristics of people who run have been identified, the adaptive skills thought to be developed through participation in this occupation are presented as they relate to the human as an occupational being.

Adaptive Skills Development

The complexity of human occupation can be organized and discussed with the use of a conceptual framework that views the human as an open system. The subsystems within the human system include the physical, biological, information processing, sociocultural, symbolic, and transcendental subsystems.[30] The adaptive skills of running are discussed in terms of their relationship with each subsystem (Fig. 26-1).

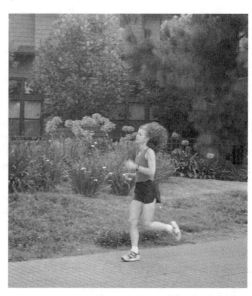

Figure 26–1. Running as an occupation has impact on all levels of the human system, from the biological to the transcendental. (Photo by John Wolcott.)

Physical Subsystem

The physical subsystem includes the physical and chemical processes required to sustain the other levels of the human system, such as the musculoskeletal system, the cardiovascular system, the nervous system, and other anatomical structures and physiological processes.[30] The single most significant physical adaptation to running is the improvement of the individual's physical fitness level. Measurable physiological adaptations occur 6 weeks into a running program.

The first changes indicate a more efficient cardiovascular system, resulting in "superior pick-up and delivery from anatomic structures."[31] They include reduction in resting and exercise heart rates and a rapid recovery to a resting heart rate value after exercise. Other effects of aerobic training are cardiac hypertrophy, increased cardiac stroke volume, an expansion of already existing cardiac capillaries and generation of new ones, increased pulmonary oxygen diffusion capacity, and increased maximal pulmonary oxygen uptake.[18,31,32] In addition to improved cardiovascular function, running enhances the capacity of the muscle to use oxygen. This appears to occur through an increase in the number of cellular mitochondria and their efficiency and by an increase in the density and generation of muscular capillaries.[31,32]

Effects of long-term training include an increase in blood volume, which acts as a reservoir for water loss from perspiration, thereby improving the ability to dissipate heat during exercise. Increased musculoskeletal endurance results from training along with a reduction of tissue adiposity and weight and an increase in lean body mass. Other effects of long-term training are changes in blood lipid levels, especially a reduction in triglycerides and an increase in cholesterol-carrying capacity of high-density lipoproteins associated with lower incidence of heart disease.[31,33,34]

Other physical adaptations less desirable than improved physical fitness are the risks of running and include minor ailments, such as blisters, muscular aches and pains, musculoskeletal injuries, and overtraining syndrome.[17,18,34] Minor ailments generally occur at the beginning stages of running programs and are part of the normal process in the transition from a sedentary to an active life-style. Treated properly, such problems tend to disappear rapidly.[17] Unfortunately, musculoskeletal injuries are common, have a long recovery time, and are frequently severe enough to require extended time off from running. Injuries of this type typically affect the tendons or ligaments of leg joints, with the ankle and knee being particularly susceptible.[18,34] Overtraining syndrome is manifested by fatigue, loss of enthusiasm for workouts, loss of sleep or weight, edginess or nervousness, change in appetite, and reduced performance. Overtraining may occur in elite runners and recreational joggers and increases the likelihood of musculoskeletal injuries. At this time, it is necessary for the runner to listen to his or her body and reduce training requirements for a couple of days.[18]

Biological Subsystem

The biological subsystem is composed "of living systems that directly relate to biological adaptation."[35] The focus is on processes that are often considered to have a biological basis. Two phenomena within the biological subsystem are discussed in relation to the occupation of running. They are the innate drive for physical activity and the competitive nature frequently found among males of a species.

The first phenomenon can be related to evolutionary selection pressures for running in humans. Human runners have a high energetic cost of transport when compared with quadrupedal animals and running birds, yet of these animals, humans are among the best distance runners.[26,36] Biological adaptations that are believed to contribute to human endurance running include an efficient heat dissipation system, consisting of highly secretory sweat glands and an absence of body hair; increased levels of circulatory hormones from relatively large adrenal and thyroid glands, needed for the mobilization and use of fuel for the muscles; an omnivorous diet with an increased potential for muscle glycogen storage; and bipedalism with the possibility for an enhanced biomechanical energy transfer system and the release of mechanical constraints on the respiration cycle.[36] Given the high energetic cost of transport and these biological adaptations, it can be hypothesized that there was strong selective pressure for endurance running during the course of human evolution. Carrier[36] suggested that early hominids may have used endurance running in persistence hunting, a method in which prey are run down by an extended pursuit of a day or two at a time. Persistence hunting may have allowed hominids to occupy a new predatory niche, specifically, "that of a diurnal predator which depended upon exceptional endurance in hot (midday) temperatures to disable swifter prey animals."[37] Although this theory has received criticism,[38] it does shed light on the innate drive for physical activity. In summary, hominids survived on the basis of their physical abilities. Successful living required running fast and long to hunt, walking far to forage and gather food, and fighting hard when necessary for self-protection.[15,17,31,36] All of these factors contributed to a strong selective pressure for a physically active life-style.

Another human characteristic that seems to have developed in response to natural selection is the strong physical competition drive among male humans. Male nonhuman primates tend to engage in a rougher style of social play than do females. It has been hypothesized that juvenile play is the forum in which the young perfect skills and strategies needed in later life, which, in the male case, includes the development of competitive abilities.[39] The asymmetry of reproductive roles is such that the female humans bear the reproductive costs and therefore limit the reproductive rate of the species. As a consequence of this asymmetry, men must compete for access to a limited resource, that of fertile women. Natural selection has favored men who can compete for female sexual cooperation.[39,40]

> Since humans represent a species that takes such a long time to mature, and since the kind of skills that characterize an adult take years for an individual to consolidate, one can expect that to the extent this holds, males would be expected to show greater interest in competitive interactions and dominance strivings with other males.[41]

Information Processing Subsystem

The information processing subsystem of the human focuses on the cognitive structures and processes used in the organization of occupational behavior. Phenomena of interest here are learning, memory, rule formation, and planning.[30] The occupation of running facilitates adaptation within this subsystem through the processes of physical training methods and orchestration of running into a daily routine of occupations. Knowledge and understanding of the scientific principles of training underlie a systematic training program. The runner must learn how his or her body responds and adapts to running to establish realistic personal goals.[42,43] Training requires the ability to think and plan ahead and to develop a realistic timetable to meet personal goals.

Orchestration of running into a busy, daily round of occupations also requires planning and scheduling abilities. Running, as does any occupation, necessitates adjustments and organization to create and maintain a harmonious balance within daily life.[22] Key elements of accommodation and adaptation to a running life-style are discipline, perspective, and realistic priorities. Once again, self-knowledge of personal variables, such as daily rhythms, physical abilities, mental discipline, daily habits, schedules and routines, and occupational role responsibilities, are essential.[22]

Sociocultural Subsystem

The sociocultural roles subsystem incorporates the influence of social and cultural expectations on occupations. Running, as a sociocultural phenomenon, has a social meaning derived from a shared cultural knowledge base. A person must assume the self-identity of a runner.[43] A large part of the socialization process occurs through the mastery of knowledge about running, including training techniques, proper clothing, and nutrition, passed along through informal contacts in a form of "oral tradition" from more experienced runners to less experienced runners.[43]

Local race events and fun runs are a part of the knowledge that is shared by word of mouth among runners. Participation in running events includes a wide range of performances, from a casual, noncompetitive approach to a highly competitive, goal-oriented effort. Individuals make judgments about their performance and therefore establish an individual meaning for a particular event based on common running knowledge. Other runners recognize and validate these judgments, thereby providing the shared social meaning of running.[43] Individual meaning is the personal interpretation of one's performance formed through an interplay of factors, including race distance, finishing time, weather conditions, course layout, and physical conditioning and preparation. Race events have an explicit organization of competition within which each runner will have his or her own individual meaning.[43]

Symbolic-Evaluative Subsystem

This subsystem "addresses the social systems used in the personal assessment of the value of an occupation."[44] These systems include language and communication, arts, sciences, value systems, and human emotion. The relationship of the occupation of running to the symbolic-evaluative subsystem is frequently discussed in the literature in terms of the effects of running on mental health. The development of psychological adaptive skills through running is thought to occur mainly in the areas of mood control, self-esteem, and creativity.[4] Also of note to the symbolic-evaluative subsystem is the concept of positive addiction to running for its beneficial psychological effects.[3]

Several studies have been conducted on the effects of running on moods, specifically depression and anxiety.[26–28,45–50] Runners demonstrated more positive mood profiles than nonrunners. Runners were described as significantly less tense, depressed, fatigued, and confused and were more vigorous.[46–49] Perceived outcomes of running as reported by runners included improved psychological health as evidenced by relief of tension, mood elevation, and feelings of well-being (i.e., pleasure and confidence).[26–28,50] Only one study[45] reported conflicting results. Based on a national probability sample using a longitudinal research method, results indicated a small positive effect on perceived health with no significant effect on mood.

Improved self-image has been associated with running. Personal control, improved physical appearance, self-confidence, self-discipline, self-respect, and feeling better about oneself are aspects of improved self-image as perceived by runners.[26–28,50] Running also has been found to have an effect on creativity.[4,51] A positive addiction to running has been described and appears to be associated with the often described "runner's high," a dreamy detached state of mind achieved during long distance runs.[3,18,28,50] Withdrawal symptoms, such as irritability, sluggishness, guilt, and increased tension and restlessness, are reported by runners when they miss a run and are put forth as evidence of a positive addiction.[3,18,28,50]

Transcendental Subsystem

The transcendental subsystem is associated with the meaning attributed by the individual to his or her life experiences. The life satisfaction, quality of life, purpose, and meaning gained by the individual through engagement in occupations across his or her life history are addressed by this subsystem.[30] It is believed that the relationship of running to this subsystem goes beyond the level of positive addiction and runner's high to the level of personal exploration and meaning. It is not a transformation of self into someone different, but rather an integration of self into a fuller sense of self. Only one reference to this subsystem was found in the literature. It is called holistic running and has been described in the following manner:

> Holistic running refers to the experience of long distance running beyond what is required for physical fitness, as a means of helping to integrate our physical and spiritual selves; our work, play, and leisure; our relations to one another and the world. To accomplish this, holistic running incorporates aspects of exercise physiology along with Western religion, biochemistry, biofeedback, yoga, and Zen. For me, holistic running—running beyond the threshold of fitness—has been a means of personal exploration. It has helped to encounter the dim, confusing isolation of my subjective self. It has taught me something about how I work, how the universe works, and how I fit in. And it continues to help me understand myself and the world. I'm learning about Nature and my own nature.[52]

So defined, holistic running seems to be a human adaptation at the transcendental subsystem level and demonstrates how engagement in occupation, in this instance, running, can provide purpose and direction for the future in harmony with the individual's hopes, emotions, and dreams.[30]

Future Directions for Study of the Occupation of Running

It is clearly evident from the scope of this paper that future directions for the study of running as an occupation are as wide and far ranging as running itself. Quantitative research methodologies will go a long way in elucidating the physical and psychological adaptations to running. An understanding of the mechanisms at the level of the physical subsystem is essential to an understanding of the occupational behavior of running at all other levels of the human system. Equally important are the relationships of the other subsystems to running. Research cannot be done in isolation because all the subsystems of the human are inter-related and have multiple effects on the occupation of running. Ethological descriptive and comparative studies at the biological and information processing subsystem levels will help to tease out genetic and environmental effects and gender differences but when applied to humans, must be considered in terms of sociocultural roles and symbolic meanings. Qualitative research methodologies, such as ethnography, life history, autobiography, and participant-observer studies, are critical to attempts to understand the impact of society, culture, and personal meaning on the occupation of running. While not wanting to fragment the human when studying occupation, the research question will determine the appropriate level of investigation and research methodology best suited to serve as a starting point for the understanding of running as an occupation.

This paper has used several different frames of reference to view the occupation of running. The history of running provided a historic perspective. The effects of society and culture on the current popularity of running within industrial and postindustrial societies were explored as a cultural adaptation. The adaptive skills developed through participation in running and their relationships to subsystems within the human as an occupational being were discussed. This paper attempted to describe fully a multifaceted occupation that has many meanings and purposes to millions of people.

Discussion Questions

1. Occupational therapists have historically drawn distinctions between therapeutic exercises that target specific motor impairments versus therapeutic activities or occupations that are part of patients' usual routines and that may provide embedded exercise. When, as in the case of running, is therapeutic exercise also coextensive with occupation? When is it not?
2. Why might exercises that are coextensive with meaningful occupations provide greater therapeutic leverage than exercises that originate from the minds of therapists, being born, so to speak, solely from a medical clinic or purpose?

References

1. Krise, R, and Squires, B: Fast Tracks: The History of Distance Running. Steven Greene Press, Brattleboro, 1982, p v.
2. Henning, J: Holistic Running: Beyond the Threshold of Fitness. Atheneum, New York, 1978, p xi.
3. Glasser, W: Positive Addiction. Harper & Row, New York, 1976, p 109.
4. Anderson, B (ed): The Complete Runner, vol 2. Runner's World Books, Mountain View, CA, 1982.
5. Staff: Who is the American runner? Runner's World 12:35, 1980.
6. Milvy, P: Introduction and Welcome. In Milvy, P (ed): The Marathon: Physiological, Medical, Epidemiological, and Psychological Studies. New York Academy of Sciences, New York, 1977, p 1.
7. Cumming, J: Runners and Walkers: A Nineteenth Century Sports Chronicle. Regnery Gateway, Chicago, 1981.
8. Cooper, B: Ann Trason's historic milestone. Running Times, 1990, p 24.
9. Staff: Memorable moments of the '80s. Running Times, 1990, p 16.
10. Higdon, H, and Higdon D: Has the running boom peaked? Women's Sports and Fitness 7:25, 1985.
11. Staff: The second stage. Women's Sports and Fitness 7:24, 1985.
12. Burfoot, A, Wischnia, B and Post, M: The American marathon: Part 1. Runner's World 1980, p 58.
13. Firebaugh, G: Gender differences in exercise and sport. Sociol and Soc Res 73:59, 1989.
14. Higdon, H, and Higdon, D, p 82.
15. Jokl, E: Running, psychology, and culture. In Milvy, P (ed): The Marathon: Physiological, Medical, Epidemiological, and Psychological Studies. New York Academy of Sciences, New York. 1977, p 970.
16. Russell, B: In Praise of Idleness. George Allen and Unwin, London, 1935.
17. Kuntzleman, CT: The Exerciser's Handbook. Arbor Press, Spring Arbor, MI, 1978.
18. Alexander, S: Running Healthy. Stephen Greene Press, Brattleboro, VT, 1980.
19. Spreitzer, E, and Snyder, EE: Correlates of participation in adult recreational sports. J Leisure Res 15:27, 1983.
20. Hughes, WA, Noble, HB, and Porter, M: Distance race injuries: An analysis of runners' perceptions. Physician Sports Med 13:34, 1985.
21. Staff: Los Angeles Marathon IV Official Results Book. Running Times, 1989, p 1.
22. Waitz, G, and Averbuch, G: If I can, you can: How to make room in your life for work, play, romance—and running. Women's Sports and Fitness, 1986, p 34.
23. Harris, MB: Runner's perceptions of the benefits of running. Percept Mot Skills 52:153, 1981.
24. Barrel, G: The running bug. Sport and Leisure 27:20, 1986.
25. Clough, PJ, Shepherd, J, and Maughan, RJ: Social-class differences in a sample of non-elite marathon runners. Percept Mot Skills 66:495, 1988.
26. Johnsgard, K: The motivation of the long distance runner: I. J Sports Med Phys Fitness 25:135, 1985.
27. Johnsgard, K: The motivation of the long distance runner: II. J Sports Med Phys Fitness 25:140, 1985.

28. Summers, JJ, Sargent, GI, Levey, AJ, and Murray, KD: Middle-aged, non-elite marathon runners: A profile. Percept Mot Skills 54:963, 1982.

29. Vitulli, WP: Manifest reasons of jogging. Percept Mot Skills 64:650, 1987.

30. Clark, F, Parham, D, Carlson, M, Frank, G, Jackson, J, Pierce, D, Wolfe, R, and Zemke, R: Occupational science: Academic innovation in the service of occupational therapy's future. Am J Occup Ther 45:300, 1991.

31. Zauner, CW, and Benson, NY: Give Us This Day Our Daily Run. Mouvement, Ithaca, NY, 1981.

32. Costill, DL: A Scientific Approach to Distance Running. Track and Field News, Los Altos, CA, 1979.

33. Leon, AS, and Blackburn, H: The relationship of physical activity to coronary heart disease and life expectancy. In Milvy, P (ed): The Marathon: Physiological, Medical, Epidemiological, and Psychological Studies. New York Academy of Science, New York, 1977, p 561.

34. Ullyot, J: Is running really the road to fitness? Women's Sports and Fitness 7:30, 1985.

35. Clark et al., p 302.

36. Carrier, DR: The energetic paradox of human running and hominid evolution. Curr Anthro 25:483, 1984.

37. Carrier, p 489.

38. Nickels, MK: Comments. Curr Anthro 25:490, 1984.

39. Periera, ME, and Altman, J: Development of social behavior in free-living nonhuman primates. In Watts, ES (ed): Nonhuman Primate Models for Human Growth and Development. Alan R. Liss, New York, 1985, p 217.

40. Draper, P: Two views of sex differences in socialization. In Hall, RL (ed): Male-female Differences: A Biocultural Perspective. Praeger, New York, 1985, p 5.

41. Draper, p 16.

42. Clarke, R: Foreword. In Humphreys, J and Holman, R (eds): Focus on Middle-distance Running. Adam and Charles Black, London, 1985.

43. Nash, JE: Weekend racing as an eventful experience: Understanding the accomplishment of well-being. Urban Life 8:199, 1979.

44. Clark et al., p 303.

45. Agnew, R, and Levin, ML: The effect of running on mood and perceived health. J Sport Beh 10:14, 1987.

46. Boyce, L: Marathoner's psyche profiled. Track Field Quart Rev 86:41, 1986.

47. Dyer, JB, and Crouch, JG: Effects of running on moods: A time series study. Percept Mot Skills 64:783, 1987.

48. Gondola, JD, and Tuckman, BW: Psychological mood state in average marathon runners. Percept Mot Skills 55:1295, 1982.

49. Gondola, JD, and Tuckman, BW: Extent of training and mood enhancement in women runners. Percept Mot Skills 57:333, 1983.

50. Summers, JJ, Machin, VJ, and Sargent, GI: Psychosocial factors related to marathon running. J Sport Psychol 5:314, 1983.

51. Gondola, JC, and Tuckman, BW: Effects of a systematic program of exercise on selected measures of creativity. Percept Mot Skills 52:153, 1985.

52. Hemming, p 23.

by Heidi McHugh Pendleton, MA, OTR

27

The Occupation of Needlework

A History of Needlework
Ontogeny of Needlework Skills
Research Methodologies
Implications for Occupational Science
Concluding Remarks

The phenomenon of occupation is the core of the emerging occupational science. In a seminal work authored by the framers of the new science, occupation refers to specific:

> chunks of activity within the on-going stream of human behavior which are named in the lexicon of the culture, for example, "fishing," or "cooking," or at a more abstract level, "playing" or "working." These daily pursuits are self-initiated goal-directed (purposeful), and socially sanctioned. They are constituted of adaptive skills which are organized and are optimally, though not always, personally satisfying.[1]

In the early developmental stages of this new science, in-depth exploration of a variety of occupations and analysis of the adaptive skills that comprise each is an appropriate first step for increasing our knowledge and understanding of the complex phenomenon of occupation and its importance in human life.

This paper addresses the occupation of needlework. Needlework is defined as the occupation of sewing with a hand-held needle. Such sewing includes both the practical application for tasks, such as mending, patching, seaming, hemming—what the historians call "plain work"—and the artistic application involved in embroidery, crewel work, needlepoint, and patchworking—what is called "fancy work."[2] The development of the occupation of needlework is traced historically (incorporating social, cultural, and environmental perspectives), ontogenetically, and from a motor learning perspective. Next, research methodologies that have been used in this area are reviewed, and suggestions for additional research are offered. Following a discussion of the implications for occupational science, the paper concludes with some personal remarks.

A History of Needlework

Although a number of resources speculate that Eve became the first needleworker when she stitched together the proverbial fig leaves, it is more likely that our early hominid ancestors developed some method of holding together animals skins, bark, or vegetation to protect them from the inclement elements. We may never find out for sure because by the very nature of fabric, the earliest specimens were lost to posterity. Scraps of embroidery believed to have been executed during the Neolithic Age have been found in early tumuli or burial mounds. Although decorative needlecraft originated in the East, one historian claims that it was perfected early, and techniques, materials, and motifs have changed little in the ensuing dynasties and centuries. The history of western needlecraft, on the other hand, sought much of its early influence from the East but changed significantly through the centuries, reflecting more dramatically the vicissitudes of politics, society, and economics.[3]

The period from approximately the 9th century to the 15th century is called the Ecclesiastical Period—a time when needlecraft found its expression in vestments and other religious trappings, executed in opulent materials using superlative techniques. During the ninth century, the Catholic church was the primary promoter of needlework—embroidery was the handmaiden of the church. The church had the most influence on design and was the primary employer of artisans.[3]

From the end of the 10th century through the 12th century, the religious crusades dictated the direction of needlework. European crusaders traveling in the Byzantine empire and the Orient brought back, among other things, new materials, better dyes, and more and varied stitches. Romantic tales of the crusades, such as King Arthur's court and Tristan and Isolde, began to influence needlework designs with military and religious themes. Tournaments inspired the need for embroidered flags, banners, and military coats of armor. Color and design took on individual symbolism.[3]

The 14th century saw a richness of dress among the European nobles (for example, King Henry VIII) requiring more elaborate needlecraft applied to clothing and accessories, such as pouches, purses, and gloves. Huge embroidered curtains were hung to partition off rooms in the drafty halls of castles, and heavily embroidered bed hangings protected the slumberer from the cold air.[3]

During the Ecclesiastical Period, needleworkers, who were considered artists, were men who belonged to guilds. These male artists designed the embroidery, completed most of the interesting work, and had women working for them to finish the details and fill-in work.[4]

The 16th century brought the Reformation, a religious revolution that began as a movement to reform the Catholic church and ended with the establishment of Protestantism. Religious grandeur was replaced with simple unadornment. English history during this time was characterized by the hundred years war with France, the Black Death, the dissolution of the monasteries, and disbanding of the craft guilds because there was no longer the need nor the money for elaborate embroideries. It seems that once the glamour and financial incentive evaporated, sewing became, for the most part, the domain solely of women.[3]

During this period, there was a rise in the popularity of secular embroidery, which coincided with growth in female education. The wealthy sought education for their daughters, and needlework was one of the primary womanly skills on which much attention was focused. These "educated" girls advanced from plain sewing to fancy needlework, producing decorative samplers cataloging their embroidery techniques. These signed, dated, and framed "masterpieces" were displayed in their parents' homes as concrete testimony of the girls' accomplishments and the parents' financial success.[5-6]

My focus on the history of needlework now shifts from Europe to the newly colonized North America of the 18th century. For the early settlers, sewing was a vital skill for daily existence. They rejected European influence and dominance and in so doing, had to rely on themselves for production of all necessities. Wool and flax were spun into yarn (homespun); dyed with homemade dyes extracted from berries, nuts, and bark; woven into cloth; and then cut and sewn into clothing. There was no time for embroidery or fancy work. In 1765, the Stamp Act (a tax on all imported goods), which led to the Revolutionary War, served as an impetus for women to protest publicly against the British oppressors. They gathered together in sewing bees to make uniforms for the colonial army.[7]

In the early 1800s, nearly all women sewed by necessity and were responsible for all the family's clothing and household linens. A woman's daily routine was composed of cooking, cleaning, spinning, weaving, and sewing. Sewing was emphasized in private schools attended by 10% to 30% of all girls. The rest learned at home. Plain work was stressed with these girls, but samplers were made with basic embroidery stitches and simple quilts made from scraps. It was customary for a professional needlewoman to be hired to come to the house and help out for a few days with larger, more complicated projects. Fancy needlework at this time was predominantly relegated to the upper classes.[2-5]

The period from 1830 to 1860 is characterized as Victorian, reflecting the influence of Queen Victoria on morality with emphasis on the strong family unit and a strict set of rules and responsibilities for women. *Godey's Ladies Book*, the first women's magazine, was in print, as were numerous pattern books. Thus, women were less cut off from the world, inspired to sew and dress with more style, and pay more attention to decorative needlework.[2,6]

Fancy work now included canvasses depicting realistic scenes that were drawn on the canvasses by commissioned artists, usually men. Other styles and stitches included glass bead work, punched paper work (similar to needlepoint), and Berlin work (wool embroidery similar to crewel imported from Germany). Stitched or embroidered mottos invoked the evangelic and secular causes espoused at the time, including temperance and abolitionism.[2]

The industrial revolution, which began in Europe in the mid-18th century, was just beginning to assert its influence in the United States. Sewing machines were not readily available to the home user, so plain work sewing was still a predominant feature in women's lives. Needlework became associated with philanthropy. Women gathered in churches to sew articles that could be sold at "fancy fairs" to raise money for charity. The Female Assistance Society (in New York, the Dorcas Society) was founded. Needlework was a pastime and a duty; women were exhorted over and over again that they should not remain idle.[2]

Partly because of the social upheaval that accompanied the industrial revolution, the schoolgirl needlework era was drawing to a close by the end of the 1820s. Ornamental needlework and domestic embellishments ceased to be of primary importance in women's education.[6]

Needlework in the United States from 1860 to the turn of the century was most influenced by the Civil War and the Industrial Revolution. During the Civil War, the sewing societies refocused their fervor on the cause, making uniforms for their side. Fancy fairs supported the war effort, and old clothing was refurbished (a la Scarlet O'Hara and the draperies).

After the Civil War, needlework significantly changed due to improvement in technology. Sewing machines were available to the masses. Although the machines were helpful with sewing, they deprived the rural homemaker of the company of her hired needleworker help, and sewing groups no longer met because the machines could not be easily transported. Garment factories were established, and chemical discoveries provided a new color palette. Changes in retail marketing and mailing (such as mail-order catalogs) led to increased distribution to a wider public.[2]

In the early 1900s, needlework became an integral part of the Women's Suffrage Movement. Parasols, handkerchiefs, and banners were embroidered with symbols and mottoes of the suffrage movement. "There was nothing naive in the suffrage use of embroidery. They understood the symbolic content of materials. Excellent stitchery was evidence both of an education in the feminine virtues of selflessness and service and of a natural feminine capacity."[8,11] They portrayed femininity not as frailty, but as strength.

During the 1930s, the arts and crafts movement emerged. This was an attempt to acknowledge the so-called applied arts as true art. The movement opened up a space for female artists. There was an impact on the teaching of embroidery—students were encouraged to invent their own designs; they even advocated equal participation of boys, with little success. Schools and art departments in some universities began offering courses in embroidery.[8]

Needlework also was a growing leisure industry but was always associated with women. Women's magazines reinforced this association. During the depression, women were urged to be thrifty and yet brighten their old clothes and linens with colorful embroidery. Embroidery supplies were scarce during World War II, and women confined their sewing to mending. After the war, there was an abundance of materials, and the magazines encouraged women to take advantage of them. Books and articles fostered the idea that embroidery could be an expression of individuality and creativity. Embroidery prospered.[8]

Embroidery prospered again during the 1960s, appearing on jackets and jeans in symbols of defiance and in support of the peace movement. In the 1970s, the women's movement continued the use of embroidery as a symbolic gesture. "The Dinner Party" by artist Judy Chicago was a multimedia piece of art. It was composed of 39 place settings, each commemorating a particular woman in western history, including goblet, cutlery, and china plate resting on embroidered runners stitched in the style and technique of the woman's time.[8-9]

The 1980s saw a revival of enthusiasm for needlework and embroidery as a home craft or hobby. Embroidery is now practiced as a fine-art medium, with many art schools having embroidery departments. Many artists now consider that embroidery offers textures and colors that would not be possible in any other medium.

Women no longer embroider as a gesture of wifely or domestic duty. However, there is still a separation of femininity/embroidery from masculinity/professionalism, preserving embroidery as the demarcator of women's sphere. It is fine to embroider as long as it is not carried across the border into masculine territory (with a few notable exceptions, such as professional athlete Rosie Greer's penchant for needlepoint as a pastime) and certainly not into the professional arena. "Despite the proliferation of professional groups and the recognition of embroidery as an art form in the 20th century, feminine ideals still dominate attitudes toward the art to an amazing extent. Embroidery continues to be seen as an emotional gesture rather than creative work."[10]

The history of needlework has been considered. Next the development of needlework skill in the individual is explored.

Ontogeny of Needlework Skills

The skills that comprise the occupation of needlework customarily develop during the life span of an individual. Whether an individual develops or chooses to develop these skills depends on a number of variables. Chief among these is the individual's ability to achieve adequate fine motor skills.

The motor precursors or subskills to the skill of sewing appear to begin at 4 months of age when the child brings her or his hands together. At 10 months, a pincer grasp develops, and the child begins picking up food morsels, practicing grasp and release characterized by crude motion. Between 2 and 2.5 years of age, the child begins to string large beads and at 3 years, can attempt lacing. At this age, the child shows a persistent and increased interest in finer manipulation, but massive muscles continue to dominate. The 4-year-old child still finds lacing an effort but has made significant and steady progress. Upper extremity motion now includes supinated grasp. The typical 5-year-old child is now skilled in using many basic self-care tools (such as a toothbrush) and can use these tools effectively in activities requiring two- to three-step sequences. She or he is able to tie knots, but tying a bow may be beyond skill level. At 6 years old, bow-tying is usually mastered, and the child begins handicrafts, such as sewing.[11,12] Sewing projects for the beginner often include making crude doll clothes or executing simple embroidery. Skill increases with further fine motor practice as does the complexity and intricacy of the project attempted. By 15 years of age, dedicated needleworkers can master most stitches and achieve an accomplished level of needlework performance.[6]

Needleworkers might well remember their first attempt at sewing—the awkward handling of the needle and cumbersome manipulation of the fabric—not knowing how much pressure to exert and invariably pulling the needle straight up, overextending one's reach until the thread was stretched out taut from the material. Typically, the thread became knotted or a finger was poked (bleeding onto the project), and the budding needleworker doubted the possibilities of ever perfecting the necessary skills.

How does the motor learning skill required for the performance of needle-work develop? According to Elliott and Connolly, skill is "an ability to achieve defined goals with an efficiency beyond that of an inexperienced person."[14] To be skilled in performing needlework, one must first master the subroutines (or performance units) that comprise it.

Basic motor acts, such as sewing, are learned. The learner has a conscious awareness of movement and visually monitors progression of the plan. The needle-worker's hands are positioned in such as way that skilled movement is promoted. Through continued repetition of movement sequences, the needleworker organizes, modifies, and refines these sewing motions into a purposeful plan in time and efficiency.[11,15]

The needlework learner may begin by observing those around her and may mentally practice the stitches she sees being performed. When she has the opportunity to hold the threaded needle and material and actually executes a stitch, further motor learning may take place as Schmidt's motor learning schema suggests. According to Schmidt's theory of motor skill learning, a generalized motor response schema (or pattern) is established for each movement. In the early motor learning stages, as each movement is performed, it is guided by and matched to information stored regarding previously learned related movements. Information previously stored corrects and monitors new movements until they are perfected.[15,16]

Sensory cues help the needlework learner to determine how much force to exert when pushing the needle through the material, how far to push the needle through the material before coming back up to accomplish the right size stitch, and so forth. Each time the needlework learner needs to repeat the stitching process or use this skill or similar skills (more advanced, varied, or intricate stitches) at another time or under different circumstances (frame-mounted tapestry, for instance), the appropriate motor response schemata are strengthened and available for future use.[15,16]

As the needleworker becomes more skilled through repetition and refinement, the sewing movements become automatic, are successful, and are memorized for later recall. Conscious motor planning is no longer needed.[14]

Because sewing requires different but complementary bilateral hand skills, motor skills and plans (schemata) need to be learned and perfected for each hand. According to Elliott and Connolly:

> A movement of one hand may only be simultaneously and purposefully combined with a movement of the other when the two components are sufficiently well practiced and do not require continuous monitoring. The movements are lawfully related within the demands of a task, which is in itself within the attention capacity of the operator, that is to say, the movements made by the two hands must comprise part of some overall task, the attainment of which is monitored.[17]

The type of bimanual combination found in sewing is what Elliott and Connolly would describe as a distribution of labor between manipulation and support across the hands. Although the nondominant hand is primarily involved in support of the material, it is frequently involved with skillful manipulation of the fabric as well. Thus, in the occupation of sewing, motor learning involves developing fine motor skills in both hands.

Research Methodologies

The major portion of the research that has been conducted on the subject of needlework has been historical, encompassing descriptive and longitudinal studies. Although the culture and customs are recorded, the studies are most often done from the perspective of an artist/needleworker and not through the eye of an impartial ethnographer. The occupational scientist, reading such histories, feels compelled to ask different questions and wants more details; for example, how precisely does the time span in needlework fit in with needleworkers' other daily occupations?

For the purposes of occupational science, the life history method might provide interesting and informative results when applied to the occupation of needlework. An individual's personal experience with developing the adaptive skills and subskills involved in needlework could be chronicled over her or his life span. Although diaries provide some of the social information available, in most instances, the man of the family was the diarist and only mentioned the woman's occupation in needlework as it affected his daily occupations. Diaries of the actual needleworker would provide a more relevant account.

In addition, the occupational scientist might find it useful to conduct experimental research to determine how the motor learning of stitchery actually takes place and the specific variables that might influence this motor learning. Comparison studies of needlework acquisition in western cultures versus other cultures might uncover valuable information regarding the development and valuing of occupation in general.

Implications for Occupational Science

Needlework is an occupation that has been used as a therapeutic activity throughout the history of occupational therapy. Sewing has been taught to patients as an independent living skill necessary for the maintenance and even the provision of clothing. Embroidery, needlepoint, and the more decorative aspects of stitchery have been used in developing a patient's leisure skills. Needlework can provide opportunities for expressing creativity and individuality and the concomitant increases in self-esteem. It has been useful in developing fine motor skills and improving cognitive and perceptual skills. Many needlecrafters claim a sense of well-being when engaged in a sewing project.

Some budding occupational scientists are interested in the development of adaptive skills in the human and the relationships of these skills to the performance of human occupation. Comprehensive investigation of time-honored occupations, such as needlework, can provide valuable information. Needlework, as this paper has shown, has been practiced for centuries, for practical and aesthetic reasons, and by some men but mostly by women. Required skills can develop in early childhood, and many needlecrafters practice their skill throughout their lifetime.

This investigation of needlework raises many questions for future research. How does the occupation of needlework fit into the needlecrafter's everyday round of occupation? What attracts people to the occupation of needlework? How does an individual generate interest in new occupations or rekindle interest in previously loved skills? If individuals claim to feel more fulfilled, industrious, even more healthy when engaged in occupations like needlework, why do they stop? Learning the answers to these questions may provide a greater understanding of how and why meaningful occupation is inherent to our well-being and provide us with ideas for therapeutic intervention when skill acquisition is impaired.

Concluding Remarks

As this paper comes to a close, I question what led me to choose needlework for a first formal quest into the realm of occupation. I realize that it has been more than 15 years since I have really immersed myself in this formerly loved occupation, and I miss it. Although legitimately able to beg a scarcity of time, I know that I harbored a secret embarrassment regarding its value as limited in the life of busy professional women. Maybe it was just a little too domestic, too unscholarly.

Interested in sewing since the age of 6, I was fortunate to have a mother who, although she did not sew herself, fostered the dreams and aspirations of her daughters. She helped me to acquire the embroidery accoutrements and then to learn the necessary skills to produce a succession of embroidered doll bibs and clothes. What fun! At 11, I began a series of summer vacations devoted to Singer sewing lessons. I made clothes for myself, and one dress even won an award. How proud I was! Spare time in high school and college found me producing numerous projects in crewel work, needlepoint, and Christmas stockings in applique. Great gifts, lovingly made, were proudly presented to friends and loved ones. My pièces de résistance were frothy bassinets for my nieces and nephew. And then to my surprise, I found myself in a graduate program preparing for a profession, which, in one semester, required that I take neuroanatomy and weaving. What a wonderful combination! How then did such interest and enthusiasm wane? In researching this chapter, good memories returned and a new pride in this skill of mine evolved. I am taking up the needle again!

Discussion Questions

1. Pendleton's chapter presents a "simple" occupation and develops its significance from both a historical and ontogenetic perspective. In so doing, she reveals how the interconnected influences of culture, economics, gender, power relations, technology, enjoyment, and aesthetics converge in one occupation. What are the advantages and limitations of such an analysis for occupational therapists?
2. Does the process of making the history of an occupation such as needlework visible help to substantiate its importance as an occupation?

References

1. Department of Occupational Therapy, University of Southern California: Proposal for a new-doctor of philosophy in occupational science. Unpublished manuscript, 1987, p 1.
2. Vincent, M: The Ladies Worktable: Domestic Needlework in Nineteenth Century America. Allentown Art Museum, Allentown, PA, 1988.

3. Jones, ME: A History of Western Embroidery. Watson-Guptill Publications, New York, 1969.

4. Bridgeman, H, and Drury, E: Needlework: An Illustrated History. Paddington Press Ltd., New York, 1978.

5. Wiczyk, AZ: Treasury of Needlework Projects from Godey's Lady's Book. Arco Publishing Company, New York, 1972.

6. Ring, B: American Needlework Treasures: Samplers and Silk Embroideries from the Collection of Betty Ring. EP Dutton, New York, 1987.

7. Macdonald, AL: No Idle Hands: The Social History of American Knitting. Ballantine Books, New York, 1988.

8. Parker, R: The Subversive Stitch: Embroidery and the Making of the Feminine. The Woman's Press, London, 1984.

9. Chicago, J: The Dinner Party: A Symbol of Our Heritage. Anchor Press/Doubleday, Garden City NJ, 1979.

10. Parker, p 213.

11. Coley, IL: Pediatric Assessment of Self-care Activities. C.V. Mosby, St. Louis, MO, 1978.

12. Erhardt, RP: Development Prehension Assessment. Therapy Skill Builders, Tucson, 1989.

13. Arnold, A: The Crowell Book of Arts and Crafts for Children. Thomas Y. Crowell Company, New York, 1975.

14. Elliott, J, and Connolly, K: Hierarchical structure in skill development. In Connolly, K, and Bruner, J (eds): The Growth of Competence. Academic Press, New York, 1973, p 136.

15. Connolly, K: The nature of motor skill development. Journal of Human Movement Studies 3:128, 1977.

16. Dickinson, J, and Goodman, D: Perspectives on motor learning theory and motor control. In Zaichkowsky, LD, and Zvi Fuchs, C (eds): The Psychology of Motor Behavior. Movement Publications, Ithaca NY, 1986, p 29.

17. Elliott and Connolly, p 144.

*by Julie McLaughlin Gray, MA, OTR,
Bonnie L. Kennedy, MEPD, OTR,
and Ruth Zemke, PhD, OTR, FAOTA*

28

Dynamic Systems Theory: An Overview

Even very simple . . . systems can display a remarkably rich and subtle diversity of behavior.[1]

It is usually their very openness to a complex environment that drives them.[2]
Behavior can be constrained by multiple influences and attributes.[3]

They simply cannot be "chopped up" into lots of simple bits and still retain their distinctive qualities.[2]

The extraordinary complexity of human occupation compels and inhibits its study. Seemingly ordinary, everyday occurrences of human engagement in occupation become elusive on close examination, emerging as the result of complex systems

297

of interaction. The previous quotes seem to characterize this phenomenal interaction, yet they refer to systems that do not appear related to the purposeful, meaningful activity of human beings; systems such as the pattern of a dripping faucet, the life cycle of slime molds.[4] These statements emerge from a relatively new perspective in science dedicated to the study of dynamic, complex systems: dynamic systems theory. Sharing a remarkable similarity to occupational science in its scope and philosophy, this material might be able to shed light on the complex process of human occupation.

The incorporation of systems theory into the study of human occupation is not a new phenomenon. General systems theory, introduced by von Bertalanffy[5] as a new philosophy of science in which systems at many levels are considered in terms of common elements, is the primary example. According to this theory, a system might be described as a complex of elements interacting in a functional way. Several models for occupational therapy and occupational science have used this general concept of open systems. Examples include the model of human occupation by Kielhofner and Burke,[6] the model of the human as an occupational being in the University of Southern California curriculum model, and more recently, the occupational science model.[7] These models acknowledge the interaction or feedback from the action itself, and the output that can be occupational. This interaction has been posited as the key to adaptation.

These and other open systems have usually adopted the concept of hierarchy for the organization of subsystems within the human and, as such, have discussed the control of higher levels and the constraints of the lower ones. Concepts of heterarchy, however, such as in the distributive systems of the functional brain, may be of greater relevance in human functioning across the life span. Without hierarchy, occupational science lacks a model for understanding how subsystem elements are ordered to produce the behavioral outcomes that we recognize as developmental milestones or occupational performance. Dynamic systems theory might provide such a model. In particular, dynamic systems theory suggests that even without hierarchical ordering of subsystems, an understanding of the formation of relatively stable patters of behavior and of the extensive change that we recognize in human function can be found within the relationships of the organism's subsystems, the task, and the content. Studies of complex, "dynamic" systems suggest that living systems are self-organizing and pattern forming. Human patterns of occupation may reflect this quality.

This paper and the one that follows explore the relevance of dynamic systems theory to the science and study of the human as an occupational being. The first paper begins with a review of the historical development of dynamic systems theory. This history is included in the hope that it will assist the reader in developing an understanding of dynamic systems theory adequate for analyzing its relevance to occupational science. This understanding is further expanded using a description of the major principles of dynamic systems theory.

The following paper explores the application of these dynamic systems principles to the science of occupation. It begins with three justifications for including dynamic systems theory in occupational science, providing additional support for its relevance. An example relating dynamic systems theory to the occupational patterns of minority women who are positive for the human immunodeficiency virus (HIV) are described. Examining other fields of inquiry in which dynamic systems theory has been used and exploring the application of the major concepts of dynamic systems theory to major concepts in occupational science and occupational therapy, the authors attempt to answer three main questions: Is it appropriate to apply the study of dynamic systems theory to the study of human occupation? What does dynamic systems theory offer the study of the human as an occupational being? What implications for research and further discussion arise from the above considerations?

A Historical Background

A scholarly investigation of the relevance of a theory to occupational science, or any field, should attempt to expose the underlying assumptions and premises of that theory for analysis as well. Often these underlying assumptions or premises are not explicitly stated, which seems to be the case with dynamic systems theory. A description of the historical development of the study of dynamic systems is included to provide some insight into the foundation of the theory.

According to Thelen and Ulrich,[4] a "classic introduction" to the study of dynamic systems is "Order Out of Chaos: Man's New Dialogue with Nature" by Prigogine and Stengers.[8] Prigogine and Stengers trace the history from Newton to the present. Through their historical account, they described a significant change of perspective within science, a change that has led to a dynamic systems view. They claimed that this shift was "not the result of some arbitrary decision. In physics it was forced upon us by new discoveries no one could have foreseen."[9]

Prigogine and Stengers outlined three major historical periods in scientific inquiry: classical science; equilibrium thermodynamics, which represents the beginning of a science of complexity; and nonequilibrium thermodynamics, which supports "the science of complex phenomena"[10] as it is studied today. They based their analysis of a scientific "conceptual revolution"[11] on two issues that science has always attempted to address: the relationship between order and disorder and the question of evolution or irreversibility. Other authors provided similar historical analyses.[12-14] An overview of this historical progression is helpful in understanding the emergence of a dynamic systems view and making an informed decision regarding its applicability to a field such as occupational science.

Classical Science

Classical science, sometimes referred to as classical mechanics,[13] was spawned by Newton's presentation of the *Principia* to the Royal Society of London on April 28, 1686.[8] Contained in Newton's work were the basic laws of motion and such fundamental physical concepts as mass, acceleration, and inertia. The assumptions of classical science centered, according to Prigogine and Stengers, "around the basic conviction that at some level *the world is simple* and is governed by time-reversible fundamental laws."[15] They suggested that science today has freed itself from these laws, which they consider to be excessively simplified. Nevertheless, classical science dominated for many years and maintained that "ultimately any set of phenomena could be reduced, completely and unconditionally, to nothing more than the effects of some definite and bounded set of fixed laws which determined completely and precisely the phenomena."[16]

The concepts of statistical and quantum mechanics are described by some as a step between classical mechanics and thermodynamics, an alteration of the view of classical mechanics by the confirmation of atomic theory.[13] In brief, Kugler et al. described the laws of quantum mechanics as "providing a precise description of micro behavior at the atomic or molecular state"[17] where the laws of classical mechanics "provided a sufficiently accurate description of behavior at the macroscopic scale."[17] Prigogine and Stengers[8] seem to place much less emphasis on quantum mechanics in their historical analysis. They stated, "it is true that quantum theory has raised many new problems not covered by classical dynamics, particularly as far as time and process are concerned."[18] They mentioned quantum theory only to "emphasize its role in the construction of the bridge from being to becoming,"[19] the second of which they claimed as their main emphasis.

Equilibrium Thermodynamics

Prigogine and Stengers labeled thermodynamics as the first "nonclassical" science.[20] Thermodynamics arose from "the two descendants of the science of heat: the science of energy conversion and the science of heat engines."[20] Prigogine and Stengers described two different processes on which thermodynamics is based. The first, reversible processes, are "independent of the direction of time,"[20] and the second, irreversible processes, "depend on the direction of time."[20] Thermodynamics involves the "transactions of various forms of energy in all of its possible forms . . . by describing a system in terms of concepts and laws derived from the study of macroscopic phenomena such as pressure, volume, temperature, concentrations, etc."[21] It involves the study of the relationships of variations in these properties.[8] According to Prigogine and Stengers, the final state of thermodynamic evolution, equilibrium thermodynamics, was the center of scientific research in the 19th century. At that time, "irreversible processes were looked down on as nuisances, as disturbances, as subjects not worthy of study."[20]

There are three laws of thermodynamics. The first and second laws of thermodynamics are included as the most relevant to a discussion of dynamic systems. The first law of thermodynamics is that of conservation of energy, whereby "in all macroscopic chemical and physical processes, energy is neither created nor destroyed but merely transformed from one form to another."[22] The second law, which Prigogine and Stengers considered "the most original contribution of thermodynamics,"[20] generalizes "any spontaneous process results in an increase in the disorder of the system plus its surroundings."[22] This disorder, also called entropy or randomness, increases to a maximum until the system is at a point of local equilibrium, in which it can no longer undergo any changes.[13] Entropy can remain constant during a process, in which case the process is defined as reversible. With this law, the unidirectional arrow of time was introduced into physics. "This law provides a criterion for predicting the temporal direction of a given process."[22] It provides some explanation for irreversible phenomena.

Nonequilibrium Thermodynamics

Out of the 20th century came nonequilibrium thermodynamics, with the recognition that in far from equilibrium situations, new types of structures may spontaneously originate.[8] These new types of structures, or new states that may emerge, reflect the interaction of the system with its surroundings. Prigogine and Stengers referred to these structures as "dissipative structures."[20] Through these processes, irreversible changes occur when entropy is not maintained but increased, and in nonlinear fashion, emergent qualities appear. Spontaneous self-organization is observed. Principles of nonequilibrium thermodynamics are being applied in a variety of fields today. These principles are explored in the following description of dynamic systems theory and further considered for application to the science of human occupation in the following paper.

The previous changes, when viewed in retrospect, demonstrate a gradual shift in science away from reductionism. Prigogine and Stengers[8] believed this was, in part, by necessity. It was their belief that in many systems, "a description of elementary behaviors is not sufficient for the understanding a system as a whole."[23] It is now being acknowledged that we live in a pluralistic world, and although there are processes that are reversible and deterministic, there also are highly complex processes that involve randomness and irreversibility. Traditional science emphasized order, uniformity, stability, and equilibrium,[24] and "our vision of nature is undergoing a radical change toward the multiple, the temporal, and the complex."[25] Prigogine and Stengers summarized this new development as "science . . . rediscovering time, due to the nonlinearity that is now acknowledged in complex systems."[11] It is this "conceptual revolution" that they set out to describe. They believed this revolution to have far-reaching implications that relate to qualitative changes in behavior or processes on a number of levels, and represent a convergence of science and the humanities. For these reasons, more recent scientific principles, specifically out of physics and relating to dynamic systems, are being applied in a number of academic areas.

Dynamic Systems Theory

Dynamic systems are systems that change with time. They are characterized by complexity, randomness, and nonlinearity.[1,4,8,12] An underlying assumption in dynamic systems theory is that biological organisms are complex, multidimensional, cooperative systems that exhibit self-organizing properties. The following is a description of the primary concepts and terminology used in a theory of dynamic systems. Despite this organizational framework, all concepts are highly inter-related.

Complexity

Increasing Complexity

A fundamental characteristic of dynamic systems is that they evolve with time, and this evolution, or change, is in an irreversible pattern, demonstrating a remarkable ordered complexity. This increasing complexity in the behavior of dynamic systems is often described through the use of relatively simple mathematical equations, representing behavior that is not simple in the least.[26] Thelen and Ulrich give the example of a dripping faucet and boiling water. Behind the apparent randomness of the clock-like drips, there is an amazing hidden self-organized order. When water is heated, there is a transition from homogeneity to rolls and layers; the rolls then dissolve, and the layers become turbulence. The authors emphasize that even very simple systems can, with time, evolve into highly organized patterns that can be mathematically defined. "Patterns generated in these conditions, while drastically more simple than the behavior of the single elements alone, can show a remarkable ordered complexity as they evolve over time . . . both the compression of the original degrees of freedom into order and pattern, and the dynamic complexity of the resulting pattern . . . is not simple at all."[26]

Multiple Degrees of Freedom

In a dynamic system, degrees of freedom represent the complexity, the multiple factors involved and options available to influence a transition phase. A significant characteristic of complex systems is their large number of degrees of freedom and components.[1] As self-organization occurs, these degrees of freedom are drastically reduced: "As the elements are 'sucked in' to play a particular role in the pattern, they are no longer free to act independently."[27] Using the fluid example again, the degrees of freedom are described as the potential ways for the water molecules to combine. Another example of degrees of freedom is provided by researchers applying the dynamic systems principles to the acquisition of movement patterns.[28] Scholz described the degrees of freedom available during the production of observable movement patterns as the "nearly infinite combinations of possible states or values that the neural, muscular, and skeletal components of the motor systems can assume."[19] This also was described by Kamm et al. as "many muscles spanning multiple joints that must be linked cooperatively for coherent action."[30]

Heterarchy

Also inherent in the dynamic systems perspective is the inadequacy of the notion of hierarchy. "A systems description of behavior does not assume any one of the contributing factors . . . has some privileged status over the other subsystems."[30] Behavior, therefore, is considered an emergent property of the interaction of many subsystems, including the context or environment. This is described sometimes as a "confluence of variables,"[30] or heterarchy.

Self-organization

As stated previously, dynamic systems theory is based on the notion that complex biologic organisms exhibit self-organizing properties. One of the most exciting findings of the study of dynamic physical systems has been the acknowledgment of the potential for self-organization (or reorganization) of a system in a destabilized state of disequilibrium. "Systems driven far-from-equilibrium tend to undergo abrupt spontaneous change of behavior. They may start to behave erratically, or to organize themselves into new and unexpected forms."[31] Through this process, a number of degrees of freedom are significantly curtailed, and a new pattern formation is evident. As discussed previously, an example of this pattern formation is given by Thelen and Ulrich[4] as the response of fluids to certain thermodynamic conditions in which several single elements act autonomously as one unit. Davies described these states as possessing a "degree of global cooperation."[32] An important aspect of this process is that a symmetry is broken down into a more complex state. Often systems organize themselves into unexpected forms. For this reason, dynamic systems are considered *nondeterministic*.

The Arrow of Time—Irreversibility

Another significant characteristic of dynamic systems, one that distinguishes them from other complex systems previously studied in science, is their relationship to time. Dynamic systems exhibit complex behavior over time and display changes that are irreversible.[4,8] This is in contrast to many simple physical systems and reflects the view of time as moving in one irreversible direction. The phrase "arrow of time" is used by Prigogine and Stengers[8] to symbolize the unidirectional change, or time-symmetry, found in many processes.

Irreversibility becomes clarified when explained in contrast to the classical view of reversibility. According to classical science, processes begin with initial conditions, and their atoms or particles follow predetermined plans that can be traced forward or backward. Irreversible processes, on the other hand, are time oriented and cannot be traced backward. An example of this in chemistry is the mixing of two liquids, such as alcohol and water. "They tend to mix in the forward direction of time as we experience it."[25] The reverse process is never observed. Davies used more familiar examples of this irreversibility. "Just think of trying to unbreak an egg, grow younger, make a river flow uphill or unstir the milk from your tea. You simply cannot make these things go backwards."[33]

Under the rubric of classical science, the idea of irreversible processes was considered, more or less, an illusion. It is precisely this notion of irreversibility and growing complexity or order that came into conflict with the second law of thermodynamics. According to this law, the system is expected to go from order to disorder. Disorder, or entropy, is expected to increase.[4] However, Prigogine and Stengers emphasized, "far from being an illusion, irreversibility plays an essential role in nature and lies at the origin of most processes of self-organization."[23] It may actually be "a source of order, of coherence, of organization."[34] They asserted that irreversible processes have an enormous constructive importance: "Life would not be possible without them."[35]

Entropy

Entropy relates directly to the notions of self-organization and irreversibility. It refers to disorder and energy loss. The physical sciences consider the laws of thermodynamics to apply to all systems, yet the second law suggests that time produces an increase in entropy, in disorder. In mechanical systems, this produces breakdowns, either gradual or, like the "one-horse shay," sudden. "It was in order to distinguish the two types of processes (reversible and irreversible) that the concept of entropy was introduced, since entropy increases only because of the far-from-equilibrium, irreversible processes."[20] Entropy is described as "the name for the quality of systems that increases under the second law-mixing, disorder, randomness."[36] Thelen and Ulrich more simply defined entropy as "disorder in the universe."[37] Basically, entropy correlates with the amount of energy spent and is usually given a positive label; it increases. Therefore, entropy applies to processes of an irreversible nature, because energy is not restored from within the system.

"Increasing entropy corresponds to the spontaneous evolution of the system . . . for all isolated systems, the future is in the direction of increasing entropy."[38]

Pattern Formation

Through this process of self-organization, new, unexpected, and more complex patterns are formed. "The detailed form of the new phase is essentially unpredictable."[39] Davies states that the simplest physical form of self-organization is a phase transition, or phase shift, such as changing the liquid to a gas. One example of a phase transition is the acquisition of new behaviors during infant development.[3] More about pattern formation is discussed under the concept of emergence.

Phase Shifts

Far From Equilibrium

These spontaneous transition or phase shifts, described as the process of self-organization, generally occur in far-from-equilibrium states.[18] While self-organization can occur in equilibrium and far-from-equilibrium states, usually the "systems driven far-from-equilibrium tend to undergo abrupt spontaneous changes of behavior. They may start to behave erratically, or to organize themselves into new unexpected forms."[31] They are characterized by "a continual throughput of matter and energy from [the] environment."[40] The far-from-equilibrium states all contain an element of instability and a tendency to seek out increasing levels of complexity and organization. Prigogine and Stengers referred to these states or structures as "dissipative structures." These dissipative structures "evade the degenerative effects of the second law by exporting entropy into its environment."[41] The emergence of life itself was postulated by Davies as having emerged from far-from-equilibrium conditions.

Emergence

No discussion of dynamic systems or complexity would be complete without addressing the principle of emergence. Emergence is inherent to all dynamic systems and is discussed by each of the previous authors. Emergence refers to the spontaneous formation of a new pattern of organization of subsystems (behavior) that is not specified by the subsystems. In other words, the original elements cooperate to produce an organization not contained within the individual units. The behavior of the system is *not* the sum of its parts.

At this point, it is important to acknowledge that emergent qualities were important in the general systems or open systems view. Emergence is not a new concept nor unique to dynamic systems. In the open systems model, it was suggested that from the lower subsystems arose the emergent phenomenon that identified the higher level, much as we feel the mind arises out of, but is more than and different from, the combined neural elements of the brain itself. What is new about the dynamic systems view is that it is nonhierarchical. No one subsystem has priority for organizing the behavior of the system as is suggested in hierarchical thinking. The subsystems relate heterarchically. Dynamic systems theory suggests that out of any combination of subsystems, with change in some parameter, the disequilibrium of living may produce spontaneous self-organization with the emergence of new, more complex levels of occupational performance. This type of emergence is the identifying property of nonlinear systems.

Nonlinearity

Nonlinear relationships prevail in far-from-equilibrium conditions.[8] Systems "become inordinately sensitive to external influences. Small inputs yield huge, startling effects. The entire system may reorganize itself in ways that strike us as bizarre."[42] This should not be confused with the issue of reversibility versus irreversibility. All nonlinear patterns are irreversible. The term "nonlinear" is used to describe the situation in which a spontaneous and unpredictable phase or pattern emerges without all the intermediate steps, or *linear* relationships, that would naturally link it to the former state. This is in contrast to a linear system in which a single cause and its effect are linked proportionately.[1] Correspondingly, a linear system is thought to be reducible to its component parts without distortion. It follows the model of reductionism in which knowledge of the component parts adds up to knowledge of the whole. On the other hand, "in a nonlinear system, the whole is much more than the sum of its parts, and it cannot be reduced or analyzed in terms of simple subunits acting together."[48]

Nonlinearity describes spontaneous self-organization.[13] As an application, Thelen[44] and Kamm et al.[3] believed that the processes of development, for example, motor development, are nonlinear. Another example of nonlinearity in behavior is the gait pattern of a horse. "When horses change their gait from a walk to a trot to a gallop, the phase relationships between the limbs are abruptly changed . . . [and] discontinuous because there is no stable intermediate gait between a walk and a trot."[45] The new stepping behavior spontaneously emerges. When one becomes aware of the heterarchical nonlinearity in a dynamic system's behavior, the possibility of any type of regularity seems remote. However, some regularity is indeed observed in emergent phenomena, and attractor states provide some means of explaining that regularity.[4]

Attractor States

An attractor is a preferred pattern of behavior or state to which the system is attracted.[1,8] According to Kamm et al., the "concept that the organism, the task, and the context self-organize behavior to a preferred form, or attractor, is central to a dynamical approach."[46] An attractor is a common but not obligatory configuration (state or behavior) of the system. It is a behavioral pattern easily fallen into and returned to after perturbation, after disruption. Complex physical systems tend to discover remarkably stable states possessing a high degree of cooperative activity and organization.[1]

Attractor states are emergent phenomena.[4] It is important to emphasize their emergence because due to the consistent nature of attractor states, they can often be misperceived as preprogrammed or determined states. Attractor states are certain patterns of behavior autonomously preferred by complex systems strictly "as a result of the cooperativeness of the participating elements in a particular context."[47] Chemical equilibrium is an example of an attractor state.[8]

Attractor states also can be described qualitatively. Sometimes called attractor "wells,"[3] they may be identified as deep or shallow, depending on "the ease with which the system returns to the attractor and on how difficult it is to move the system away from or out of the attractor."[48] In terms of the system's behavior, while in a shallow attractor, behavior is preferred but flexible. Within a deep attractor, behavior is limited and often considered hard-wired or obligatory.[3]

The Parameters

Certain variables of the dynamic system involved in phase shifts have been described as order and control parameters. The terms "order parameters" and "control parameters" seem to have arisen out of synergetics, "the study of physical, chemical, and biological systems that are composed of a large number of components or degrees of freedom" by Haken.[4,49] These terms, as applied to components of dynamic systems, provide additional conceptualization of the complex processes.

Order Parameters

Order parameters are variables that express the compression of the multiple degrees of freedom by apparently ordering the previously disorganized system.[4] As Thelen and Ulrich described, "when the multiple degrees of freedom of complex systems are compressed, *under certain physical and thermodynamic conditions*, the resulting system can be described more parsimoniously in terms of one or several variables that express this compression."[47] These variables are usually called the order parameters (or by Thelen and Ulrich as the collective variable). The order parameter is simply "the dimension of the system that expresses the underlying pattern that emerges from the cooperation of the elements."[47] The notion of order parameters or collective variables is used to provide a framework for research into these complex systems. According to Scholz,[26] through identifying the order parameters of a system, conditions precipitating change and the effects of parameter manipulations can be discovered, and formal modeling of coordinative patterns and predictions about a system's behavior can be accurately generated. The order parameter is the variable of interest in many studies. For example, alternating leg movements on a treadmill is identified by Thelen and Ulrich as the order parameter in their study on newborn infant stepping behavior.

Control Parameters

A control parameter is the variable responsible for moving the system through its collective phases or stages. It can be organic or environmental. When changing, the control parameter "leads to corresponding changes . . . in the collective behavior of the system."[50] The control parameters are considered "nonspecific" in that "the variable being changed does not specify to the system what pattern it should adopt . . . [but] a change in such a variable is seen to provide a sufficient condition for pattern change to occur."[51] Another important aspect of the control parameter is that a small change in a control parameter may have large effects on the behavior of the system, and different control parameters may influence the phase shift or pattern formation at different times.[3] This is precisely why dynamic systems are described as nonhierarchical. A change in the control parameter, often a seemingly insignificant one, causes and defines the emergence of a new pattern in the behavior of the collective system.

The concept of control parameters is useful for research models. Scholz explains "observing the behavior of candidate variables in the region of a pattern transition may allow one to determine which of these variables is an order parameter (or control parameter) for the behavior."[51] Van Geert,[52] in his model on cognitive and language growth, described the control variable as a "timing device for the dependent variable. . . . The dependent variable cannot start growing until the control variable starts growing or until the latter has reached some threshold level."[53] Fat gain among infants was identified as a control parameter in a study on infant stepping behavior.[3] As Kamm et al. described, although it is not specific to stepping, fat gain "specifically reordered the assembly of the stepping behavior."[46]

Conclusion

In summary, this paper represents a thorough review of the theory of dynamic systems. At this point, it is hoped that readers familiar with occupational therapy and occupational science have begun to consider the possible relationship of this theory to the study of human occupation. There is no doubt one is faced with incomparable complexity when studying the human as an occupational being and attempting to bring about changes in the behavior patterns of people who are affected by illness or injury.

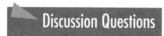

Discussion Questions

1. How is dynamic systems theory similar to general systems theory? How does it differ? In other words, what important aspects of complex systems behavior does dynamic systems theory uncover?
2. Do you agree that dynamic systems theory could benefit occupational science? What might be some possible applications?

References

1. Davies, P: The Cosmic Blueprint. Simon & Schuster, Inc., New York, 1988, p 25.
2. Davies, p 22.
3. Kamm, K, Thelen, E, and Jensen, JL: A dynamical systems approach to motor development. Phys Ther 70:763, 771, 1990.
4. Thelen, E, and Ulrich, BD: Hidden skills: A dynamical systems analysis of treadmill stepping during the first year. Monographs of the Society for Research in Child Development, 223(1), 1991.
5. von Bertalanffy, L: Perspectives on General System Theory. Braziller, New York, 1975.
6. Kielhofner, G, and Burke, JP: A model of human occupation, part I. Conceptual framework and content. Am J Occup Ther 34:572, 1980.

7. Clark, FA, Parham, D, Carlson, ME, Frank, G, Jackson, J, Pierce, D, Wolfe, RJ, and Zemke, R: Occupational science: Academic innovation in the service of occupational therapy's future. Am J Occup Ther 45:300, 1991.
8. Prigogine, I, and Stengers, I: Order Out of Chaos: Man's New Dialogue with Nature. Bantam Books, New York, 1984.
9. Prigogine & Stengers, p 8–9.
10. Prigogine & Stengers, p 105.
11. Prigogine & Stengers, p. xxviii.
12. Gleick, J: Chaos: Making a New Science. Penguin Books, New York, 1987.
13. Kugler, PN, Kelson, JAS, and Turvey, MT: On the control and coordination of naturally developing systems. In Kelso, JAS, and Clark, JE (eds), The Development of Movement Control and Coordination. Wiley & Sons, New York, pp 5–78.
14. Laszlo, E: The Systems View of the World: The Natural Philosophy of the New Developments in Science. Braziller, New York, 1972.
15. Prigogine & Stengers, p 7.
16. Kugler et al., p 23.
17. Kugler et al., p 24.
18. Prigogine & Stengers, p 11.
19. Prigogine & Stengers, p 219.
20. Prigogine & Stengers, p 12.
21. Kugler et al., p 27.
22. Kugler et al., p 29.
23. Prigogine & Stengers, p 8.
24. Toffler, A: Foreword: Science and change. In Prigogine, I, and Stengers, I (eds): Order Out of Chaos: Man's New Dialogue with Nature. Bantam Books, New York, 1984, pp xi–xxvi.
25. Prigogine & Stengers, p xxvii.
26. Thelen & Ulrich, p 8.
27. Thelen & Ulrich, p 7.
28. Scholz, JP: Dynamic pattern theory: Some implications for therapeutics. Phys Ther 70:763, 1990.
29. Scholz, p 827.
30. Kamm et al., p 770.
31. Davies, p 83.
32. Davies, p 73.
33. Davies, p 14.
34. Prigogine & Stengers, p 15.
35. Prigogine & Stengers, p 125.
36. Gleick, p 257.
37. Thelen & Ulrich, p 13.
38. Prigogine & Stengers, p 119.
39. Davies, p 84.
40. Davies, p 183.
41. Davies, p 85.
42. Prigogine & Stengers, p xvi.
43. Davies, p 25.
44. Thelen, E: The (re)discovery of motor development: Learning new things from an old field. Dev Psychol 25(6):946, 1989.
45. Thelen, E, Kelso, JAS, and Fogel, A: Self-organizing systems and infant motor development. Dev Rev 7:39, 1987.
46. Kamm et al., p 772.
47. Thelen & Ulrich, p 10.
48. Kamm et al., p 771.
49. Scholz, p 829.
50. Thelen & Ulrich, p 11.
51. Scholz, p 832.
52. van Geert, P: A dynamic systems model of cognitive and language growth. Psychol Rev 98:3, 1991.
53. van Geert, p 41.

by Julie McLaughlin Gray, MA, OTR,
Bonnie L. Kennedy, MEPD, OTR,
and Ruth Zemke, PhD, OTR, FAOTA

29

Application of Dynamic Systems Theory to Occupation

Is Application Appropriate?

It has been suggested by occupational science founders that occupational science will necessarily incorporate material and research from other fields.[1] Nevertheless, materials should not be assimilated indiscriminately. As responsible investigators, occupational scientists must consider the potential relevance and usefulness of various outside theories to their area of inquiry. Three ways of justifying the use of dynamic systems theory as a complement to the study of human occupation are discussed here: examination of its application in other fields, direct recommendations for application by dynamic systems theorists, and last, its goodness of fit with occupational science.

The use of dynamic systems theory in other fields of inquiry may provide some justification for its application to occupational science. The dynamic pattern theory, or dynamic systems theory, has been used within several disciplines outside of physics as a model for explaining and adding understanding to complex behavior. Dynamic systems theory has been used to understand and study motor development by such scholars as Kamm and her colleagues.[2] Thelen and Ulrich[3] used a dynamic systems model to identify the multiple elements involved in infant locomotion. These individuals recognized that although human motor development is characterized by milestones, there also is a degree of fluidity and unpredictability within those parameters. Dynamic systems theory is used to study and explain the complexity of this development process. Dynamic systems theory also was used by van Geert[4] to examine cognitive and language growth and by Kelso and Tuller[5] and others to explore the behavior of action systems. A defense for inclusion of dynamic systems theory in occupational science can begin with these examples. While all of this research seems to support the import of dynamic systems theory into occupational science studies, they are not sufficient reasons in and of themselves. After all, the profession of occupational therapy has learned through history that it can be compromised by simply attempting to mirror the important work of others.

Another strong endorsement for the application of dynamic systems theory to the study of human occupation comes from encouragement by primary sources within the mathematical and physical sciences. Prigogine and Stengers,[6] considered a classic reference for this material, believed these new developments in science represent a coming together of science and the humanities, a "conceptual revolution" with far-reaching implications related to qualitative changes in behavior or processes on a number of levels. They acknowledged that there are different classes of dynamic systems; in other words, they are not all molecular. Likewise, Toffler believed the Prigoginian model lends itself to what he calls "analogical extension"[7] and stated that these ideas are beginning to spawn research in economics, human geography, ecology, urban studies, and several other disciplines. Therefore, if encouragement by those considered "grandparents" of this theory is justification, perhaps application is appropriate.

Finally, and most importantly, the goodness of fit between dynamic systems theory and occupational science goals must be considered in a decision to use this material. Common to other applications of dynamic systems theory is the acknowledgment by the researchers of the complex nature of dynamic systems, including the multiplicity of possible contributing and inter-related variables of the phenomenon under study, the emergence of spontaneous state changes, and the importance of context or environment as an essential consideration in processes of change. Behavior is considered an emergent property of the interaction of many subsystems and is not explainable in the mechanistic terms of classical science.

Likewise, occupational therapists have recognized that the occupational behavior of their clients cannot be predicted or explained by analysis of any single underlying system. Range of motion in a joint cannot, in and of itself, predict an individual's likelihood of playing the guitar after surgery, for example. Clients have surprised therapists in innumerable ways. Occupational science founders admit that because "occupational science deals with universals, it must necessarily be abstract at the conceptual level."[8] Therefore, it would seem appropriate to use an admittedly abstract model, such as dynamic systems theory, in the study of human occupation if it will shed light on the complex processes involved. It is the authors' shared belief that application is a worthwhile enterprise.

Application to Human Occupation

How might this theory help explain and understand occupation? This application is organized around four major features of dynamic systems as discussed by Thelen and Ulrich[3] in their monograph on a dynamic systems analysis of infant locomotion. These features are complexity, self-organization, phase shifts, and collective variables and attractor states. A discussion of the relevance of this material to human occupation raises more questions than provides answers, but nonetheless, the hope is to inspire a stimulating discourse.

It is important when applying any of these concepts that occupational scientists identify their "unit of analysis." What is the outcome, or pattern, they are attempting to explain and understand? The authors propose that human engagement in occupation is the emerging pattern of interest in the dynamic system studied in occupational science. A deeper understanding of the processes involved in human occupation from a dynamic systems perspective also may prove valuable to occupational therapists because efforts in therapy attempt to create changes in the occupational behavior of others, and occupation is used to create change.

Complexity

Complexity may possibly be considered the signature feature of dynamic systems. Dynamic systems are characterized by remarkable levels of complexity, both in terms of the multiplicity of variables involved and the behavior of the system over time. As mentioned in the previous paper, all of these complex elements are arranged in a nonhierarchical fashion. Occupational scientists and occupational therapists investigate an extremely complex phenomenon, the interaction between the human and the environment on multiple levels within human occupation, and occupational scientists aim to illuminate this complex phenomenon from a nonreductionistic view of human activity and health. Zemke, in her paper in this book, asserted, "with the interdisciplinary nature of the development of occupational science, we must search for and use scientific knowledge which rejects . . . dualism and supports the complexity of the human as an occupational being."

The significance of context and environment is consistently addressed when describing the complexity of dynamic systems. Thelen and Ulrich, in their descriptions of early limb coordination, discussed the importance of what they call "facilitative contexts."[9] In their example and within dynamic systems in general, no particular component alone could influence this developmental behavior; "all together are necessary."[10] Likewise, occupational therapists and occupational scientists have consistently recognized the importance of environmental context in their theories and treatment approaches. Dynamic systems theory might provide a framework for examining just how environmental contexts interact with other factors in the formation of occupational patterns and which types of environmental contexts are most conducive to participation in certain occupations.

As an example, dynamic pattern theory may offer a way of conceptualizing the processes involved in adaptation through occupation. Literature on adaptation acknowledges several possible influences on adaptive behavior, such as cognitive processes,[11] support networks,[12] and social ideologic constraints.[13] When one considers the range of potential combinations between internal and external components, the complexity of adaptation through occupation can be appreciated. Dynamic systems theory may provide a means of sorting out the patterns and relationships amidst this complexity.

Self-Organization

Closely related to this feature of complexity is the tendency for dynamic systems, as they evolve over time, to demonstrate a propensity for self-organization. Pattern formation is the classic example of self-organization. Self-organizing systems are characterized by multiple degrees of freedom (the many different ways in which they might combine and form a pattern) and irreversibility. The pattern to be formed is not predetermined. As a pattern is formed, however, the degrees of freedom are reduced because their role then becomes determined by the emerging pattern.

Occupation may play a significant role in self-organization. The self-organization that occurs through the interaction of the organism with the environment over time is one that has, through evolutionary success, become a particularly strong element in human function. From the seemingly random behavior of the infant, recognizable patterns of the individual within a particular cultural and physical milieu emerge. The variety of competent and skilled occupational performances increases with time until one has a potentially satisfying repertoire from which to orchestrate his or her daily round of activities.

Degrees of freedom are evident in the number of ways the elements or components of human occupation may combine to form a pattern of engagement in particular occupations. The elements possessing multiple degrees of freedom might be likened to performance components and contexts, as outlined in the American Occupational Therapy Association's Uniform Terminology.[14] In a dynamic system, such as the occupational human, the complexity of the possible behaviors is almost overwhelming to consider, yet at any given moment, one sees behavior representing a particular combination. In fact, combinations are recurrent such that we can recognize them across people as states, such as an infant sleeping, a toddler throwing a tantrum, a student alert and attentive, a couple expressing their love, and the mourning of an elder at the loss of a lifetime partner. In spite of the complexity and apparent infinite variety of possible combinations of human subsystems, task, and context, occupational behavior takes relatively stable forms. The stable states are as interesting to occupational science as the processes of change.

The belief that the behavior is not predetermined but actively evolves from the interaction of many processes is in concert with occupational scientists who also state that "humans are not preprogrammed to engage in a planned round of activities."[15] Occupational therapists and occupational scientists hold that individuals make decisions regarding their engagements in occupations. This suggests the limit of nondeterminism. What does this model tell us about occupation? Can we use this model to identify patterns in the increasing complexity of human occupation? Some interesting parallels can be drawn.

Self-organization or pattern formation, like occupation, occurs within the stream of time. The processes are irreversible; in other words, they "depend on the direction of time."[16] Discussions of time and time use have existed in occupational therapy since Adolph Meyer,[17] and temporality has been recognized as an important component of occupational behavior and within the study of occupational science. This irreversibility of time and change in living systems is one of the reasons that traditional reductionistic scientific approaches are not sufficient to study occupation. One cannot break an egg down to its constituents and then put it back together again, even with all the queen's horses and men of the traditional scientific establishment.

It seems that occupational therapists have been examining irreversible processes without labeling them as such. The physicist Paul Davies[18] used components of daily occupations to exemplify irreversibility, such as breaking an egg and stirring milk into tea. Occupations are described as occurring within the stream of time. Within the course of a day, humans as occupational beings are thought to "configure activities within time that can be chunked and correspondingly labeled."[19] The human as an occupational being displays irreversibility, or time-oriented, unidirectional change. Across time, individuals develop their individual histories of experience. One begins the narrative journey that is the description of self and carries out the actions by which an identity is formed, recognizable to oneself and others. Even most of the repeated daily rituals, the fairly simple task of taking a sip of coffee and returning the cup to a desk, for example, cannot be reversed, in the physical sense, especially when the numerous interacting components must be considered. Irreversibility in human occupation becomes painfully evident in the scenario described below, that of women who have been infected with HIV.

The concept of entropy poses some interesting questions when related to occupation. Perhaps the aging and death of living systems represents this irreversible loss of energy, but within a lifetime, it may represent a positive force, not just a negative one. Although entropy, or increasing disorder with energy output, is a fact of life from infancy on, occupation offers the opportunity to take in energy and increase order within the system. Czikszentmihalyi and Larson[20] discussed the energizing or negentropic effect of challenging activity, such as that in which we can develop the state of flow. For example, they described that certain occupations, which they labeled negentropic, may help adolescents overcome the destabilizing effect of puberty and the anxiety of losing the familiar historical narrative of childhood and facing an unknown future of adulthood.

Phase Shifts

Prigogine and Stengers summarized dynamic systems theory as a whole new development in which "science . . . [is] rediscovering time, due to the nonlinearity that is now acknowledged in complex systems."[21] To reiterate, nonlinearity relates to the notion that small events can create large changes in the system's behavior. This means that a small change in a subsystem or a change in a small subsystem may have a large effect on the individual. It is in contrast to reductionism, the model of traditional physical science that has been inadequate to explain much of human behavior. In a nonlinear relationship, the whole can be more than the sum of its parts, the life more than constituent chemicals and structural features. As Toffler[22] described, when a system reaches a far-from-equilibrium condition, it is inherently impossible to know in advance how the system will change or adapt. When nonlinear changes occur, the new behavior pattern is described as emergent. New types of structures may spontaneously originate that reflect the interaction of the system with its surroundings.

According to dynamic system theory, the disequilibrium resulting from increasing entropy with time, such as aging, or from a nonlinear change in a control parameter, such as disability, does not have to produce any given pattern or outcome. On the other hand, a fairly linear view would suggest that a person who has had a spinal cord injury will produce a phase shift or reorganization into a more limited group of attractor states, with less variety of occupational performance (somewhat predictable from the functional cord level) and in general, a less satisfying and complex life than that which had been previously experienced. Thus, our developmental view of an infant's or child's discontinuity and even temporary disruption in performance with development of a new motor or other milestone performance also can be reflected in an occupational therapy view of the individual's potential response to disease, impairment, or disability. That is, in the complex dynamic human system, the disequilibrium produced by these potential control parameters may be the source of new self-organization, stimulated by control parameters from within the occupational therapy treatment process. A new, more complex, reorganization of the individual as an occupational being may occur.

Again, we see many examples of nonlinearity in human occupation. Bateson,[23] in her work *Composing A Life*, described a similar spontaneity and unpredictability in the discovery or creation of one's life goals. Occupational patterns do, at times, appear to be emergent phenomena, the result of the interaction of many variables on multiple levels, usually unexplainable by simple reduction to the component parts. Florence Cromwell, in a Spring 1995 occupational therapy history lecture given at the invitation of the members of Pi Theta Epsilon at the University of Southern California, gave a beautiful example of an unexpected, emergent pattern as the result of occupation. She described a significantly disabled and dependent woman who, with the help of her occupational therapist, elected to sew and make a bathrobe for her brother. She was able to do very little with her arms and therefore several adaptations had to be made. Nevertheless, she completed the bathrobe and gave it to her brother, and in Florence Cromwell's words, "that bathrobe was a transforming event in her family."

It seems that therapists frequently see similar responses and changes in and as a result of occupational therapy with their patients in treatment. The experience of the onset of disability may be a destabilizing element, disrupting stable attractor patterns of occupation in the individual and demonstrating a major increase in entropy, or energy loss, and increased disorder. However, out of such a major life perturbation, occupational therapy and dynamic systems theory posit the possibility of reorganization that is not only stable, but more complex than that which existed before the disability. Experiences acquired through engagement in activity are often transforming, frequently in ways one cannot predict. An example might be the ability of the experience of caring for one's physical body to lead to changes in the emotional state of someone who is depressed. Another example is the observation that a person who is recovering from a stroke who refuses to work on self-care activities in treatment displays spontaneous and unexpected increases in self-care independence after a few sessions of working on his or her ability to swing a golf club, their chosen occupation. The concepts of nonlinearity and emergence may help occupational therapists and scientists further understand these processes of change, particularly unpredictable change.

Order and Control Parameters and Attractor States

Finally, examination of the notions of attractor states, collective variables (also called order parameters), and control parameters in relation to human occupation may prove useful. As mentioned, these components are most helpful in the research of a dynamic system. Specifically, identification of attractor states and control and order parameters assist in organizing and studying the regularity of behaviors witnessed in dynamic systems.

These regularities are called attractor states. Complex systems seem to "prefer patterns of behavior strictly as a result of the cooperativeness of the participating elements in a particular context."[24] In a sense, the notion of attractor states may provide a rationale for studying such complex behavior as human engagement in occupation. It seems inherent in the choice to develop a profession such as occupational therapy and similarly, a science of occupation that some regularity in terms of occupational behavior has been observed.

Attractor states might refer to occupations themselves or perhaps patterns of occupation that emerge with regularity through the interaction of various components within a particular context. Zemke, in the recent American Occupational Therapy Association Self-Study series,[25] has considered attractor states as a potentially useful concept in studying habits, for example. In relatively deep attractor wells, such as routines and habits, common patterns of occupation, such as self-care activities, are observed almost universally. Possible degrees of freedom are reduced or compressed by routine and habit. Occupational behavior is so complex and multifaceted that examination on multiple levels seems essential to determine what might be an attractor for a given individual.

Order and control parameters are helpful in sorting through this complex multiplicity of variables. Essentially, order parameters define the variable of interest, meaning the dependent variable. In other words, the order parameter is a dimension or attribute of the system that measures or describes the pattern. In occupational science, an order parameter might be some aspect of occupational performance that one wishes to examine and understand in relation to several variables, such as independent use of public transportation by an individual with schizophrenia or adoption of new daily routines on retirement.

Control parameters are variables that are responsible for moving the system through phases or stages. In other words, the control parameter is identified as the variable that when changed, elicits the larger change in the behavior of the whole system. What is significant about control parameters is that there is not a cause and effect relationship between the variable and the resultant change. The change occurs only as a result of a shift in the control parameter within the confluence of several other variables.

An examination of the control parameters in occupation might yield information as to what specifically causes changes in occupational behavior and within occupational therapy, for that matter. It seems that occupational therapists attempt to influence control parameters. It would be helpful to explore the elements involved in the interaction of the human with the environment and the interaction between patient and therapist to identify the components (including contexts) that lead to change with some regularity. Are occupational therapists convinced that it is their current interventions, or do they sometimes wonder, in the sea of components involved in occupation and occupational therapy, what most influences a transformation in behavior? Is the occupational therapy the control parameter? In human occupation, is choice or decision a prevailing control parameter? Likewise, knowledge of the control parameters in occupational patterns that are less "healthy" or functional in a particular context may be helpful as well in terms of prevention.

An Example: Women and HIV

This example is a beginning effort to apply dynamic systems thinking to occupation on a relative macroscopic level of socially constructed systems. In comparison, the work of developmental theorists[3] focuses on the development of motor skills in individuals, which is on a level of relative microsystems. Precedent has been set for the application of dynamic systems theory to macrosystems with the work of Vallacher and Nowak,[26] who examined dynamic systems in human social behavior.

What follows is an outline of contexts of occupation. These contexts are taken from demographic descriptions of people with AIDS provided by the Centers for Disease Control and Prevention (CDC).[27] Early in the AIDS epidemic, demographic variables were considered risk factors. However, the term "risk factors" was misleading because it placed the focus on groups, such as homosexual men, Haitians, and heroin users.[28] The focus now is on risk behaviors that expose a person to bodily fluids carrying HIV, such as sharing needles for intravenous (IV) drug use or unprotected sexual intercourse. This conceptual shift is the focus of health education and disease prevention information from the CDC and the American Red Cross.

Interestingly, the analysis of risk factors for a variety of human illnesses did not demonstrate the expected additive linear process in the work of Milsum[29] who used relative risk analysis. Milsum suggested the need to apply nonlinear systems thinking to the analysis of health and disease. Likewise, Vallacher and Nowak[26] suggested that while dynamic systems theory may not become a unified theory to explain everything about behavior, its value does lie in the shift in thinking to consider a variety of nonlinear processes in building and testing theory in human social behavior. Feminist theorists have challenged linear and hierarchical thinking in their own field, and this work appears highly compatible with the analysis presented here of the contexts of occupation of women with HIV infection.

The work of black feminist theorists, such as Patricia Hill Collins,[30] posits that the relative lack of privilege or what might be interpreted as the lack of access to resources and health-promoting occupations for black women is the result of an intersection of social systems of race, class, and gender that structures opportunities in society. Audra Lorde,[31] a black feminist, brought sexual orientation into the discourse of oppression, citing the denial of rights to women who are lesbians. No one system—race, class, or gender—is credited as the cause of social conditions that deny many women of color access to adequate health care, education, and employment; safety for themselves and their families; and respect.

In short, these intersecting systems of race, class, and gender compress the degrees of freedom to engage in a wide variety of healthful occupations and to derive the benefits of satisfaction and adequate support, those associated with productive living. Women can be denied access to opportunities for health care, housing, jobs, and control of their daily occupations through the intersection of environmental systems of race, class, gender, sexual orientation, and disability status. This discussion uses the experience of women who are infected with HIV, which is associated with AIDS, as an example of systems that collectively intersect and compress the degrees of freedom of women, creating phase shifts in patterns of health.

As previously described, dynamic systems theory recognizes that change in a system, such as a human, results from a confluence of intersecting variables. So many variables are involved in the health status of women with HIV that for the purpose of this brief presentation, focus is on the performance contexts of occupation as examples of potential control parameters initiating change in a system. A brief background on HIV and women is followed by the application of dynamic systems theory to this complex scenario.

Overview: HIV and AIDS

Based on 1992 data from the CDC,[27] AIDS is the fourth leading cause of death among 25- to 45-year-old women in the United States. There was a 9% increase in AIDS cases in women between 1991 and 1992, while the increase in men was only 2.5%.[27] HIV is the necessary but not sufficient cause of AIDS. HIV disease is a chronic condition manifested by a spectrum of opportunistic diseases and declining CD4 and T-cell counts.[32]

The CDC has created a hierarchical, categoric diagnostic system for HIV infection.[32] A two-dimensional grid is used to classify the disease process, using descending categories of T-cell counts along the vertical axis and symptoms of immunosupression along the horizontal. Once a person is classified, she or he can only move into a more severe category. If the person experiences an improvement in health, he or she cannot be placed in a less severe category. The model used to develop this diagnostic system uses a linear conceptualization of the disease process, from the point of infection to the point of death. This model is not consistent with the life experience of people with HIV. In their experience, health appears as a fluctuating pattern across time of all parameters, including T-cell counts, symptoms, and occupational function.

HIV is a blood-borne pathogen that is transmitted primarily through occupations such as IV drug use and sexual contact. Unlike the polio epidemic, which spread as an airborne pathogen, HIV spreads from body to body across the globe through human activity. That is one reason that HIV disease is the clinical application chosen for this example of dynamic systems application to occupation.

The routes of transmission also have been outlined by the CDC. Once again, a hierarchical model (Table 29-1) is described with transmission categories listed at the top automatically taking precedence over other transmission categories listed at the bottom. This means, for example, that if a woman has used injectable drugs once, this is assumed to be her transmission category regardless of sexual contacts. This hierarchical thinking obscures the high rate of sexual transmission and creates a pattern of data reporting that may be misleading. Injectable drug use is the listed largest category of transmission because it is automatically assumed to be the mode of transmission if the individual has ever engaged in that occupation. This presentation of data can create a false sense of security that puts a woman's health at risk. For example, in a dating situation, a woman may assume that "HIV is a disease that happens to people who use drugs. So I'm safe. This guy looks clean." A doctor may assume that "This is a nice lady; she doesn't need an HIV test." It also should be noted that there is no transmission category for sexual contact between women, which has led directly to the myth that "lesbians do not get AIDS."

A Dynamic Systems Analysis

Women, particularly black and Hispanic women, draw attention to a dynamic systems analysis of HIV disease because they are over-represented in the epidemic. This over-representation may be associated with the proposed compression of degrees of freedom available to them to engage in health-promoting occupations. As mentioned previously, the writings of black feminists[30, 33-34] have pointed out that the limited opportunities, resources, and power available to black women is the result of the intersection of systems of race, class, and gender, which provides structure for much social activity. These black feminist writers have rejected linear, hierarchical models previously proposed by predominantly white feminists (for example, liberal and radical) that proposed gender as the variable that was the cause of the underprivileged status of all women.

Table 29-1   Exposure Categories

Men who have sex with men
Injecting drugs
Men who have sex with men and injecting drug use
Hemophilia/coagulation disorder
Heterosexual contact
Receipt of blood products
Other, not identified risks

Adapted from Centers for Disease Control and Prevention, HIV/AIDS Surveillance Report (6)1, 1994.

In addition to race, class, and gender, disability status, such as being HIV positive, is itself a socially identified status variable used as the basis of discrimination. After their HIV-positive status was discovered, both women and men have lost their homes, jobs, friends, and family contacts. Some have lost their doctors, who have refused to treat them, and a few have even been denied access to airline flights. The contexts of occupation contain many control parameters that compress the degrees of freedom available to HIV-positive women engaging in occupation. The application of dynamic systems theory in this paper is a biopsychosocial view of health that takes a multidimensional stance on the causes of disease, disallowing unitary cause disease models, like germ theory, which typically recognizes only a single pathogen as the cause of disease.

Potential Control Parameters

Concepts from dynamic systems theory, such as potential control parameters, can be identified in contexts of occupation related to women with HIV. To reiterate, a control parameter, according to dynamic systems theory, would be the variable in which change engenders a change or phase shift in the entire system. A phase shift in this example would be a change in the pattern of health of a woman in relation to HIV infection status.

The performance contexts of occupation from the Uniform Terminology of the American Occupational Therapy Association[14] are used as a helpful tool in organizing this example. These performance contexts are the temporal aspects, including chronologic, developmental, life cycle, and disability status, and the environmental aspects, including physical, social, and cultural components of performance contexts of occupation. The following is an outline of those performance contexts as they relate to women and HIV. These contexts represent some of the multiple variables, each with multiple degrees of freedom, interacting in this dynamic system.

Temporal Aspects

Chronological Age

Most women diagnosed with AIDS are between 25 and 35 years of age. Because HIV is present in the body 10 to 15 years before the onset of AIDS, these women became infected between 15 and 20 years of age.

Developmental Stage

Young women are becoming infected with HIV at the highest rate in their late teens and early 20s. Heterosexual contact, an occupation, is the most rapidly rising mode of transmission for women in the United States.[35] A difficulty accepting personal mortality, portrayed by thoughts, such as, "It can't happen to me" or "not just this once," characterizes this developmental stage. Important occupational science questions are what are the occupational patterns of these young women? What opportunities are there for them to engage in health-promoting occupations? What knowledge is accessible to them? Considering that some middle and high schools do not teach anything about sex, much less safer sex, to attempt to prevent transmission of HIV to this vulnerable group, what power do these young women have to demand information or to negotiate for safer sex?

Life Cycle

Many women find out they are HIV positive in the course of pregnancy or shortly after having a baby. Women of childbearing age (15 to 44 years) accounted for 84% of the cases of women with HIV in 1993.[35] Multiple caregiver roles are a fact of life for most women in this age group. Health care providers find that many women do not keep appointments for themselves nor even make appointments in the absence of available child care. They also have observed that women take care of their own health care last, attending to others in the family before themselves.

Disability Status

HIV serostatus has been the basis of discrimination for housing, education for children, employment, transportation, child custody, and access to marriage partners. The performance context of the disability status of being HIV positive operates as a stigma. Women with HIV are selective about who and when they tell about their HIV status because of fear of discrimination, which may lead to losses of social contacts, day care for their children, and generally freedom to continue their usual round of daily activity, including their jobs.

Environmental Aspects

Physical

Geographic location is one aspect of the physical environment that bears a relationship to women and HIV. The AIDS epidemic in the United States from 1983 to 1993 has grown substantially and is concentrated in urban centers, primarily in coastal areas.[27] As would be expected, the presence of HIV in the environment does increase the likelihood of exposure to the virus through engagement in occupations. There also is a high prevalence rate among women in Africa and in certain areas of Asia. If one asserts that there is nothing biologically, morally, or intellectually weaker about the women in areas with a high incidence of the virus, then these data suggest the importance of the physical contexts of occupation.

The presence of micropathogens associated with opportunistic infections vary across the globe. These opportunistic infections generally lead to death in people with HIV. The most common cause of death in women with AIDS in the United States is pneumonia,[27] while in Africa the most common cause of death is gastrointestinal diseases from parasites, resulting in dehydration and malnutrition.

Community resources also might be included as an environmental variable in the disease process. Historically, women have been excluded from clinical trials of drug treatment in the United States. The National Institute of Health guidelines for research projects has changed, and women are beginning to be included. Generally, participation involves access to free medications and medical care. It is suggested that this access to free health care may influence health. Clinical trials and medical personnel who specialize in HIV care are concentrated in cities. Rural women have less access to these services.

The availability of occupations for social and economic support can be considered part of context. At the Ninth International Conference on AIDS in Berlin, Dr. Karen Hein reported a sharp rise in the number of young adolescent girls diagnosed with AIDS around the world.[36] Many of these cases have resulted from what Hein called "survival" sex: unprotected heterosexual intercourse in exchange for food, clothing, and shelter, not drugs. She distinguished between survival sex and commercial sex, from which we can infer that form, function, and meaning in context[15] influence the engagement in occupation and ultimately the health status and immunocompetence of these women.

Social

A survey of the living conditions of women with AIDS revealed that 51% have children, 90% are unemployed, 83% live with a household income of less than $10,000, and only 14% of these women are married, compared with the national average of 50%.[37] This study suggests a large number of very sick women are raising children alone under conditions of extreme poverty in American cities. Women with HIV are poorer than men with HIV, and these women have less access to medical insurance and experienced health care practitioners.

The focus of this example has been on women and the unique intersection of potential control parameters. In repeated studies, women have been found to die sooner than men from HIV. With heterosexual transmission being the most rapidly rising route of transmission, many of the women care for husbands and children with HIV. Clinicians have repeatedly observed that women seek care for themselves later, last, or not at all, leading to more serious conditions when they do seek care.

The social construction of the disease as a gay man's disease or a disease of injectable drug users led to assumptions that have influenced women's health. The diagnostic criteria changed for AIDS in 1994, but prior to that, women's prognosis was based on definitions developed for men. Many women with HIV died of pneumonia and cervical cancer before being actually diagnosed with AIDS. Early in the epidemic, women were told that the disease would not affect them, that heterosexual transmission was unlikely. Doctors still do not routinely offer HIV testing along with gynecologic examinations, believing that the disease does not affect women. Women who ask their doctors about the test are routinely discouraged from having it done because "nice ladies do not get this disease." This is, of course, not true. Many women with HIV report three or less lifetime partners.

The modes of transmission tracked by the CDC do not include sexual contact between women. Although there are lesbians with AIDS who have not had any history of injectable drug use, heterosexual contact, or other transmission risk identified by the CDC, transmission between women is not recognized and tracked by the CDC. This is due to the hierarchical transmission categories discussed previously. If a lesbian has had sex with a man even once, and she has AIDS, her case is reported in the heterosexual transmission category, no matter how many times she has had unprotected sex with women. The description of this disease process is socially constructed in a way that obscures transmission between women and can give lesbians a false sense of security that they are safe from AIDS.

Cultural

Ethnic minorities are disproportionately represented in AIDS cases among women. While 21% of women in the United States are black and Hispanic, 74% of women with AIDS were from these two groups in 1993.[27] The disproportionate burden of this epidemic on women of color is growing, with an over-representation of women and men of color in the AIDS epidemic. If race and ethnicity were not a potential control parameter, these numbers would not be disproportionate.

Culture may play an important role in this distribution. For example, in some Hispanic cultures, it is not considered appropriate for women to be knowledgeable about sexual practices. A woman who asks her male partner to use a condom or have an HIV test is suspected of having poor moral character. Fear of reprisal may prevent women from insisting on safer sexual practices.

Summary

This case example has focused on the performance contexts of occupation to discuss briefly potential control parameters that may initiate a phase shift in the attractor state of health. The purpose was to demonstrate the intersection of several variables that may initiate a change in health status to describe the role that occupation may play among those many variables, and to stimulate thoughts about nonlinear, nonhierarchical models of change. Many more potential control parameters must be described to develop and test models of human occupation and health in the case of women with HIV and AIDS. Dynamic systems theory applied to occupation reaffirms a multidimensional view of health and disease as a pattern arising from the confluence of variables. This presentation has been limited to the performance contexts of occupation for women with HIV in the interest of brevity; however, it should stimulate thinking about all levels of analysis through the lens of occupation.

Conclusion

The study of dynamic systems theory illuminates an evolutionary process that is changing the meaning of science and the notion of complexity. This paper is intended to begin to draw parallels between the behavior of dynamic systems and engagement in occupation and suggest possible applications of dynamic systems theory to the science of occupation. It seems that dynamic systems theory holds potential for increasing the understanding of the complex processes and states involved in engagement in occupational patterns.

Dynamic systems theory also has the potential to inform directly the practice of occupational therapy and contribute to the current efforts to demonstrate and understand treatment outcomes. A dynamic systems approach to treatment might suggest that treatment should create a phase shift in the pattern of health and occupation by focusing on control variables and shallow attractor wells, for example. Evaluation would then focus on identifying order parameters, potential control variables, and shallow attractor wells.

Researchers also need to find a way to identify and support the dynamic, non-linear effect of engagement in occupation as a control parameter in the desired changes of the occupational therapy process. One challenge will be to identify order parameters, measures that can describe the changes in occupational patterns occurring as the result of occupational therapy participation. Development of appropriate outcome measures versus just doing any available outcome measure will be an essential task. Much of the profession's future may depend on identifying the parameters of occupation and finding measures that will grasp the complexity of occupational therapy's work and its effects on the dynamic system that is life.

In conclusion, these attempts at applying dynamic systems concepts to human occupation and the process of occupational therapy are only a beginning. It is the authors' hope that they have evoked acknowledgment that exploration of dynamic systems principles with respect to our studies is a worthwhile enterprise and have aroused in the reader some interest and ideas in exploring this application further.

Discussion Questions

1. How might researchers in occupational science design a study using dynamic systems theory?
2. What are some appropriate order parameters and possible control parameters involved in daily occupations?
3. Do you agree that dynamic systems theory might help with outcome studies requested in occupational therapy? Do you consider the Functional Independence Measure an appropriate outline of order parameters?
4. What are your general observations of nonlinearity in occupation or occupational therapy?

References

1. Yerxa, EJ, Clark, F, Frank, G, Jackson, J, Parham, F, Pierce, D, Stein, C, and Zemke, R: An introduction to occupational science, A foundation for occupational therapy in the 21st century. In Yerxa, EJ, and Johnson, JA (eds): Occupational Science: The Foundation for New Models of Practice. The Haworth Press, New York, 1990, pp 1–17.
2. Kamm, K, Thelen, E, and Jensen, JL: A dynamical systems approach to motor development. Phys Ther 70:763, 1990.
3. Thelen, E, and Ulrich, BD: Hidden skills: A dynamical systems analysis of treadmill stepping during the first year. Monographs of the Society for Research in Child Development 223(1), 1984.
4. van Geert: A dynamic systems model of cognitive and language growth. Psychol Rev 98:3, 1991.
5. Kelso, JAS, and Tuller, B: A dynamical basis for action systems. In Gazzaniga, MS (ed): Handbook of Cognitive Neuroscience. Plenum Publishing, New York, 1984, pp 231–356.
6. Prigogine, I, and Stengers, I: Order Out of Chaos: Man's New Dialogue with Nature. Bantam Books, New York, 1984.
7. Prigogine and Stengers, 1984, p xxiii.
8. Yerxa et al., p 4.
9. Thelen and Ulrich, p 81.
10. Thelen and Ulrich, p 82.

11. Cohen, F, and Lazarus, RS: Coping and adaptation in health and illness. In Mechanic, D (ed): Handbook of Health, Health Care, and the Health Professions. The Free Press, New York, 1983, pp 608–635.
12. Corbin, JM, and Strauss, A: Unending Work and Care: Managing Chronic Illness at Home. Jossey-Bass, San Francisco, 1988.
13. Goffman, E: Stigma: Notes on the Management of Spoiled Identity. Prentice-Hall, Englewood Cliffs, NJ, 1963.
14. American Occupational Therapy Association Terminology Task Force: Am J Occup Ther 48:1055, 1994.
15. Clark, FA, Parham, D, Carlson, ME, Frank, G, Jackson, J, Pierce, D, Wolfe, RJ, and Zemke, R: Occupational science: Academic innovation in the service of occupational therapy's future. Am J Occup Ther 45:300, 1991.
16. Prigogine and Stengers, p 12.
17. Meyer, A: The philosophy of occupational therapy. Archives of Occupational Therapy 1:1, 1922.
18. Davies, P: The Cosmic Blueprint. Simon & Schuster, New York, 1988.
19. Clark et al., p 301.
20. Csikszentmihalyi, M, and Larson, R: Being Adolescent: Conflict and Growth in the Teenage Years. Basic Books, New York, 1984.
21. Prigogine and Stengers, p xxviii.
22. Toffler, A: Foreword: Science and change. In Prigogine, I, and Stengers, I (eds): Order Out of Chaos: Man's New Dialogue with Nature. Bantam Books, New York, 1984, pp xi–xxvi.
23. Bateson, MC: Composing A Life. The Atlantic Monthly Press, New York, 1989.
24. Thelen and Ulrich, p 10.
25. Zemke, R: Habits. In Royeen, C, (ed), American Occupational Therapy Association Self-study Series: The Practice of the Future: Putting Occupation back into Therapy. AOTA, Bethesda, MD, 1994.
26. Vallacher, RR, and Nowak, A: Dynamical Systems in Social Psychology. Academic Press, San Diego, 1994.
27. Centers for Disease Control and Prevention. Women with AIDS Slide Series L-264 (5). Division of HIV/AIDS, National Center for Infectious Diseases, Centers for Disease Control and Prevention, Atlanta, GA, 1993.
28. Shilts, R: And the Band Played On. Penguin Books, New York, 1987.
29. Milsum, JH: Health, Stress, and Illness: A Systems Approach. Praeger, New York, 1987.
30. Collins, PH: Black Feminist Thought: Knowledge, Consciousness, and the Politics of Empowerment. Routledge, New York, 1990.
31. Lorde, A: Sister Outsider. The Crossing Press, Freedom, CA, 1984.
32. Centers for Disease Control and Prevention. MMWR 41 (no. RR-17). CDCP, Atlanta, GA, December 18, 1992.
33. Combahee River Collective: A black feminist statement. In Jaggar, A, and Rothenberg, P (eds): Feminist Frameworks. McGraw-Hill, New York, 1984, pp 202–209.
34. King, DK: Multiple jeopardy, multiple consciousness: The context of a Black feminist ideology. Signs 14:42, 1988.
35. Centers for Disease Control and Prevention. MMWR (44)5. CDCP, Atlanta, GA, February 10, 1995.
36. Pearlman, D: Alarming rise in youth with HIV. San Francisco Chronicle, San Francisco, June 7, 1993, p A2.
37. Chu, SY, and Diaz, T: Letter to the editor. J of Acq Immun Syn 6:431, 1993.

Occupational Science: Mapping New Directions for Occupational Therapy

In Section IV, Zemke discussed Edelman's theory as a framework for understanding the relationship of biology to meaning. She points out that in Edelman's view, neuronal selection determined largely through everyday experiences, is responsible for the emergent quality of higher order consciousness, or in common parlance, the mind. Of course, because humans possess minds, they are able to imbue their occupations with meaning. Higher order consciousness is composed of such elements as language, an awareness of the self as a conscious being acting on things, assimilation of cultural meaning, and a sense of past and future.

How is occupational science most apt to impact occupational therapy? In Ottenbacher's short paper entitled "Academic Disciplines: Maps for Professional Development," he claims that if occupational science and occupational therapy are truly integrated, new clinical approaches may emerge that are derived from the occupational science knowledge base. In this section, we have included papers in occupational science that suggest some new or expanded directions for practice. The papers as a group focus largely on the "mind" and occupation, or on the symbolic dimension of occupation. The topics thus include how individuals give their lives meaning through narrative interpretation, how personal themes of meaning are used to guide choices of occupation, and how notions of time can be used to improve patient care. Finally, a grounded theory of therapeutic techniques to elicit occupational story telling and story making is described that was inspired by occupational science.

The first paper by Knox emphasizes social order. Using three generations of her own family as a case study, Knox illustrates intergenerational transmission spanning a periods of approximately 70 years of certain values that were presumably first held by her grandparents. Therapists will be dazzled by the numbers of individuals in this family who carved out occupational foci centered on the values of learning, interest in others, and service. Importantly, Knox introduces the reader to Harré's concept of the moral career, which he defines as "the social history of a person with respect to the opinions others have of his qualities and worth and the attitudes to and beliefs about himself that he forms on the basis of his readings of the attitudes and beliefs of others."[1] What if therapists began to assess the sense of social worth patients possess about themselves and then assisted patients to engage in occupations that would be consistent with the patients' moral careers? Such an approach would constitute an innovative strategy for working with the symbolic dimension of occupation in the therapeutic context.

Jackson's paper on meaningful existence in old age reports on a qualitative study that identified the adaptive strategies used by a group of elderly people who were living successfully in the community. She found that eight categories of adaptive strategies were used by her respondents, many of which were expressions of the symbolic dimension of occupation. Personal themes of meaning, which Jackson called motifs of occupation, emerged as a powerful factor contributing to overall life satisfaction. Jackson defined these themes as "complex cognitive contracts that emerge from the values and expectations embedded in one's particular sociohistorical circumstances, the opportunities available throughout one's life, and most importantly, the idiosyncratic way an individual interprets his or her life events". These themes, Jackson proposes, are the building blocks of an evolving self-identity that is continually being revised "in light of present circumstances." Religion, productivity, generosity, and effective familial bonds were some of the themes that gave meaning to the activities in which Jackson's respondents engaged. Other adaptive strategies included risk and challenge in occupation; activity patterns and temporal rhythms; control; maintaining continuity through spatial, social, and cultural connectedness; technology; support networks; acknowledging identity through the celebration of occupations; and advocating social change.

In Section II, Frank defined adaptation as the process of maximizing one's life opportunities. Jackson's respondents were selected as exemplars who were adapting optimally to old age through the strategies they had invented to deal with physical decline, losses of loved ones, and a potentially compromised sense of social worth. In a sense, they are "experts" on coping with change, decline, and unexpected life circumstances. The eight domains of adaptive strategies that Jackson identified can be thought of as a potential map for new models of practice. Adaptation of our patients may, in fact, be facilitated by attending more vigilantly to the occupational motifs that thread the lives of our patients, to the risks and challenges that they take, to temporal rhythms, and to the celebration of occupations and the other domains identified in Jackson's study. The detailed examples of adaptive strategies that Jackson reports provide a variegated landscape of potential avenues of practice.

White's paper pointedly concentrates on the application to practice of a key concept in occupational science, temporal adaptation, a concept to which Jackson's paper also referred. White begins by asking the question of how we can use notions of time to their full value in practice. The remainder of the paper is a beginning attempt, using a qualitative design, to answer this question in relation to the experience of patients in intensive care units. Using "environmental mapping, checklists of temporal cues, interviews with staff, and participant observation," White was able to document the distortions in temporal rhythms that characterized the intensive care unit setting. He then makes specific recommendations on what therapists can do in the future to rectify the situation. This paper stands out as a particularly compelling example of how grounded research applied to one aspect of a clinical setting can result in innovative treatment ideas. Unlike the prior papers discussed in this section, in relation to which therapists will need to devise their own clinical applications. White's is the first of the group in which an occupational scientist becomes specific in proposing changes within the context of practice.

Just as White's study of the intensive care unit resulted in specific practice recommendations, Clark, Larsen, and Richardson's study reported in the next paper illustrates how a comprehensive practice theory can emerge from qualitative research designed in accord with concepts from occupational science. The grounded theory that they present delineates specific techniques that therapists can use to evoke occupational story telling and occupational story making. Here, as in the case of White's paper on the intensive care unit, therapists need not ask, "How can I derive clinical applications from the abstract ideas presented in this paper?" Instead, they need to make a judgment on whether or not they wish to use the grounded practice theory that is detailed and if they choose to do so, assess how such use would be feasible in the settings in which they work.

The last paper in this section contains the closing remarks made by Jerry Johnson at Occupational Science Symposium IV. We have included the paper in this section because its overall message is that the existence of a knowledge base on occupation produced by occupational scientists challenges therapists to explore ways to incorporate it in practice. While occupational science focuses on all aspects of occupation from the physical to the symbolic, Johnson emphasizes its contributions on the "meaning of occupation" in her talk. She states, "It is difficult for an individual therapist who seeks to balance subjective meaning in a [health care] system that values objective outcomes". We realize that applying concepts from occupational science in clinical settings will take flexibility, creativity, practicality, and innovative problem solving. We believe, however, that occupational therapy stands to benefit, because more refined knowledge about the multiple dimensions of occupation is bound to stimulate the development of potent therapeutic techniques, result in better prepared therapists, and launch the profession on a trajectory that is in keeping with its time-honored recognition of the importance of human occupation to health and well-being.

Reference

1. Harré, R, Clarke, D, and de Carlo, N: Motives and Mechanisms: An Introduction to the Psychology of Action. Methuen, New York, 1985.

by Kenneth Ottenbacher, PhD, OTR/L, FAOTA

30

Academic Disciplines: Maps for Professional Development

The process of establishing an academic discipline is different than the continuing development of an academic profession. Training and education for occupational therapy have occurred in academic environments for more than 50 years. It is only recently, however, that our field has begun to consider itself an academic discipline. The purpose of a profession is to provide a service needed in society. The purpose of an academic discipline is to generate and refine a body of knowledge.

As an academic profession we frequently expect information derived from educational environments to have direct clinical application. Much of the information related to the development of an academic discipline, such as occupational science, will have clinical implications but not direct clinical applications. As professional practitioners, we should not be discouraged if the information presented here or in future studies of occupational science does not suggest a specific new treatment technique that can be immediately used in the clinical setting. The information contributes to the evolving body of knowledge that is the foundation for the academic discipline of occupational science.

The emphasis on the development of an academic discipline does not mean that professional skills are being ignored, however. In any applied field, practitioners must be taught technical skills to become competent clinicians. The question is not whether students should be taught clinical skills. The more important question follows: From where do the technical skills come, and where will they lead professional practice? When an academic profession and academic discipline are truly integrated, the skills emerge from a clearly defined and well-developed knowledge base—a knowledge base generated by members of the academic discipline. This knowledge base is used to guide and refine professional practice. The knowledge base also provides the justification for many components of a true profession, i.e., professional autonomy, the ability to set standards for practice, and many others.

The knowledge base associated with an academic discipline provides a map for professional development. It tells us where we are and points out directions for future development. Without a clear understanding of the geography associated with professional development, we are like the famous U.S. Supreme Court Justice Oliver Wendell Holmes, Jr., who one time found himself on a train but could not locate his ticket. While the justice searched through his pockets, the conductor told him not to worry, "Don't worry, Mr. Holmes," the conductor said, "You'll probably find your ticket when you get off the train, and I'm sure the railroad will trust you to mail it back." Justice Holmes looked at the conductor with some irritation and said, "My dear man, that is not the problem at all. The problem is not where my ticket is. The problem is—where am I going?"

Professional skills are the ticket we need to provide effective therapeutic service, but only a research-supported knowledge base that is part of a defined academic discipline can provide us with direction and tell us where we are going. If you have any question about where we are going, I suggest you ask one of the authors in this book.

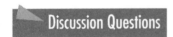

Discussion Questions

1. Do you agree with Ottenbacher's view of why occupational therapy would benefit from developing a science of occupation?

by Susan H. Knox, MA, OTR, FAOTA

31

Shared Moral Careers and Occupational Choice in a Family

Family Demographics

The Grandparents

Children of Nathan and Kathleen

Grandchildren

Discussion

Like father, like daughter . . .
Like mother, like daughter . . .
Like grandparents, mother and father, like children . . .
Genes or example?[1]

During a recent family reunion, five cousins were discussing the careers and activities of their families. They were struck by the number of them who were at that time or earlier in their lives employed in public service or involved in volunteer work. They wondered about the influences that led them all to pursue service roles and traced these back to their grandparents.

What influences a person's choice of careers or occupations? This question has long been of interest to occupational therapists, particularly as it relates to the individual's unique sequence of activities and choices that ultimately leads to careers and other choices of daily occupation. However, another way of analyzing occupational choice might be to look at patterns of occupations in groups of individuals. This approach might shed light on some of the more subtle factors influencing choice, such as sociocultural beliefs, values, and motivations. In this paper, the choice of occupations in a family unit spanning three generations is examined to see how family values and activities have influenced the occupational choice of individual members. The framework for this analysis is largely action theory, as described by Harré and his associates and von Cranach.[2-4] In this theory, moral career is defined as "the social history of a person with respect to the opinions others have of his qualities and worth and the attitudes to and beliefs about himself that he forms on the basis of his readings of the attitudes and beliefs of others."[5] These moral careers make a person aware of the social patterns and cultural values on which they are based. Harré maintained that often members of a society or group share ideals and concepts of worthiness and hence moral careers and that they structure their lives toward those values. In this paper, I will illustrate how members of the Smyth family seemed to be shaped by the moral careers of their ancestors so that there seems to be cross-generational transmission of a certain kind of moral career.

In undertaking this analysis, a methodology that Harré[2] presented for the study of the psychological aspects of a human life was adapted. Harré recommended that life forms be studied through the analysis of the lives of diverse individuals. Suggested methods for this type of study are two kinds of life documents, the biography and the diary. He described the diary as a contemporaneous record of the psychological life course, whereas the biography is not only a historical accounting, but a representation of an individual's psychological structure. Harré suggested analysis of the biography for themes of behavior, which could be further explored.

This study used a variation on the methods proposed by Harré. Themes depicting shared values and beliefs of several generations of a family were extracted using content analysis from biographical accounts, historical documents, and interviews. The purpose of the analysis was to gain a sense of how the moral careers of individuals affect the occupational choices of family members in successive generations. The family I have selected is my own, and the generations chosen include my maternal grandparents, their offspring, and their grandchildren (my generation). Material has been gathered from a number of sources: an extensive family genealogy compiled by Charlotte Blaney,[6] books written by two of the children,[7] books written by the grandfather Nathan,[8,9] and a videotape of a family reunion in 1985, which included recollection by two of the daughters and a conversation among five of the grandchildren.[10] Many of the quotes are from this videotape. Specifically, the methodology used was analysis of the written and genealogical material and conversations from the videotape to provide evidence of values and beliefs that appear consistently throughout the three generations.

Family Demographics

The Smyth family genealogy shows a rich history of service-related occupations, including ministers, missionaries, physicians, and teachers.[6] Three generations are considered in this paper. The grandparents are Nathan and Kathleen (Fig. 31-1). They had five children: Bill, Elizabeth (Betke), Anna (Nancy), Kay, and Winnie, and 20 grandchildren.

Nathan and Kathleen were married in 1907, and their children were born between 1908 and 1918. They reared their children in Englewood, New Jersey, between the two world wars. The children married between the years 1933 and 1942,

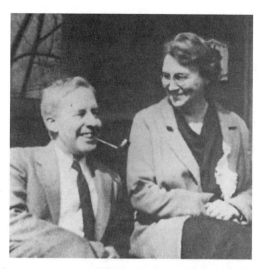

Figure 31–1. Nathan and Kathleen Smyth seem to have influenced the moral careers of both their children and grandchildren. (Photo courtesy of Susan Knox.)

and the grandchildren were born between 1935 and 1957. All but four of the grandchildren are married.

All of the children of Nathan and Kathleen and most of their grandchildren have worked or are working in public service or have volunteered for public service agencies. Tables 31-1 and 31-2 depict the family occupations. A brief description of the grandparents and their offspring illustrates their values and beliefs.

The Grandparents

Nathan was the son of a minister. His father was a prolific writer and published 16 books, including his autobiography. Nathan attended Yale University, received his law degree in 1900, and throughout his life, wrote many books on philosophical topics. He worked for many years in the District Attorney's office and held a fed-

Table 31–1   Children of Nathan and Kathleen

Kay: Teacher; missionary. Married Len, a minister, who did missionary work.

Bill: Involved with what is now United Way; executive in the Eberhard Faber Pencil Corp. Married Helen.

Elizabeth (Betke): Speech pathologist; director of education at state school for the mentally retarded; PhD in special education; was awarded the Governor's service award as volunteer of the year. Married Fred, a physician.

Nancy: Journalist; worked with planned parenthood and family planning; volunteer work. Married Milton, a newspaper reporter and publisher.

Winnie: Secretary; active in volunteer organizations; was awarded a state award as volunteer of the year. Married Grant, an attorney.

Table 31–2   Grandchildren of Nathan and Kathleen

Children of Kay and Len
  Winnie: Owns a personnel relations, job placement, and management consulting firm
  Kathy: Early religious work; caterer; involved with hunger programs
  David: Early religious work; consultant in city planning
Children of Bill and Helen
  Bill: Headmaster of a private boys' school
  Whitney: Public relations in telecommunications
  Theo: Former Peace Corps volunteer; interior decorator
  Linda: Professional artist; teacher
Children of Betke and Fred
  Fred: Computer programmer; active in religious organization; volunteer work
  Susan: Former Peace Corps volunteer; occupational therapist
  Peter: Has autism; works in a sheltered workshop
  Bill: Construction worker; volunteer for social causes
Children of Nancy and Milton
  Mary: Sex equity coordinator; active in treatment and care of abused children; teacher
  Richard: Director of an inner city development agency
  Peter: Director of a youth agency dealing with child abuse and other problems
  Kathy: Psychiatric social worker
Children of Winnie and Grant
  Judy: Textbook publishing; former social worker
  Polly: Rehabilitation counselor; involved with workers' compensation litigation
  Nancy: Owns own copy business; director of volunteer services for United Way
  Wendy: Mother; active in church
  Beth: Works in a sheltered group home for mentally retarded

eral post with the U.S. Employment Service helping to find employment for returning soldiers after the war. He was active in volunteer work, such as serving as director of the Legal Aid Society and as chairman of the Voluntary Defenders Committee. In addition, he helped draft state legislation relating to children's courts and domestic relations.

Nathan had a strong belief in education and encouraged the value of learning in his daughters and son. His daughter, Betke, stated, "Dad was a wonderful teacher."[10] One of the grandchildren, David, recalling his mother's comments, said, "Granddad had a great interest in all of his daughters' and son's scholastic work and he used to have wonderful conversations with them, which was as much a part of their education as the formal side."[10] Another grandchild, Judy, stated, "Granddad gave every daughter a choice, either a debut or college, and to their credit, every one chose college."[10] Nathan's daughter, Betke, related this about him: "His interest in words and writing, in poems and in puns certainly rubbed off on me. . . . He helped me with homework, not by giving the answer but by asking me what was the question. I then figured out the answer. His legacy to me is curiosity, sense of humor, interest in words, and all that implies."[10]

Nathan also ingrained the ideal of public service in his children. Not only were his career and volunteer activities in this area, but he expressed these ideals in his writing. In his book *Lest Freedom Fail*,[8] he stated:

If we are to survive as an individualistic democracy we must revise our American Dream; make it a dream not only of equal rights and opportunities but also one of fulfillment of social obligations. Grover Cleveland popularized the aphorism that "public office is a public trust." We must come to see also that private property is a public trust. . . . The concepts of individual social responsibility and voluntary co-operation are not mere products of speculative morality. They express laws of human life revealed by experience.[11]

Kathleen was a descendent of Peter Bulkley, a clergyman who escaped England, came with his congregation to America, and founded the city of Concord, Massachusetts. Her father was a physician and missionary. Three of her siblings were physicians. Kathleen did not attend college nor did she have a formal career; however, she was actively involved in volunteer work throughout her life. In the 1930s, she became interested in the teaching of the Moral Re-Armament religious group, and for the rest of her life she was active in that group. During the war, she organized women's groups to raise money for the war effort, and she worked in hospitals. One of her daughters, Betke, stated, "She indoctrinated us with the idea that you were supposed to volunteer."[10] Another daughter, Nancy, stated, "Mother's legacy was a deep-rooted need to help others."[12]

Many of the values embodied by the grandparents are expressed in this quote by Nathan:[11]

All of us know that the interested life is the happy one. He who ventures, labors, and endures to enlarge his interests, rejoices in life. He who glides the easy slope of self-indulgence, indolence, and vacuous amusements, descends into the gulch of narrowing interests at the bottom of which runs the sour cream of boredom, cynicism, self-pity and unhappiness. Thus, by the sanctions of pleasure and pain, does the cosmic design impel man to climb to ever higher ranges of interesting experiences. The basic laws of ethics thus derived may be stated very simply: Be interested. The second is: Be interested in others. Neither, however, is an easy commandment. Few are they who wholly succeed in obeying either of them.[13]

Children of Nathan and Kathleen

Nathan and Kathleen had five children. All of them graduated from college, two with advanced degrees, and all had careers while involved in volunteer activities.

After their marriages, the children of Nathan and Kathleen no longer lived in close proximity to each other. Except during World War II, when for short periods some of the sisters lived together or with their parents while their husbands were stationed overseas, the children scattered across the United States and the world.

One daughter, Kay, and her family lived in Burma, teaching and doing missionary work. For the next 20 years following the war, Kay and her husband and their children worked for the Moral Re-Armament movement in America, India, China, Japan, and Taiwan.[7]

Bill died early in life (at age 39) in an airplane crash.

Betke worked actively as a health professional most of her life. After her third child was born with autism, she earned a second master's degree in speech pathology and a doctorate in special education. After retirement, she continued to be actively involved in volunteer work of all types, and she was a strong advocate for individuals with developmental disabilities.

Winnie spent most of her married life in volunteer work. She also worked for various health agencies in her city. She earned a master's degree late in life also.

Nancy worked for many health agencies in her area and for public welfare and departments of health resources. After retirement, she still volunteered for many groups.

The value of work and public service was evident in this second generation. Betke stated, "We were really modern; they talk now about how mothers never thought about getting jobs, but all of us worked or planned to work."[10]

All of the children exemplified the value of "volunteerism." Two of the daughters were honored by their respective state governors as "volunteer of the year." Winnie stated, "I do think volunteerism is the backbone of American society, and I'm just glad we were all brought up to believe in it and become involved in it."[14]

Grandchildren

Nathan and Kathleen had 20 grandchildren. Eighteen of them graduated from college, eight with advanced degrees. One of the grandchildren, Peter, has autism, lives with his mother, and works in a sheltered workshop. The other 19 have been involved in public service in some way, either by profession or volunteer service.

When reviewing the occupations of the grandchildren, the values of education and public service are certainly evident. One of the grandchildren, Nancy, when talking of volunteerism, stated, "I know, I got that from Mother, too; it's a part of what you do."[10] Peter, son of another daughter, stated, "What I remember about Mother is that she has this very powerful social conscience . . . that was reinforced to all of us throughout our lives. All of us have gone into various aspects of social work or social development."[10] My family was always involved in some organization advocating for individuals with developmental disabilities.

Nancy closed her book with the following statement: "Caring for others and an abiding interest in people and the world around us—these are the qualities which enriched Nat's and Kathleen's lives, and those around them. It is a rich legacy they gave their children and those who come after. It is one we can all cherish."[15]

Discussion

Analysis of occupational choice in this family highlights some of the sociocultural values and ideals that are passed through generations. Although there is a great deal of variety reflected in the professional choices seen in this family, the themes of learning, interest in others, and service are evident. These themes exemplify Harré's concept of shared moral careers, and in this paper, I have shown how such careers can ultimately influence occupational choice.

When analyzing my own family, I have been fortunate to have a legacy of writings and personal recollections on which to draw. However, a limitation of this analysis is certainly that my interpretations are influenced by my own values and beliefs. As Fulghum stated, "In a sense, we make up all our relatives, though. Fathers, mothers, brothers, sisters and the rest. Especially if they are dead or distant. We take what we know, which isn't ever the whole story, and we add it to what we wish and need, and stitch it together into some kind of family quilt to wrap up in on our mental couch."[16]

In spite of the bias inherent in studying one's own family, this paper illustrates one method of analysis that would be useful to the occupational scientist studying occupational choice. The biographical analysis of a social group has the advantage of revealing values and beliefs that might not be as apparent in more traditional interviews or questionnaire techniques. Qualitative analysis of family data such as this enriches our understanding of the complex issues that influence who individuals become as occupational beings.

Discussion Questions

1. Drawing on action theory, Knox has used the family as a social context that profoundly influences the values, beliefs, occupations, and moral careers of its members. How does or does not the social context of the many different medical and educational settings in which occupational therapists work similarly influence these same phenomena in practitioners and patients or clients?
2. How might the occupation of autobiography be used as a therapeutic occupation?

Reference

1. Berliner, NS: A Legacy in Kind. Privately printed, Birmingham, AL, 1988.
2. Harré, R: Social Being: A Theory for Social Psychology. Rowman and Littlefield, Totowa, NJ, 1979.
3. Harré, R, Clarke, D, and DeCarlo, N: Motives and Mechanisms: An Introduction to the Psychology of Action. Methuen, London, 1985.
4. von Cranach, M: The psychological study of goal-directed action: Basic issues. In von Cranach, M, and Harré, R (eds): The Analysis of Action. Cambridge University Press, Cambridge, 1982.
5. Harre, p 316.
6. Blaney, C: The ancestors and descendants of Lucius Duncan Bulkley. Privately published, Sherborn, MA, 1985.
7. Allen, LB, and Allen, KS: People, Pagodas and Pyramids. Privately printed, Stamford, CT, 1985.
8. Smyth, NA: Through Science to God. Macmillan, New York, 1936.
9. Smyth, NA: Lest Freedom Fail. Dodd, Mead and Co., New York, 1940.
10. Smyth Family Reunion, 1985, videotape.
11. Smyth, 1940 p 40.
12. Berliner, p 32.
13. Smyth, 1936 p 146
14. Berliner, p 195.
15. Berliner, p 197.
16. Fulghum, R: All I Really Need to Know I Learned in Kindergarten. Villard Books, New York, 1989, p 184.

by Jeanne Jackson, PhD, OTR

32

Living a Meaningful Existence in Old Age

In the book *The Courage to Grow Old*,[1] Phillip Berman sets out to explore his fundamental conviction that aging in American society requires a certain kind of courage—a courage to continue life with excitement and vitality among the unknown yet inevitable challenges that arise. His intent was to contradict the conventional image of aging held by what he called our youth-obsessed society. This conventional perspective, for the most part, conjures up pictures of canes, walkers, convalescent hospitals, and Alzheimer's disease. It represents what no one can escape—physical decline. The deceptive element in the above image is that it simply reduces aging to a physical representation, neglecting to acknowledge the richness of a lifetime of experiences. Nevertheless, to camouflage the increasing physical disabilities that accompany growing old is equally disrespectful.

For Berman,[1] listening to the voices of 41 prominent men and women between the ages of 68 and 92 provided a rich variety of reflections on growing old—reflections that captured the diversity of experiences and seemed to negotiate between loss and the tenacity for life. These impressions ranged from those who quite simply stated, "I have come to approach the last years of my life with an attitude of irony and pity. For me there is no dignity in growing old,"[2] to those who claim, "We who are old have a great responsibility to live our lives fully; to do what can be done and bring to it something of what we have learned, to show that life is still rich and good; to face reality and discover our own strength."[3] Regardless of their particular responses to aging, the stories told by the men and women with whom Berman spoke honestly and clearly illustrated the process by which they struggled with life decisions that accompany growing old. Berman summarized this process in a singular message, a common wisdom expressed overtly and subtly by many—that of living life creatively and continuing to create throughout life.

It was within this framework that this research project was undertaken. A primary goal of occupational therapists has been to foster creative adaptation, enabling individuals to continue a meaningful existence following disability. Adaptive equipment, energy conservation techniques, and training in activities of daily living are all traditional methods used by occupational therapists to promote successful adaptation. In this paper, I intend to build on the existing traditions and by listening to the voices and stories of one group of elderly individuals, to discover the adaptive strategies that they deemed most influential in maintaining a meaningful life. Like Berman, I wished to tap into the worlds of meaning in which these individuals exist and to draw out their expertise on the creative aging enterprise, specifically with respect to their adaptive responses to disability.

The primary purpose of the pilot study discussed in this paper was to discover the adaptive strategies used by one group of elderly people with disabilities who were living successfully in their community. To accomplish this purpose, adaptive strategies are viewed as the complex system of methods and plans used by individuals to overcome obstacles and live satisfying, meaningful lives. This particular group, the Health Care Advocates (HCA), was asked to participate in this study because they were identified by health care professionals and themselves as exemplar individuals who could provide valuable information on aging with a disability and constructing meaningful lives.

The study is presented in four sections. First, the theoretical foundation provided by occupational science is discussed. Second, the HCA is described. Third, the data collection process is described. Finally, each of the seven categories of adaptive strategies found as the study's results are analyzed.

Theoretical Foundation

Occupational science is the theoretical foundation for this research project, providing its conceptual framework. Because this science is in its beginning years of development and has yet to be fleshed out, its underlying assumptions provided guidance for the study. Five of these assumptions are briefly summarized below.

Yerxa et al.[4] conveyed the most fundamental assumption of occupational science in the statement, "Individuals are most true to their humanity when engaged in occupations." Occupations are defined as culturally and personally meaningful activities in which individuals partake on a daily basis or at various times throughout their lives. As Yerxa et al. pointed out, occupational science is grounded in the notion that the human is an occupational being and that the drive to be occupied has evolutionary, psychological, social, and symbolic roots.

Second, occupational science honors the human as an author of his or her life story.[4,5] Individuals make choices as to which occupations comprise their day and in doing so, create themselves as occupational beings. Although human agency is valued, occupational science equally respects the social-historical condition under which individual choice is expressed. People's choices for action are impelled by personal passions and convictions, yet these commitments are embedded within a particular social-historical community of beliefs.[6] People do not act in isolation of others nor do they automatically assume the particular cultural traditions and beliefs into which they are born.[7] Rather, they engage in an ongoing negotiation between their personal vision for an acceptable life and the enabling and constraining forces of their particular social traditions. The resolution of the above tension is expressed in the occupational configuration that emerges on a daily basis and throughout one's life.

The third assumption underlying occupational science addresses the notion that people engage in storied actions. Not only do they participate in a regimen of daily occupations, but they create narratives of meaning about what they actually do with their time and the symbolic significance of their occupations. Bruner[6] claimed that the impetus for action lies in a tenacious human desire for meanings and that through engagement in symbolically significant occupations, people negotiate an evolving story about their life events and how their lives fit or contradict the world around them. Yerxa[8] echoed the importance of attending to the symbolic significance of occupations, stating that "humans live by and for symbolic causes." People "do occupations" for reasons. Whether their reasons are fueled by passionate convictions or complacent justifications, they are as much a part of people's actions as is the physical doing of an activity. Thus, the subjective experience of engagement in occupations is an essential component of this study.

Fourth, occupational science respects the adaptive nature of the human. Reilly[9] aptly reflected this notion in her statement, "Man through the use of his hands as they are energized by mind and will can influence the state of his own health." Here she conveys her belief that humans have the capacity to respond to the challenges presented in life and the potential to create a life that is healthy and meaningful to themselves and their society. Furthermore, Reilly claimed that the adaptive nature of the human has evolutionary roots and is embedded in the drive for exploration and competence as one interacts with his or her environment.

The fifth assumption on which occupational science rests is that occupations are carried out within a particular physical, social, political, and historical environment. As stated previously, the environment acts to enable and to constrain engagement in certain occupations. Furthermore, through human action, the environment is transformed, as are its social traditions.

In summary, occupational science influenced both the direction of the study and the interpretation of the findings in a number of ways. My intent to study the adaptive strategies of elderly individuals was grounded in the belief that individuals adapt to the changes they encounter throughout their lives. The notion that humans are authors of their lives who actively reconstruct their occupational involvement and transform their environmental situations following disability is embedded in the study. I therefore expected my elderly subjects to have stories to tell about their successful and failed attempts at adaptation. My concern with the subjective and objective dimensions of occupations influenced the choice to use a qualitative approach in this study. Finally, my concern with not only the actual carrying out of adaptive strategies, but with the symbolic significance of those strategies emanated from the assumption that individuals imbue their actions with meanings.

The Health Care Advocates

A group of 20 elderly individuals with varying degrees of physical, cognitive, and emotional disabilities participated in this study. The group was composed of 18 women and two men ranging in age between 60 and 90 years. During the group sessions that I attended, only 14 members were present. Absences were not taken lightly by the members and for the most part, occurred only in case of severe illness or if a member was forced to move to a convalescent hospital.

Prior to the formal organization of the HCA, each of its founding members had been active participants in a short-term adult day group, which provided counseling, activity, and exercise. When the adult day group ended, approximately 12 of its members, the psychologist, and the social worker expressed a commitment to continue meeting yet change the direction of the group to address self-help advocacy concerns. This new focus was spirited by a passionate desire of the members to improve health care for the elderly. In particular, they sought to enlighten health care providers about growing old and the experiences of elderly patients. For each member, past attempts to receive proper evaluation and treatment for their disabilities had led to extensive battles with the medical system. Most had become disillusioned and mistrusting of health care professionals who had rushed members through appointments, spending little effort to understand their complaints or explain treatments. Thus, the experiences of these individuals, together with their commitment to change the system, prepared them to assume a position of teacher for health professionals and advocates for the elderly.

For the last 6 years, since the inception of the group, the members have gathered every Tuesday. The 1st hour of their meeting is reserved for socializing, during which each member shares special weekly events. The 2nd hour is devoted to an educational experience. The weekly meeting ends with lunch.

Educational activities include posing as patients for interviews with different health professionals, such as psychologists, medical doctors, and occupational, physical, and speech therapists; participating as an audience for lectures given by recreation therapists; and participating in research projects. In addition to teaching others, speakers occasionally present information on topics of interest, such as health care for the elderly in other countries. Beyond Tuesday meetings, members also participate in classes for health care professionals where they may discuss topics such as coping with aging, health care and the older patient, and life-styles and aging.

Initially, the group was dedicated to "getting the message out." Efforts were spent developing a manual in which the members discussed the doctor–patient relationship, attitudes and helping style of the health care professional, communication, and humor in the medical clinic. Opportunities for presentations at the National Gerontological Association, publications in gerontology journals, and appearances on television were organized by the group liaisons. Members speak of those days with much excitement. Stories of their travels "up north" for a conference presentation and personal fears about their abilities to speak in front of a crowd were told not only by the original players, but secondhand by other members. In the last couple of years, these opportunities have waned.

Membership in the group carries significant meaning for its affiliates. One becomes a member only through invitation, following a 3-week trial period, which ensures compatibility. Once invited to join, death or severe illness appear to be the sole reason people terminate. The importance of membership was exemplified in one person's life when, at his funeral, "being a Health Care Advocate" was mentioned among the 10 things for which he'd like to be remembered. In addition to the explicit group purpose, many HCAs attribute to membership maintaining friendships, commitment to a cause, and the acceptance of disability. An attitude of acceptance of disability seems to distinguish this group from other organizations for the elderly. One member stated that the relatively small group size and slow pace enable her to move around with a walker and participate in activities. Adapted vans are provided for outings, and encouragement is given to those whose cognitive disabilities interfere with self-expression.

Methodology

Data Collection

Gaining insight into the adaptive strategies used to meet the challenges of aging with a disability required an ethnographic approach to data collection and analysis, in particular, participant observation and semistructured interviews. On three occasions, I attended the HCA weekly meetings. On one additional occasion, I accompanied members on a luncheon outing in celebration of St. Patrick's Day. The combination of observations during the semiformal meetings and participating in an informal outing allowed me to become sensitive to the personalities of those whom I would be interviewing and to understand the general purpose of the group.

Concurrent with these four observation sessions, semistructured interviews were conducted with eight members: seven women and one man. Participants were chosen from a list of volunteers, with an attempt to interview people with varying disabilities. Thus, the sample included two women with arthritis, one of whom had limited use of her hands and one who used a walker; two women with emotional problems, one of whom had memory problems due to a history of depression and a suicide attempt and one who previously experienced panic attacks; three women with a combination of back problems, arthritis, and cerebrovascular accidents, one used a wheelchair and the other two used walkers; and one man who had a history of reactive depression and is presently experiencing a hearing loss and memory problems.

In addition to focusing on disabilities and functional impairments, I attempted to select people with different living situations, because I hypothesized that place of residence would influence independence, activity levels, and adaptive strategies. Two women owned their own homes, one of whom shared it with her daughter who had a disability. One woman owned a mobile home. Three women and one man rented; one lived in a regular apartment, two in homes, one in a senior citizen apartment complex, and one in a retirement home.

Limited finances were discussed by four members; however, they expressed satisfaction that their financial situation did not interfere with medical treatment, housing, or equipment needs. Social activities, such as travel, were most restricted. Housing subsidies were provided for two individuals, and three were eligible for subsidized workers.

Interviews were informal and usually lasted approximately 2 to 2.5 hours, loosely divided into three sections: a brief account of the individual's life stories, a description of daily activities and strategies used to maintain important activities in their lives, and information on values, goals, life philosophy, and the meaning of growing old. Although I posed questions, I encouraged the interviewees to take a leading role in the discussion and freely narrate their lives.

Because the social situation influences the type of information obtained, interviews were conducted at the member's place of residence. Homes were chosen because they would provide a relaxed, familiar environment conducive to exploring somewhat personal issues. My intention was that within their own place of residence, the interviewees would feel most comfortable to share their problems and joys of aging. In retrospect, observing spontaneous interactions and phone calls with neighbors, family members, and workers provided powerful insight into hidden issues of dependency and the individual's support structures and home environment as forms of adaptive strategies.

In addition to participant observations and interviews, I was able to secure minutes from seven of the meetings that I was unable to attend, a videotape of the group that was aired on television, and articles published by the group members and psychologist. These were supplementary material providing a sense of history to the group.

Data Analysis

Data analysis occurred throughout the process in accordance with the grounded theory approach.[10] Interviews were taped, enabling me to quote verbatim and preserve the informant's own wording. Immediately following each interview, I summarized the information obtained, trying to isolate my impression of the interview process, the important themes in the individual's life that stood out, the activity flow of their day, and the most prominent adaptive strategies. After the audiotapes were transcribed, I listened again to the interview and began initial coding procedures, identifying overall general insights and adaptive strategies. As certain categories reappeared, a more focused coding procedure was used in which redundant categories were collapsed. The interviews were then searched in a more selective manner to develop the categories of adaptive strategies that were emerging in finer detail. Memos were used to elaborate on the ideas by teasing out the patterns of adaptation that were occurring and by examining relationships that existed between categories. Of course, the analysis maintained a cyclical process in that, as categories were more defined, the interviews became more focused, at least during the last half hour.

This pilot study reflects the adaptive strategies of one select group of elderly individuals who are white, come from middle to lower income brackets, and for most of their lives, lived in a traditional heterosexual marriage. This particular standpoint may have influenced the type of adaptive strategies that emerged, such as the composition of social networks. It is troublesome to lump people together as "the elderly," assuming that a universal "role" or "model" exists. It is even more detrimental to assume that a universal model rests on the voices of white, middle income, heterosexuals because they have often been given the dominant voice. Nonetheless, this group constitutes a particular viewpoint and one that has valuable insight into the process of growing old. By acknowledging their particular backgrounds, a broader foundation for their responses is laid, and the reader can avoid assuming universality.

Adaptive Strategies

Adjustment to change and loss was universally experienced by each of the eight HCA members who shared their stories with me. Loss presented itself in many forms: physical decline; emotional instability; death of a spouse, parent, or child; and financial devastation. Regardless of the loss, these individuals attempted to adapt, calling on their resources and redesigning their daily activities to meet their needs. This is not to imply that all the HCA members were completely successful in their attempts to find satisfaction. Liza, confined to a retirement home, desperately wants release. Charlie longs for his deceased wife and wistfully complains of severe loneliness. Others expressed contentment and happiness. In all cases, adaptation was present.

Adapting to loss for the elderly is often a subtle and continuous challenge. Constant negotiations between resources and limitations against a background of personal meaning occurred. In my 4 months of knowing the HCAs, three of the informants experienced falls and loss of workers that once again disrupted their lives and demanded reorchestration of daily activities. The findings presented in this paper do not necessarily address the subtle, adaptive responses unique to the individual but rather attempt to elucidate seven broad categories of adaptation that were extracted from the data. These include personal themes of meaning as motifs for occupations, risk and challenge in occupations, activity patterns and temporal rhythms, control, identity through occupations, maintaining continuity, and promoting social change.

Personal Themes of Meaning as Motifs for Occupation

Aging brings an awareness of the passage of time and the diversity of life experiences that have occurred within that time. Successful adaptation to aging is characterized by a reinterpretation of these diverse events into meaningful stories that provide a sense of coherency to life experiences and their relationship to present circumstances.[11] Through the creation of life stories, individuals select among their experiences, organize them into a logical sequence, and imbue them with symbolic meaning.[11] A current interpretation of life emerges out of this process, providing a sense of unity between an individual's self-identity and his or her actions in the world.

Kaufman[11] identified life "themes" as a medium through which elderly individuals often unknowingly reflect on their past and share their life story. Themes, in this sense, are complex cognitive constructs that emerge from the values and expectations embedded in one's particular sociohistorical circumstances, the opportunities available throughout one's life, and most importantly, the idiosyncratic way an individual interprets his or her life events. Themes become the building blocks for an evolving self-identity that is continually being created in light of present circumstances.

For the HCAs, personal themes of meaning emerged as a strong and effective strategy for organizing and interpreting the present events in their lives. The choices they made about how to spend their time and energy on a daily and weekly basis often reflected their personal themes of meaning. No one individual described his or her activity patterns in terms of personal themes; however, within the interview process, individuals often chose to link past and present activities through themes of meaning. Furthermore, as each individual discussed his or her daily and weekly routines, many of their occupations were important because they symbolically expressed personal themes of meanings. It is this last notion—how themes of meaning influence daily and weekly occupations—on which I elaborate.

Religion was the most common theme discussed by the members of the HCA, although the way in which religion held meaning and was woven into their lives differed. For some members, religion was an overriding theme that organized and permeated their experiences. June, who considers herself to have always "believed in God," mentally organized her daily and weekly schedule around religious events. Sunday morning begins with "choir practice" and "Sunday school" and ends with "an evening church service." Wednesday is spent preparing for and attending "evening church supper." Saturdays, although only occasionally, include "special church lectures." Religion also is manifested in her daily activities. Her day begins with prayer time and reading the Bible. Neighbors, friends, and even her landlord with whom she interacts daily are members of her church.

For others, the theme of religion gave guidance to one or two occupations in their week. Charlie, who is still deeply mourning his wife's death, relies on the promise of eternity with his wife to guide his remaining time on earth. According to his faith, it is not enough to believe in God; one must perform good works to better the world. Thus, he designates his time to serve on church and community service committees. For Charlie, the theme of religion was expressed in only a few weekly meetings and Sunday service. However, these specific occupations encompassed deep symbolic significance and gave meaning to his existence.

Although the focus of this adaptive strategy is how themes of meaning influence participation in occupations, the theme of religion also influenced the members' overriding philosophy and attitude toward life, old age, and death. Those who spoke of death described their religious beliefs as providing peace and contentment with the prospect of dying, a promise of eternal life:

> And we trust in God and hope, let him take care of us. . . When my time comes, I'm ready to go; I've nothing to fear by dying. (Rosa)
>
> Being a Christian . . . don't have to worry about dying . . . gives a sense of peacefulness and security. Knowing you're never alone, the Lord is always with you. (June)
>
> And I hope that at the time I'm called home to be with God, that I'll do it right here in that bed. (Dana)

To them, death simply served as a time marker separating earthly time from heavenly time. The theme of religion functions not only as a foundation for tying together the values and events of their earthly life, but also provides a continuity between their presence on earth and their spiritual existence in heaven.

Finally, the HCAs relied on religious themes to make sense of the losses and miracles in their lives. In three cases, the informants experienced severe grief and pain over the death of their loved ones. Although these individuals were devastated by their losses, their belief in God facilitated an acceptance of their loved one's death:

> Charlie spent the last 2 years of his wife's life caring for her. "I mean she was right with me, depended on me. . . . In fact, when she first went to the hospital, I had to take care of everything for her; she couldn't go to the bathroom, she couldn't bathe, she couldn't do anything, and I took care of her that way."
>
> Although following his wife's death, Charlie experienced a severe case of depression, he now retells the event as "The last week . . . she didn't hardly know me the last week. To me, it was a good time. She had to die. Instead of praying for her to get better, I prayed for her to be relieved from her suffering, and the Lord would relieve her suffering."

Margaret experienced three deaths within 1 year of each other: first her son, then her nephew, and finally her husband. As she looked back on the experience, Margaret explained,

> "I couldn't have made it to get through what I went through with my husband and son if I hadn't had the Lord. . . . It was just after my husband died that I got off the track" (referring to years of alcoholism). Referring to her son she stated, "after God gave him to me for 17 years, he loaned him to me and he needed him, so he called him home no matter how horrible it is."

Although religion emerged as the most common theme for the group, each individual's life account was filled with a variety of other symbolic themes of meaning. Productivity, generosity, generativity, creative expression, caregiving, affective familial bonds, and independence were among other personal themes that framed and gave meaning to the HCAs' daily activities. The restricted scope of this pilot project prevented me from securing a complete life history; however, even within the limited 2.5 hour discussion, at least two to three significant themes emerged for each individual. The following cases exemplify a few of these themes and how they drove present occupations.

Prominent themes in Bertha's life were productivity and generosity. Her concurrent worker, mother, and volunteer endeavors contributed to this identity in her early life. She spoke proudly of the products that were made by the factory where she was employed. Memories of the elaborate dinners she prepared for families and friends were treasured: "I used to cook some awfully big meals. All my life . . . I've had as high as 17 to cook for." She also described numerous volunteer projects she took on with a sense of accomplishment. "I've made 87 afghans for the convalescent home there at the circle." Presently, she spends the majority of her day restricted to one chair in a small mobile home as a result of back pain and arthritis. Productivity and generosity still guide her activities, although on a restricted basis. Teaching health care professionals as a member of the HCA provides her an opportunity to continue giving of herself and helping others. "I think the reason I'm still doing the HCA is because I've helped so many people when I was young."

Rosa dedicated her life to her husband and children. Two years after her husband's death, he is still very much alive in the memorabilia that fills her house. Feeling satisfied that she has completed her mission to provide a solid, healthy upbringing for her children, she devotes her time to talking with her grandchildren and taking short trips with her daughter. One child still living with her provides familial affiliation.

Edith, whose life was built around raising "foster children," now offers her back bedroom to a woman she calls her "adopted adult daughter." Company helps alleviate the loneliness of an empty home following the death of her husband and maintains her image as "caregiver."

Again, in these three examples, the fit between personal themes of meaning and present activities and relationships is present. In Edith's case, her past image as a caregiver and mother is reconstructed into a symbolic mother image and gives meaning to renting out her back room. For Bertha, her present occupation of volunteering was symbolically meaningful because it remained congruent with her past identity as productive and generous. For Rosa, the theme of familial affiliation is continued with her grandchildren.

Similar to Erikson et al.'s[12] work, the themes that emerged from the HCAs' stories were either grounded in convictions that were developed and refined throughout their lifetimes, as exemplified in Bertha's story, or surfaced from a dramatic emotional event. As previously stated, Charlie's story exemplifies the second situation. He was devastated by his wife's death and continues to mourn for her companionship and love. The time spent caring for his wife in the hospital was cherished. "In a way it was a pleasure just to be with her all the time." However, he painfully recalled her treatment by the medical professionals. "Now, you know they try to get these people [health care professionals] to treat them nice. But back in those days they didn't." Referring to the physician, he said, "There are still a lot of doctors that kind of think they're God, you know, and you're supposed to kow-tow to them." The pain that Charlie experienced due to the detached hospital personnel and his sense of helplessness at watching his wife be pulled away from him fueled his passionate commitment to making the health care system a more empathic place for elderly individuals to receive care. This commitment is realized both through his enrollment in Toastmasters to master speaking and through his membership in the HCA. In this sense, his wife's death was the catalyst for his present action.

Regardless of whether themes of meaning were developed over a lifetime or due to a specific event, the HCA exemplified how certain themes embodied powerful convictions that are woven into occupations. Additionally, the stories of the

HCAs exemplified how some convictions are translated into visible and easily articulated goal-directed social actions, as in Charlie's case, whereas other convictions nurture less noticeable actions, such as baking lemon cakes for friends as an expression of the belief that one must care for one's neighbor.

In sum, the relationship between personal themes of meaning and one's daily and weekly itinerary was clearly depicted in the stories told by each member. For these people, disability and aging have interrupted the amount and type of daily activities in which they typically engaged. One powerful method by which members of the HCA negotiated the loss of an activity imposed by disability was to weave a present motif of activities with threads of meaning from the past. For this group, it was not enough to reinterpret the past into life themes. They searched out specific opportunities that allowed them to continue to express personal themes of meaning in their daily or weekly occupations.

Although an avenue of expression through the actual doing of occupation was clearly essential to members of the HCA, they did not spend all their time engaging in symbolically meaningful occupations. The actual time spent pursuing those occupations deemed most relevant to their themes of meaning was, for some, rather small, despite their importance. What emerged as more significant than the time spent in such occupations was, first, that an opportunity existed. Second, how these individuals framed certain meaningful occupations within their overall patterns of daily and weekly activities appeared to be more important than the amount of time spent in a particular occupation. One might conclude that for these individuals, the relationship between themes of meaning and occupations was similar to a figure-ground situation. The occupations that are most symbolically significant in their lives emerged to the forefront of their consciousness and thus their stories; whereas, other occupations that made up their day receded into the background of insignificance.

Risk and Challenge in Occupation

The desire for an engaged life was expressed by all members of the HCA. Complaints about growing old reflected their resentment at experiencing restriction in their activity level. Even a discussion of pain was framed as an interference with being active.

> Both my wrists are sore today to where I can't use my hands very easy, you know. And it's being laid up to where you can't enjoy going out . . . going on a trip with senior citizens. (Edith)

Although activity was relished, the degree and type of occupations for which individuals longed for varied. As discussed in the last section, because occupations that embraced themes of meaning were essential in their lives, a prominent adaptive strategy was to ensure the opportunity for such occupations. However, quiet satisfaction also was found in mundane household activities. "But when I go in and clean them up and they look real nice, when I get through it makes me feel good." For others, playing with grandchildren, taking walks, or reading was experienced with fondness and contentment. Sometimes gazing outside or meditating provided a sense of peace.

Among these prosaic occupations, though, the HCAs yearned for challenge and excitement. Similar to the incorporation of themes of meaning into occupations, this quest for challenge was not necessarily desired on a daily basis, but every so often, tucked away somewhere in their activity patterns, they craved excitement. If it wasn't present, reliving memories became an alternative. This urge was best expressed in the instances in which members shared with pride the memory of their excursion "up north" to present their opinions on aging at a National Gerontology Conference. Regardless of their insecurity ("I didn't think I could talk in front of all those people, but I did") the chance to take a risk was relished.

The challenge of developing a new skill was equally cherished. Charlie struggled with his desire and many failed attempts to write articles about the realities of caring for loved ones with Alzheimer's. Despite failure, Charlie was driven to continue in this new endeavor and searched out others to help him.

Proponents for the Independent Living Movement[13,14] claim that human dignity exists in the opportunity for risk and failure, yet when individuals are disabled, they are often deprived of such opportunities. Risk deprivation leads to stagnation not only for the individual, but for society as a whole. It is argued that when forced into safe existences, people with disabilities actively struggle to reintroduce elements of typical arousal into their daily practices. Some theorists believe that as people age, they purposefully disengage from their activities and social systems to prepare for their eventual death and thus would treasure an absence of challenge in their lives.[15] The experiences of the HCAs suggest the opposite. Neither age nor disability takes away their desire for opportunities to test their abilities and risk failure. Clearly, these individuals strive to remain challenged in their lives, regardless of their age and disability.

Activity Patterns and Temporal Rhythms

The third adaptive strategy relates to the way in which the members established temporal rhythms through routines and pacing. Engagement in activities set a tempo or rhythm to the lives of the HCAs. As each member described a day or week, he or she tended to chunk activities into routines, often associating a particular activity with a day of the week or a period in a day:

> So she'll wash on Wednesday, clean house on Friday, and on Thursday, why we go over and get groceries and things . . . that we need. (Bertha)
> The first thing I did was take my shower, and then I came down and had breakfast, and went outside and cleaned the patio. . . . I washed off the plants and then [I waited for you]. (Rosa)

Additionally, one or two prominent occupations were often recounted as providing the overall structure to their day. For example, Margaret discussed her Fridays in terms of three occupations: doctor's appointment, lunch, and shopping. It is as if these occupations provide temporal intervals throughout her day. Within that structure, she completed other occupations, such as opening the mail, answering the phone, talking to a friend, or reading a book. Occupational routines appeared to be an adaptive strategy that provided the members with a security in what was experienced as a natural, subconscious rhythm to their day.

Zemke (in this book) proposes the term occupatiotemporality to depict a temporal order defined by the flow of activities that regulates individuals' lives. This notion suggests that although a natural biotemporal order and a socially constructed sociotemporal order contribute to one's perception and use of time, the experience of time also is embedded in the bodily movements and shift of consciousness that occur between various occupations. Clearly, the examples discussed previously demonstrate the degree to which the HCAs experience their days and weeks as a flow of occupations. Occupations seem to be the reference point that frames their day-to-day existence.

This was not consistent for every member. Liza, who resides in a retirement home, is bound by a sociotemporal order exhibited in a rather strict meal schedule. "Breakfast is at 8 o'clock, lunch is at 12 o'clock, and dinner is at 5 o'clock." Zerubavel[16] points out that sociotemporal regularity is managed effectively by the driven schedule. Perhaps using a socially constructed time frame (i.e., hourly clock schedules and calendars) becomes more important when the temporal order of collectives must be regulated, as in a retirement home, than when someone is focused on her or his own schedule.

Socially constructed schedules, such as those imposed by work or having children who attend school, were virtually nonexistent in the HCAs. As retired individuals, they experienced significantly less external demand on their time and attention. Although occupations such as medical appointments or church activities required coordination with social institutions, for the most part, the HCAs needed only to coordinate with one or two friends. An internalized daily rhythm determined by daily occupations seemed to be adaptive for the HCAs. Zerubavel[16] supported this notion in his comments that westernized individuals are compelled to schedule their days, and when that schedule is not imposed by social demands, they will seek to impose it on themselves.

The HCAs used temporal pacing to carry out their daily occupations and their social interactions. For example, preparing to go on a luncheon excursion demanded much more time than it had in the past. Whereas many people would jump into their cars, choosing their destination en route, the members of the HCA had become experts at perceiving potential problems, especially with reference to architectural and mobility barriers, and allocated extra time to prepare for the event. In addition, Liza paced herself by shifting her own time clock and scheduling her luncheon outings on the "off hour," slightly out of synchrony with the fast-paced business world. "I always let those people who work eat, and then [I] go a little bit early or later. . . . Then I don't need to worry about the crowd and falling." Thus, she remained active in her community at her own pace.

Control

The spirit of independence is a tenacious American value that permeates many social institutions in this country and was clearly embedded in the personal ethos of most members of the HCA. The importance of retaining independence and autonomy was expressed in comments, such as "I got my freedom" (referring to living in her own home); "I don't want to be sick on them; I'd rather pass away as quick as I can" (Rosa); and "When I leave it's going to be feet first" (Dana, referring to dying in her own home). Regardless of their love for and involvement in networks of family and friends, their desire to remain autonomous was strong enough to warrant a wish for a peaceful death rather than dependence. These wishes are best understood when placed within the context of their age, feelings that they have lived fruitful and complete lives, and their sense of peace with respect to an afterlife. Dependency to some degree, whether on family or friends, was characteristic of most members' lives because they appreciated interconnectedness with family and friends. Nonetheless, threads of this enduring value for autonomous control in one's life was present in all the stories.

Five members of the HCA maintained a somewhat restricted existence, requiring assistance with personal grooming and hygiene care, home tasks, and community mobility. Although these women dealt with dependency issues in many areas of their lives, they have creatively maintained autonomous control over their environments and activities. For example, Rosa shared her home with her youngest daughter. Although she relied on her daughter for all meals and transportation, Rosa retained decision-making control over her environment. She did so by hanging on to memorabilia, furniture, and gifts from her deceased husband, even though her children told her to "get rid of that." In this instance, control stemmed from the fact that Rosa marked her own environmental surroundings through the arrangement of symbolically meaningful objects and in doing so, retained ownership over certain spaces in the home, especially those that were communal. Furthermore, by maintaining control over the objects in her environment, she created a home that was a symbolic expression of the essential events and themes of meaning in her life.

Another way in which HCA members maintained control over their daily lives involved the innovative use of hired workers. Traditionally, "workers" are employed to perform personal care tasks and household chores that are necessary to enable the individual to remain in his or her place of residence. However, Edith and Bertha creatively managed to maintain a sense of autonomy in what was otherwise a dependent situation. They did this by directing their workers toward occupations they deemed most important to their lives, rather than toward traditional expectations.

In Edith's case, creative expression through artwork was a prominent theme throughout her life. Arthritic pain and deformities of her hands rendered her unable to fabricate quilts, one of her most cherished artistic endeavors. However, to retain this occupation in her life, Edith and her hired worker, Susie, carried out the project together. Edith used her creative abilities to design quilt patterns, select material, and verbally direct Susie to perform the physical task of cutting and sewing the quilt patches.

Likewise, Bertha, who relished cooking but did not have the physical strength or endurance to manage meal preparation, maintained control by verbally directing her worker, Kathryn, through the process. Bertha expressed this technique stating, "Oh I can't cook; it burns me up. . . . Now I tell her how to do it. . . . I know the tastes and flavors I want it to be." Regardless of physical dependency, Bertha was able to maintain control over her preferences and tasks.

In each of these situations, physical limitations prohibited "doing of these activities." However, through Edith's choice to direct Susie to meet her real interests and through Bertha's and Edith's cognitive participations in their respective activities, autonomy was affirmed.

Finally, individuals maintained control by engaging in occupations that allowed them to be alone and at peace with their own thoughts. Liza resided in the most restrictive environment, a retirement home in which she had to share a room with an assigned roommate and eat meals at scheduled times. Although least successful in her attempt to maintain a sense of control, she created a world of privacy by working in the garden or playing the piano. "The disadvantage, I feel, is that you really don't have that much privacy [referring to living in a retirement home]. I work out on the patio every so often so that I can get into myself and so that I can look within myself and know what the hell my thoughts really are."

The western notion of independence is grounded in the ability to be physically self-sufficient in carrying out personal and social tasks and economically sovereign. Independence and autonomy have become an indication of social worth and for many, a sign of personal achievement. However, these values are often at odds with the situations in which people with disabilities find themselves. Because the notion of independence and autonomy embodies physical ability, people with disabilities who may need assistance are often relegated to a passive, dependent social position and assumed to be incapable of contributing to their social community in a substantial and meaningful way. Advocates for the disabled[14] challenge this concept of independence, claiming that independence cannot be measured by the quantity of tasks one is able to perform without assistance but by the degree of freedom one has to choose his or her own course of actions. Self-direction and participation in day-to-day decision making about when and how things will be done to one's body, to one's environment, and with one's time become the crucial distinctions between dependence and independence and ultimately lead to a sense of personal and social worth. The stories told by the HCAs provide added evidence to support a definition of independence that encompasses a mental choice rather than physical action. Self-direction and control may be viewed as adaptive strategies that enabled members to retain a sense of authorship over their daily occupations despite physical dependencies.

The relationship of control to meaningfulness in daily occupations can be further teased out by the findings of this study. In her book *The Ageless Self*, Kaufman[17] commented that "What people do, the content of the activities themselves, does not determine the meaningfulness of daily life. Rather, the determining factor seems to be the sense of being able to choose to do what one wants." In this quote, Kaufman underscores the importance of control as a factor in determining meaningfulness on a day-to-day basis. However, in this study, it appears as if control alone does not determine meaningfulness of daily life. The content of the activity, what one was actually doing, was equally important as control. Edith's story exemplifies this point.

It was evident that Edith had creatively managed to maintain a sense of autonomy in what is otherwise a dependent situation by directing Susie to perform the step of quilt making that she was unable to complete. However, creative hobby work provided more fulfillment than watching her soap operas or directing Susie to make a dinner, both of which were under her control. It can be hypothesized that the importance of quilt making as an expression of a significant theme of meaning in her life was a factor that rendered the control of this activity to be particularly meaningful and desired.

Liza provided another example. She resided in a retirement home where many activities were available to her. Although the environment was restrictive, serving meals at a set time and conducting activities on schedule, she had a choice of whether or not to participate. In Liza's situation, the content of the activity was primary. She was bored by the sing-alongs, barbecues, and luncheons. To combat her boredom, she attempted, although unsuccessfully, to conduct her own activity groups, a theme consistent with her volunteerism earlier in life.

Again, control was definitely an issue for Liza; however, the opportunity to engage in an activity that was meaningful and challenging was equally, if not more, important. In Liza's case, organizing activity groups provided a new challenge for her present situation yet one that was connected to the past and allowed her to exercise control. The findings of this study suggest that the determining factors in constructing meaningful daily experiences entail not only self-direction and control, but available options for engaging in activities that provide a sense of challenge and are consistent with themes of meaning in one's life.

Maintaining Continuity Through Spatial, Social, and Cultural Connectedness

Illness or financial devastation is a disruptive force in the lives of some elderly, causing them to be dislocated from their homes or friends. Studies have shown that elderly individuals who respond to these disruptive situations by recreating a sense of continuity through maintaining stability and connectedness with society adapt more readily to their situation.[18]

Continuity or interconnectedness is described by these authors as a complex process that can be experienced as cultural, social, or spatial. Cultural continuity refers to the availability of notions, ritual, values, and symbols that have been ingrained throughout one's upbringing. Social continuity is established through the maintenance of relationships either vicariously or face-to-face. Spatial continuity refers to a sense of connectedness with a real or imagined place. All three interact to provide a temporal continuity throughout one's lifetime and even into death. Thus, even with displacement from one's home, community, and friends, continuity in the form of rituals, memories, activities, or friendships can offer stability and interconnectedness with the world.[18]

In this pilot study, most of the HCAs maintained some contact with family, even though all but two changed their place of residence following disability. Regardless of an element of stability in their lives, disability and loss led to a changing relationship between the person and his or her physical, social, or cultural environment. Maintaining temporal continuity through cultural, social, and spatial connectedness was a valued adaptation in each individual's life. The most prominent means for maintaining connectedness and stability were familial bonds, objects of meaning, fantasy, occasional acquaintances, and technology.

Familial Bonds

Of all the social relationships, the quality of the mother- or father-child-grandchild bond emerged as the most powerful, providing enduring emotional support and a sense of connectedness with past and future generations. Many members praised their mothers as being one of the most influential people in their lives, symbolizing love, caregiving, and gentleness. "Well, my mother had a lot of love and she showed it to us!" (Bertha). When talking about their mothers, the respondents expressed a sense of security and stability during their upbringing. Irrespective of the accuracy of those memories, a symbolic mother image as a stabilizing force in their lives shaped their present understanding of early childhood. This image was then carried forward into the next generation when they brought up their children.

The enduring bond between these members and their future generations was apparent in the repeated expressions of respect for their children and grandchildren. "Oh, I'm proud of this daughter over here. . . . she's a real good artist." A letter from a child was priceless. Members were quick to share the arrival of a letter with others during their meetings, often gloating over the length, for example, "nine pages long; that's a book!" One woman placed raising her children as the central theme of her life, "Well, you know my family is the most valuable [possession]. They were all my life, my husband and my children." Grandchildren were just as cherished. "My granddaughter is having a baby, I'll be a great-grandma. It makes me happy!"

With respect to temporal continuity, generations of families anchor a person in the past and future (see Knox's paper in this book). In a sense, the HCAs experienced their own accomplishments and confrontations through their children's lives. Children represent an extension of the self from past to present. However, more important for those reaching the end of their lives, children provided a sense of connectedness with this world even after death. Thus, on a biological level through genes and a symbolical level through memories, the HCAs were intimately connected with their children and through them, experienced continuity of time.

Objects of Meaning

A second strategy for providing a sense of continuity had to do with the presence of objects of meaning. Objects of meaning were collected by the HCAs and displayed around their homes to represent their life narratives. By so doing, members preserved the past as they continued to create the present. Six out of seven of the homes that were visited were filled with "objects," many discussed in the context of a story that carried deep layers of symbolic meaning. For example, Bertha proudly displayed years of certificates honoring her volunteering work, an accomplishment she held in high esteem. Rosa used objects of furniture that her deceased husband built to evoke memories. The presence of this furniture enabled her to transcend the present and reexperience the emotions of past events and at other times, to infuse those past events into her present existence. For Rosa, the furniture and other objects of meaning, embodied her personal historicity, that is, her evolving experience of self. As with all the HCAs, Rosa's home was a storehouse of memories with each object able to call forward a reservoir of sentiments that gave access to past places and times. Objects of meaning maintained the integrity of their lives over time. During her interview, she specifically identified each object, associating it with a person or special occasion.

> See this chair that's here. It's an old chair. It's a chair from my wedding; I had a lovely dining room [set]; it was from my mother; Like that chair there, going with the rocker I had in the den. When we were married 25 years he gave me that.

Pictures of family and friends, artifacts from memorable vacations, and trophies of accomplishments not only adorned their homes, (Fig. 32–1) but in one apartment complex, were placed along window sills as if to share "who they were" with friends and neighbors. In this sense, objects also broke down barriers and invited connection among neighbors.

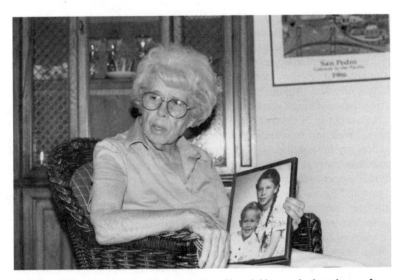

Figure 32–1. This woman has many photographs of her children and other objects of meaning throughout her home that provide continuity and share who she is with guests. (Photo by John Wolcott.)

Csikszentmihalyi and Rochberg-Halton,[19] in their book *The Meaning of Things*, pointed out that household objects not only perform a utilitarian purpose, but also constitute a symbolic reflection of the owner's identity. In the home, the owner can carefully select those objects that reflect a significant part of the self. For the elderly, household objects are an important means of preserving the past and "establishing a sense of personal continuity." Surrounded by objects that are imbued with past emotions and memories, individuals are able to fuse the past and the present in their day-to-day existence. The importance of objects as symbols of meaningful life events was certainly evident in the homes of the HCAs.

Fantasy

The third method that was used to maintain cultural, social, and spatial continuity was fantasy. Fantasy was identified by Rowles[20] as a method used to experience geographical spaces beyond one's physical abilities. As Rowles pointed out, in fantasy "the individual is unlimited. Physiological decline, ill health, economic constraints, social alienation or environmental barriers provide no limitations."[21] Fantasy, in the form of reminiscing about past trips and vacations, was used by one HCA to project himself back into what Rowles has termed "beyond spaces," that is, significant locations associated with one's past:

> Like when I retired, I got . . . a little truck and a little trailer, that was up around the Bay Area, San Francisco; in March I packed all my stuff and in my little trailer and hit the road in March. I went down California, and across in Arizona, and up into Iowa and across and back down to Alabama and up into Washington, DC, and to Toronto, Canada and Calgary, Alberta. When I got home, it was October. . . . Oh, that was the

best money I ever spent was on that year on the road. Oh boy, just like the old days when I was a kid and get out in all that flat prairie and all snow white. (Charlie)

As illustrated in this quote, Charlie remained linked with a place in his distant past through imagination. Likewise, for Bertha, fantasy provided a vicarious pleasure that had previously been part of an activity in her life.

You know when you get up at a certain age, why naturally your body grows weaker, and I'd love to get out in the yard and dig in the yard with flowers and things, but I do it in my mind. (Bertha)

By evoking the emotional sentiments, visual imagery, and perhaps even the physical sensibilities once experienced by gardening, fantasy allowed Bertha to continue this activity in her life.

In summary, fantasy was a powerful strategy to transcend the present and create a sense of continuity with past places, events, and people. All but one invited me into their past through shared memories. The stories told were so rich and detailed that it became obvious they had ventured into environments beyond the confines of the room.

Occasional Acquaintances

Brief encounters with acquaintances or even strangers emerged as the fourth method to provide continuity. In particular, this strategy connects people with their social present. Two notable methods to remain interconnected with others, the manipulation of one's environment and participation in certain occupations, emerged as particularly inventive adaptations.

Margaret, who is relatively immobile in her home, spends most of her day sitting in a chair carefully positioned so that she is visible to anyone who walks by. Her front door is conveniently propped open to invite entrance. During our interview, on three occasions, apartment workers or neighbors informally popped their heads in with a quick hello and good-bye. Each time, Margaret acknowledged them in a warm and friendly voice. Although Margaret had the greatest mobility restrictions of all the HCAs and was at risk for isolation, through a creative manipulation of her environment, she remained connected with her world on a daily basis.

Participation in certain occupations also emerged as a medium for maintaining social connections. Liza, who was able to venture out of her retirement home, yet considered herself socially isolated from her community, adeptly used this strategy. Frequent visits to the post office to "mail a letter" or the grocery store to "get a few things" were described by Liza, not so much in terms of the instrumental purpose of the venture, but more as an opportunistic interlude in which she connected with tellers and cashiers over a brief remark regarding some current event or personal happening. In these instances, the occupation served as an occasion for which superficial encounters are requisite. For Liza and many older individuals who are relatively isolated, the interactions that are integral to certain occupations take on the additional meaning of linking one socially with their present everyday world.

Rowles,[20] in a qualitative study that examined the geographic space of five elderly individuals, noticed the same type of social interaction as described previously in the life of one of his informants. Rowles[22] suggested that these quick contacts by acquaintances are a source of "self-reaffirmation and identity." People experience pleasure in connecting with others and being recognized. Both in Rowles' study and this research project, these types of interactions occurred for people who are somewhat isolated because of age and disability. For adults who work outside the home or for whom child care is constantly thrusting them into relationships with others, the opportunity to connect with others may be unnecessary and at times a nuisance. However, for Margaret and Liza, daily reaffirmations were actively sought by drawing others into their worlds.

Technology

Technology was another method by which the HCAs maintained social connectedness with their world. Television was the most frequently used to remain aware of the political and social happenings in their own city and country. Newspapers and magazines served the same purpose, but were used less frequently. Again, for individuals who were restricted to their own residences, television, newspapers, and magazines allowed them to remain part of their community. This, in turn, reaffirmed their identity as members of the collective society and grounded them in the present. The telephone was another piece of technology that enabled the members to have direct contact with their personal and social worlds. Because many of the HCAs were physically or financially unable to travel and visit friends and family, this piece of equipment mitigated isolation and preserved emotional commitments in some instances.

In summary, a sense of continuity and connectedness was desired by all members of the HCA. Although not concretely articulated as important or consciously pursued, the variety and creative nature of the five methods discussed give evidence to the importance of maintaining continuity in old age.

Acknowledging Identity Through the Celebration of Occupations

Another strategy used by the HCAs was maintenance of a sense of self-worth through the celebration of occupations. As stated previously, one of the purposes of the group was to create an accepting atmosphere in which socializing and nurturing friendships were encouraged. To accomplish this goal, the first hour of their weekly meetings was devoted to a ritualized sharing ceremony, during which each member was given an opportunity to, in the words of Myerhoff,[23] dramatize what he or she considered to be a significant event of the past week. Most shared what appeared on the surface to be somewhat insignificant, commonplace occurrences, such as getting one's hair done, eating at a restaurant, making a potholder, attending a movie, or reading a book. However, when examined within the context of a particular member's life, these occupations held great importance and were often an expression of personal themes of meaning. Thus, the meeting provided an arena to celebrate what may look to others as mundane activities but in actuality, were salient occurrences in present life that often embodied meaningful themes from members' personal histories.

Simic and Myerhoff[18] discussed the notion of "dramas of honor" as a phenomenon in which elderly individuals, especially those who are culturally or spatially disconnected, gather and formally or informally share their accomplishments as a way of establishing a sense of self-worth. Dramatization of one's accomplishments satisfies a "fierce human drive to be noticed"[24] for the things that one has done with one's life and on that basis, remembered and respected in an honorable fashion.

The HCA meetings encompassed dramas of honor in that each individual was able to share weekly accomplishments and to receive supportive public recognition from the other members. Although Myerhoff[23] focused on recognition for past endeavors, for the HCAs, present actions warranted celebration. In a sense, their meetings elevated everyday occupations, acknowledging their significance in each individual's present life. What the member did on a daily and weekly basis was "noticed" as important and an integral component to who they were in old age.

Advocating Social Change

A final adaptive strategy was that of members advocating for social change, the fundamental mission of the HCA. This strategy, unlike the others, centered on changing the environment, specifically the medical institution, which had become a central social structure in their lives. In an essay entitled "Uses of Anger," Audre Lorde[25] wrote, "But anger expressed and translated into action in the service of our vision and our future is a liberating and strengthening act." The HCAs funneled anger into an active crusade to transform the health care system—a system that often unknowingly oppresses the disabled and the elderly.

The HCAs had firsthand experience with receiving poor health care. They had watched loved ones die in convalescent homes with care that they perceived incompetent or disrespectful. Presently, their most frustrating complaint was that they felt deprived of accurate information about their health status. Health care professionals failed to spend the time or to explain thoroughly the tests, findings, or remedies for their ailments. Their future vision, a "respectful" health care system for older people in America, inspired their commitment to promote change. Dedication to this cause was apparent in their perseverance in relating their stories and concerns repeatedly as new health profession students arrived at their doorsteps. Welch[26] commented in *A Feminist Ethic of Risk* that social causes or attempts to change the injustices of the world have a temporal life in which despair and discouragement of its resistors often set in as the magnitude of problems is realized. She specifically relegated this despair response to American middle class. Some members of the HCA have commented about the difficulties in changing physicians' attitudes and wonder how far their efforts will go. These comments were transient and easily overridden by a request for another educational experience. They did not stop. For this group of individuals, although gains were not usually apparent, the resistance continued.

Summary

In summary, the findings of this study illustrate the extent to which adaptation to aging becomes a creative enterprise. Each member of the HCA was adept at inventing ways to deal with the changes that come with the passage of time. The purpose of this paper has been to bring into the forefront the very ingenious, yet often underemphasized, strategies that one group of elderly people adopted to enhance their lives. It is important that we, as occupational therapists, take the messages and important insight about adaptation that these people offer to heart.

First, it is essential that occupational therapists respect patients as occupational beings, supporting their attempts to create themselves through the inclusion of meaningful occupations in their lives. This requires an appreciative understanding of the symbolic meaning that patients attach to various occupations, whether they are as simple as reading a poem or as complex as organizing a dinner party. Most importantly, it requires that we begin to enter their worlds of meaning, assisting them in weaving past themes of meaning into present activities. Second, we need to listen intently to where and how our patients want to maintain authorship over their lives and assist them in this endeavor by fostering self-directive skills and exploring other methods for retaining control. In other words, our own definition of control and authorship needs to be broadened to avoid falling into the trap of equating control solely with physical doing. Third, it would behoove us to support our patients in their exploration of innovative methods to maintain temporal continuity and social connectedness with their families, friends, communities, and the world around them. Fourth, a broader definition of activity must be embraced if we are to meet the needs of our patients fully. This new definition must not only include the actual doings, but also respect the richness that reminiscing and fantasy can offer. Occupations can be "done in one's mind." Fifth, occupational therapists need to cherish patients' drive to be noticed for their everyday accomplishments and their potential urges to take risks and experience new successes and failures. Finally, we need to consider adaptation not only as the development of individual skills, but also in terms of our patients' abilities to manipulate their personal environments and transform their social and political situations.

Discussion Questions

1. How might practitioners determine which occupations of patients carry particular symbolic meaning, even if infrequently performed, and therefore bear an important organizational and motivational influence over their overall activity patterns?
2. If the freedom to take risks is routinely denied to people with disabilities, thereby denying them an essential aspect of their humanity, how might occupational therapists offer therapeutic activities differently than what is traditionally done to ensure appropriate levels of challenges and risks?
3. Jackson proposed that occupational therapists need to consider adaptation not only as the development of individual skills, but also in terms of patients' abilities to manipulate their personal environments and transform their social and political situation. How might we help our patients accomplish these ends?

References

1. Berman, P: The Courage to Grow Old. Ballantine Books, New York, 1989.
2. Diamond, D: Dark years and difficult questions. In Berman, P (ed): The Courage to Grow Old. Ballantine Books, New York, 1989, p 85.

3. Yates, E: Always ahead. In Berman, P (ed): The Courage to Grow Old. Ballantine Books, New York, 1989, p 250.
4. Yerxa, EJ, Clark, F, Frank, G, Jackson, J, Parham, D, Pierce, D, Stein, C, and Zemke, R: Occupational therapy in the twentieth century: A great idea whose time has come. Occup Ther Health Care 6(1):7, 1990.
5. Clark, F, Parham, D, Carlson, M, Frank, G, Jackson, J, Pierce, D, Stein, C, and Zemke, R: Occupational science: Academic innovation in the service of occupational therapy's future. Am J Occup Ther 45:300, 1990.
6. Bruner, J: Acts of Meaning. Howard University Press, Cambridge, MA, 1990.
7. MacIntyre, A: After Virtue (ed 2). University of Notre Dame Press, Notre Dame, 1984.
8. Yerxa, E: Seeking a relevant, ethical, realistic way of knowing for occupational therapy. Am J Occup Ther 45(3):199, 1991.
9. Reilly, M: Occupational therapy can be one of the great ideas of the 20th century medicine. Am J Occup Ther 26:87, 1962.
10. Charmaz, K: The grounded theory method: An explanation and interpretation. In Emerson, R (ed): Contemporary Field Research. Little, Brown Press, Boston, MA, 1983.
11. Kaufman, S: The Ageless Self. University of Wisconsin, Madison WI, 1986.
12. Erikson, E, Erikson, J, and Kivnick, H: Vital Involvement in Old Age. W. W. Norton Co., New York, 1986.
13. De Jong, G: Defining and implementing the independent living concept. In Crewe, N, and Zola, I (eds): Independent Living for Physically Disabled People. Jossey-Bass Publications, San Francisco, 1983, p 4.
14. Zola, I: Toward independent living: Goals and dilemmas. In Crewe, N, and Zola, I (eds): Independent Living for Physically Disabled People. Jossey-Bass Publications, San Francisco, 1983, p 344.
15. Lewis, SC: Elder Care in Occupational Therapy. Slack, Thorofare, NJ, 1989.
16. Zerubavel, E: Hidden Rhythms: Schedules and Calendars in Social Life. University of California Press, Berkeley, 1981.
17. Kaufman, p 108.
18. Simic, A, and Myerhoff, B: Conclusion. In Myerhoff, B, and Simic, A (eds). Life's Career—Aging: Cultural Variations on Growing Old. Sage Publications, Beverly Hills, 1978.
19. Csikszentmihalyi, M, and Rochberg-Halton, E: The Meaning of Things: Domestic Symbols and the Self. Cambridge University Press, Cambridge, MA, 1987.
20. Rowles, G: Prisoners of Space? Exploring the Geographical Experience of Older People. Westview Press, Boulder, CO, 1978.
21. Rowles, p 181.
22. Rowles, p 7.
23. Myerhoff, B: A symbol perfected in death. In Myerhoff, B, and Simic, A (eds): Life's Career—Aging: Cultural Variations on Growing Old. Sage Publications, Beverly Hills, 1978.
24. Simic and Myerhoff, p 183.
25. Lorde, A: Sister Outsider. The Crossing Press Feminist Series, Freedom, CA, 1984, p 127.
26. Welch, S: A Feminist Ethic of Risk. Fortress Press, Minneapolis, MN, 1990.

by *John A. White, Jr., MA, OTR*

33

Temporal Adaptation in the Intensive Care Unit

Centrality of Time and Occupation

Time is an extremely influential aspect of our lives that shapes the things we do and hence the kind of lives we live. In his 1922 address, Adolph Meyer recognized the critical role that time played in life and its influence on how people establish balance in their occupations.[1] He suggested that occupational therapy would be most successful by recognizing "a full meaning of time as the biggest wonder and asset of our lives."[2] That's a bold statement from one of our most influential founders! He encourages us, as occupational therapists, to explore human temporality in more depth. How can we get at the full meaning of time? How can we use time to its full value?

Occupational science is looking for answers to questions like these. In particular, occupational scientists are examining how time influences the individual's adaptation to life's demands through occupation. Much of the science of human occupation has evolved from clinical and theoretical questions derived from occupational therapy practice. The link between occupational therapy and temporal adaptation becomes evident when we treat patients whose temporal flow is disrupted by accident or illness.

Temporal Disruption

When, through the misfortune of disease or injury, a person assumes the role of patient, he or she steps out of the normal flow of time. The exemption from normal social obligations, responsibilities, and even daily life tasks is an essential element of the "sick role" as defined by Talcott Parsons in 1951.[3] The schedule demanded of a person keeping a household in order or performing a job is shaped by the sociocultural milieu in which that person lives. Hospitalization usually results in separation from individuals' occupational routines, thereby detaching them from normal temporal anchors. This process of isolation is greatly exacerbated when an individual enters an intensive care unit (ICU).

Temporal Cues and the Human Biological Clock

There are many common ways in which people remain oriented to time in their daily lives. Clocks, of course, are a powerful tool for orientation.[4,5] Most people wear a watch and if not, have a good idea where clocks can be found at home, work, or in the car to keep them on their schedule. Daylight is even more of a significant entrainer or synchronizer of daily circadian[4,5] rhythms (approximately 24-hour cycles). Although few of us know the exact moments of sunrise and sunset, we have a good idea of when those events will occur in relation to our daily activities.

Social cues also play an essential role in setting the schedules people will keep.[6-8] How strong an entraining influence does a work or school schedule play in synchronizing biotemporal clocks, thereby influencing the occupations people choose to pursue at different times of day? When I worked for 1 year in an Islamic country where Friday, the holy day, was the one day of the week off from work, I was constantly confused. Waking up on Saturday morning, I always felt that it must be Monday; after all, it was the first work day of the week. At first, my Malaysian coworkers thought I had learned the wrong Malay word for Saturday, but then they just found it amusing that I could not keep the days of the week straight.

Occupation and Temporality

Occupational therapy and occupational science are concerned with temporal adaptation because of the intimate relationship of activity, or occupation, to the passage of time.[1,9,10] Patients in the ICU are not only removed from the temporal stream and environmental cues that signal the passage of time, but, due to physical constraints, also are cut off from their customary occupations that structure the flow of their time. Therefore, the value of understanding temporal adaptation in an ICU environment is in how that insight helps us restore to our patients control over their daily life activities.

The Experience of Time in the ICU

Various studies have shown that between 25% and 40% of the patients admitted to ICU experience significant levels of disorientation.[11] A number of factors combine to create an environment alien to a person's normal life experience.[4,5,11-13] The literature on the influence of environmental factors on ICU patients suggested a number of cues that may affect their temporal orientation.

In ICUs, day merges imperceptibly into night with no way for the patient to know the passage of time. Sleep is chronically disrupted by pain and procedures, such as intragastric feeding, respiratory therapy, and blood pressure recordings. Light floods the room constantly. The unit is rarely quiet due to the noise of staff, other patients, and the ventilators and cardiac monitors.

Almost all of the studies concerned with ICU environments identified the effects of light and lighting on patients' mental status.[14,15] This is not surprising, considering how strongly our circadian rhythms depend on periodic light exposure to maintain a 24-hour cycle of alertness and sleep. Most of these studies then listed in their recommendations, the placement of an easily viewed window in patient rooms to promote exposure to diurnal changes of light and dark.[12,16-18] An ICU nurse reported that there was a significant decrease in disorientation of cardiac patients after the cardiac ICU was moved from a windowless to a windowed environment.

ICU Pilot Study

A major focus of this pilot study was to identify cues in the environment that impact circadian rhythms of the ICU patients, including social or lighting cues. The primary question framing the study was, what factors lead to temporal disorientation in patients in the ICU? The design of the study combined methodologies from several research projects that investigated aspects of the ICU setting.[4,19] The resulting method included environmental mapping (detailing characteristics of the environment), checklists of temporal cues, interviews with staff, and participant observation in collection of narrative ethnographic data.

In the data collection process, approximately 12 hours were spent in a unit that primarily admitted patients with surgical, neurological, or transplant-related medical crises. Observation time was divided into two segments that intentionally coincided with the nursing staff change. The focus on shift changes was because personal experience and the literature suggested that these are the busiest times on the unit. It also included the time between 11:00 PM and 3:00 AM, the unit's most quiet time.[4] The checklist used to guide observations of time cues was formulated into major categories after reviewing the ethnographic data. Without direct patient feedback or retrospective review of the medical record, it is impossible to say which of these factors had the most significant influence on how well or poorly the patients adapted to this environment.

Surgical Intensive Care Unit

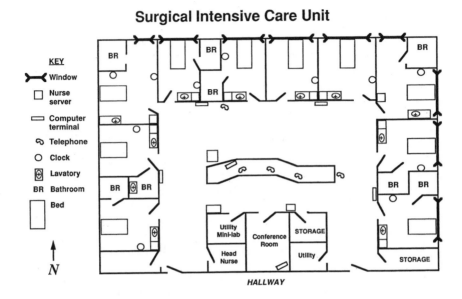

Figure 33–1. Basic floor plan of the surgical intensive care unit.

ICU Environmental Map

The physical environment seemed to be fairly typical of intensive care units. Figure 33-1 shows the basic floor plan of the 10-room unit. The nursing desk is central, and the rooms are arranged around it. Symbols are included for the more important pieces of equipment or furnishing, such as clocks, windows, telephones, and computer terminals used for patient data collection. Patient rooms included those with and without outside windows. Each room had a number of interior windows. Although necessary for adequate observation of patients, they made it more difficult to darken the room. The top two feet of glass in the rooms had been covered with a dense translucent frosting that reduced but did not occlude light coming in from other rooms. Every interior window was equipped with louvered blinds that could be operated from either side of the window.

Temporal Cues in the ICU

There were several sources of artificial lighting in each room; the only one that can be operated by the patient is the over-bed light. Lights in the nursing station area were on constantly, but at about midnight, half of these overhead lights were turned off (Fig. 33-2). Nurses made an effort to darken patient rooms during the night by turning off all the room lights when not needed for patient care. Oddly enough, the highest number of darkened rooms during this observation occurred at 6:00 AM when six of the 10 rooms had the lights out. Many patients, therefore, experienced

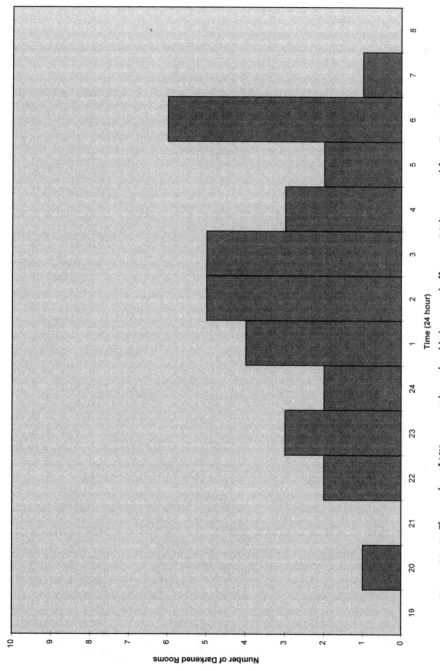

Figure 33–2. The number of ICU rooms with overhead lights turned off over a 12-hour period from 7 PM to 8 AM.

daylight conditions most of the night with most darkness at an hour when individuals begin to rise. Thus, the temporal cue of a normal light-dark cycle was not made available to them.

These rooms were not equipped with television sets or radios. A portable television was available for patient use at appropriate times, but it did not have a remote control and therefore required that staff be called to change channels or volume. Radios could be used by patients if supplied from home, although no radios were in use in patient rooms during my observations. Televisions and radios provide remote contact with the temporal rhythms of a larger social world; news and traffic reports are in the morning, soap operas in the afternoon. This mass media access can provide cues about time.

Personal care was provided for the patients by the nurses, primarily during the night shift. Baths were usually given between 2:00 PM and 4:00 AM due to the heavy work requiring two nurses. Other grooming and hygiene tasks were performed on an ad hoc basis in relation to the individual nurse's interest and availability and the patient's need. This provision of daily care is asynchronous with common self-care routines and may be disruptive to the patient's sense of time.

Each room has a clock that is usually placed at a right angle to the patient's bed. Since the clocks had a 12-hour analog face, the patient lacked clues as to whether it was morning or night. No calendars were evident at the time of this observation, and nurses reported that they did not use calendars with their patients. Calendars, like clocks, inform about the passage of time. ICU patients may "lose" time due to lack of dark-light indicators or variation in daily schedules (weekdays being the same as weekends) and may be reoriented to time by using calendars.

When I asked nurses about how they oriented patients to time and date, I received a range of answers. The range is represented by a nurse who said that he always talks to the patient, even if comatose. He explains his purposes and actions and gives the patient full orientation information as he begins each shift. At the other extreme, another nurse said that she rarely talks to her patients unless they speak first, stating that she is too occupied with patient care to talk to the patient.

Possible Areas for Occupational Therapy Intervention in the ICU

The temporal cues discussed so far could be manipulated by an occupational therapist treating or consulting in an ICU. To review them briefly, the cues of artificial and natural light and the use of television or radio to provide temporal cues for patients were discussed. Personal care activities do not occur with a regularity that would help orient patients, but this area is ripe for intervention by occupational therapists. Finally, clocks and calendars, with the implied importance of using materials that are easy for patients to read and easy for the staff to update, were mentioned.

In this pilot study, several other events or stimuli in the ICU that may serve as temporal cues were identified; however, these cues would not easily yield to an occupational therapist's intervention. Regular events, such as medical rounds, blood draws, and chest x-rays, occurred with predictability. Meals arrived dependably at 7:00 AM, 12:00 noon, and 6:00 PM but the distribution of the patients' trays may be delayed up to 2 hours, depending on their care needs. The nursing staff took their meal breaks as the workload allowed, if at all. It was fascinating that the night nurses referred to their midshift meal break as "lunch." This is in contrast with the meal at the end of their shift. At 7:30 AM they had breakfast, not dinner. Could references to this midnight lunch break be heard by patients, and if so, would it serve as a false temporal cue?

Occupational Therapy Strategies in the ICU

The results regarding temporal cues identified in this brief study suggest that the control of light in relation to day-night scheduling is one of the cues that could be most importantly modified in a concerted plan to improve patient orientation. Shifting the time of providing basic hygiene and grooming to early daylight hours also would provide temporal cues. More easily, television or radio cues might be incorporated on a routine basis.

The occupational therapist also could help educate the nursing staff about the importance of temporal orientation to patient outcomes. Brief videotaped techniques for orienting patients to time and patient-care procedures could be developed in collaboration with the nursing education department. Effective use of calendars or orientation boards requires clearly defined responsibility on the part of the therapist or nurse. These responsibilities should be negotiated between the department managers and staff involved in program implementation. The use of clocks that prominently display day and date in combination with an orientation board may improve the ease of use, and efficacy of this orienting technique.

Each hospital has unique problems and opportunities to challenge a therapist's creativity. It is hoped that this brief introduction to this methodology and the tentative study results will be helpful in directing others to study temporal adaptation in the ICU. Patients in the ICU, like some patients in convalescent centers and other long-term care institutions, are largely dependent on caretakers to shape their experience of the world by setting up their environment and framing the ways in which they can interact with it. As agents influencing the temporal experience of patients in the ICU, therapists should facilitate patients' adaptation to this alien environment. Can this influence lead to further adaptation so that patients might resume more of their chosen occupations?

Applying Occupational Science Constructs to the ICU

The outcome depends on many factors, many of which are out of our control. However, a careful look at the individual will reveal what life elements are most important to be introduced into his or her environment. Which environmental cues will most effectively reacquaint them with their temporal stream?

If you were my ICU therapist, I hope you would turn on the radio every morning to National Public Radio's "Morning Edition." That would be my link to the past through a daily habit of flipping on the radio news first thing every morning. It would be a connection to the present through reports on events of the day. It would cause me to think about the future as I wondered where this crazy world is headed. I would be connected to time through a personal occupation.

What are your most meaningful time cues? Could you translate them into an event, an environmental stimulus, or occupation in a room on an ICU? More importantly, what are the most meaningful cues for the patients you serve, and will those cues help prompt that person to action? Their act may be as simple as turning their head toward the sunshine streaming through the window, but occupational therapists celebrate the simple acts of life through our philosophy and practice.

In closing, I would like to share a brief case history written by a critical care nurse. I feel this story eloquently illustrates the major focus of my presentation:

> While caring for a patient in her late 50s who was comatose as a result of metastatic carcinoma of the brain, I carried on a one-sided conversation about many things, including a daily introduction of myself, explanations of care to be given, and discussion of the day and the weather. There was no perceptible response from the patient. Her condition appeared to be slowly deteriorating. I lost contact with her after 4 days because of an assignment change.
>
> While boarding a train about 2 months later, I was approached by a woman on crutches who called me by name and asked if I was a nurse. I answered "Yes" and eventually recognized her. Our discussion revealed much about our initial relationship. The patient expressed how she had felt during the days she lay in the hospital bed, totally defenseless, and at the mercy of those on the nursing team. She said it was very important to her that I had identified myself and talked to her each day. Of particular interest to the patient was information about when I would leave and when I would return. When I said I would be leaving for another assignment, she said she cried because she anticipated receiving no further information about the outside world. The patient recalled much more about the interactions than I did.[16]

Discussion Questions

1. White's study revealed many temporal markers and cues within an ICU environment. How might research such as his be built on in the interest of addressing how patients in ICUs and other hospital units actually reconstruct their sense of time, gradually learning how to orchestrate rounds of daily occupations?
2. Based on the results of this study, how might occupational therapists assume a consultative role within ICUs and step-down units where reorientation to time is often a critical component of recovery?

References

1. Meyer, A: The philosophy of occupational therapy. Am J Occup Ther 31(10):639, 1977.
2. Meyer, p 642.
3. Parsons, T, and Shils, E (eds): Toward a General Theory of Action. Harvard University Press, Cambridge, MA, 1951.
4. Dlin, BM, Rosen, H, Dickstein, K, Lyons, JW, and Fischer, HK: The problems of sleep and rest in the intensive care unit. Psychosomatics 12(3):155, 1971.

5. Gleck, HG: ICU syndrome: Onset, manifestations, treatment, stressors, and prevention. Critical Care Quarterly March:21–28, 1984.
6. Kielhofner, G: Temporal adaptation: A conceptual framework for occupational therapy. Am J Occup Ther 31(4):235, 1977.
7. Moore-Ede, MC, Sulzman, FM, and Fuller, CA: The Clocks That Time Us: Physiology of the Circadian Timing System. Harvard University Press, Cambridge, MA, 1982.
8. Zerubavel, E: Patterns of Time in Hospital Life: A Sociological Perspective. University of Chicago Press, Chicago, 1979.
9. Clark, F, Parham, D, Carlson, ME, Frank, G, Jackson, J, Pierce, D, Wolfe, R, and Zemke, R: Occupational science: Academic innovation in the service of occupational therapy's future. Am J Occup Ther 45:300, 1991.
10. Yerxa, EJ, Clark, F, Frank, G, Jackson, J, Parham, D, Pierce, D, Stein, C, and Zemke, R: An introduction to occupational science, a foundation for occupational therapy for the 21st century. Occup Ther Health Care 6(4):1, 1989.
11. Weber, RJ, Oszko, MA, Bolender, BJ, and Grysiak, DC: The intensive care unit syndrome: Causes, treatment and prevention. Drug Intelligence and Clinical Pharmacy 19:13, 1985.
12. Gowan, NJ: The perceptual world of the intensive care unit: An overview of some environmental consideration is in the helping relationship. Heart and Lung 8(2):340, 1979.
13. Kornfeld, DS: Psychiatric problems of an intensive care unit. Med Clin North Am 55(5):1353, 1971.
14. Campbell, J: Winston Churchill's Afternoon Nap: A Wide Awake Inquiry in the Human Nature of Time. Simon and Schuster, New York.
15. Ornstein, RE: The Psychology of Consciousness. Viking Press, New York, 1972.
16. Hudak, CM, Gallo, BM, and Benz, JJ: Critical Care Nursing: A Holistic Approach. J.B. Lippincott, Philadelphia, 1990.
17. Taylor, DEM: Problems of patients in an intensive care unit: The aetiology and prevention of the intensive care syndrome. International Journal of Nursing Studies 8(47): 1971.
18. Wilson, LM: Intensive care delirium—The effects of outside light deprivation in a windowless unit. Arch Int Med 130: 1972.
19. Jones, CL: Environmental analysis of neonatal intensive care. J Nerv Ment Dis 170(3):130, 1982.

by Florence Clark, PhD, OTR, FAOTA,
Bridget Larson Ennevor, MA, OTR/L, and
Penelope L. Richardson, PhD (Posthumously)

34

A Grounded Theory of Techniques for Occupational Storytelling and Occupational Story Making

Building a Communal Horizon of Understanding

Collaboration

Development of Empathy

Inclusion of the Ordinary

Listening

Reflection

Occupational Storytelling

Evocation of Stories of Occupation

Story Analysis and Synthesis

Occupational Story Making

Occupational Coaching

Evoking Insights

A Broadened View of Activities of Daily Living

Cultural Place

Inopportune Moments

Conclusion

Human beings constitute themselves through occupations; they evolve as occupational beings and evolve into who they shall become through immersion in daily practices, habits, and activities. We know about the hours that young gymnasts put into training for the Olympics, we can imagine the infinite number of sketches that Rembrandt must have made in childhood to hone his artistic technique, and we can be assured that Edith Wharton developed her encyclopedic vocabulary by hearing English spoken with precision and eloquence during daily activities in her home or while dining, attending theater, or going shopping with her family. Moreover, the themes that are emphasized in Wharton's novels or expressed through Rembrandt's art were influenced by these artists' experiences of engagement in a broad array of occupations that filled the stream of time in their lives. Within the context of occupation, they may have discovered that what mattered to them was worthy of being the subject of their works.

In the usual course of life events, people encounter many obstacles to the development of themselves as occupational beings. In most cases, we are able to negotiate and find solutions to overcome the obstacles and continue with self-construction. These solutions, in a sense, can be thought of as bridges that traverse difficult periods and events. Usually, we are capable of bridge construction with little or no outside assistance. However, in some cases, an individual may encounter an obstacle of such enormous proportions, a disability perhaps, that no clear direction for the next step is apparent, let alone an attempt at construction of a bridge. The enormity of the obstacle may displace the individual to a position from which escape seems impossible and which seems to extract from the person a sense of self as an occupational being. The survivor of such situations ("survivor" is a term Penny Richardson preferred to patient) then gazes over to a previous life of well-constructed bridges and traveled paths with a sense of bewilderment. The prospect of returning to life's previous path from the new position seems daunting, yet, the person longs to reclaim the old life and sense of self as an occupational being.

An occupational therapist may assist in enabling a survivor grappling with a disability to reconstruct a bridge to rebuild life again. However, the therapist must use care to ensure that the individual incorporates previously constructed paths and bridges, so that the survivor regains a sense of continuity of himself or herself as an occupational being. What is meant by an occupational being? We use this term to mean a person fully engaged in the world of activity—work, play, and leisure—who is productive and feels a sense of self-worth. Decoupling from this aspect of the self, we believe, results in poor functional ability, ill health, and depression.

In Clark's Eleanor Clarke Slagle lecture,[1] Penny Richardson, the stroke survivor with whom Clark collaborated, is quoted having eloquently stated that occupational therapy involved "recycling the old me into the new me." This paper, in a sense, resumes where the Eleanor Clarke Slagle lecture ended, using detail supported by ethnographic data. It describes the approach Clark used to evoke Penny Richardson's story and assist her in reconstructing her life—a process labeled occupational storytelling and occupational story making in the Slagle lecture. Originally, Penny Richardson was to coauthor this paper. However, 5 weeks after presentation of the 1993 Eleanor Clarke Slagle lecture, she died of a second cerebral hemorrhage. Dr. Richardson did, however, contribute to the early stages of this paper's conceptualization.

As was described in the Slagle lecture, between October 1992 and March 1993, Clark and Richardson collaborated on an ethnographic project in which Richardson described her childhood and adult occupations and her experience of rehabilitation following stroke. It became clear that the process of telling her story was therapeutic for Richardson, and this process led to an unfolding, innovative approach to occupational therapy. Through this approach, survivors can learn to use occupation as a means of connecting their former selves with their evolving selves, of becoming more productive, and of enjoying a better quality of life. This process was described in detail in Clark's 1993 Slagle lecture, a paper based primarily on coding of the 200 pages of transcripts by Clark with considerable input from Richardson.

This paper expands a second facet of the project, only touched on in the Slagle lecture. Once the interviews had been completed and transcribed, Richardson and Clark employed Bridget Larson (the second author of this paper), who had not been involved in the interviews, as a research assistant to code independently the transcripts for the techniques that Clark used during the therapeutic process. Concurrently, Richardson and Clark also coded the transcripts for techniques as a way of potential triangulation. In a peer debriefing session, Larson presented the initial categories she had identified to both Richardson and Clark, and in subsequent sessions, after Richardson's death, Larson and Clark met to refine the categories further until consensus between them was achieved. The grounded theory that emerged (the coded categories of which are depicted for heuristic purposes in Figure 34-1) provides a thick description of the techniques Clark used and that other occupational therapists can use to evoke a similar therapeutic process in their patients. Broadly speaking, the approach involves three aspects: building a communal horizon of understanding, occupational storytelling, and occupational story making. The purpose of this paper is to describe this theory of practice and provide ethnographic data as needed to illustrate its particular elements. Figure 34-1 depicts the organizational framework of the paper. In the remainder of this paper, these three focuses of the treatment approach are described in detail.

Building a Communal Horizon of Understanding

Initially, this category was difficult to label. How does one capture the sense that therapists will have to disarm themselves and leave themselves vulnerable in this therapeutic approach? Rather than standing apart from and evaluating their patients, in this approach, therapists must engage themselves fully and inextricably in a dialogue with their patients. We realized after reading an article by Chessick[2] that this coded category of acts could be conceptually framed under the label "building a communal horizon of understanding." This term, which we have borrowed from Chessick, was originally extracted from the writings of Godamer and Heiddeiger in the hermeneutic school of thought. Hermeneutics is most simply defined as the art and science of interpretation. It emerged in the 17th century as a

Building a Communal Horizon of Understanding	Occupational Storytelling	Occupational Story Making
a. Collaboration	a. Evoke stories of occupation	a. Occupational coaching - encouragement positive remake - offering occupational strategies - reaffirming and marking progress
b. Building empathy	b. Analysis and synthesis - time - value	b. Evoking insight - problematiques/solutions
c. Inclusion of ordinary		c. Broadened view of activities of daily living - emotion handlings - friendship/intimacy - symbolic dimension of occupation
d. Listening		d. Image reconstruction
e. Reflection		e. Cultural place

Figure 34–1. Grounded theory on the techniques of occupational storytelling and occupational story making.

discipline to establish accurate interpretations of biblical text, but by the end of the 18th century, it was applied to literary works and historical periods. By the turn of the 19th century, its application was expanded to the understanding of human motives and acts, and it was introduced as an alternative to the "objective" methods of inquiry emanating from the social sciences.[2]

A central tenet of the hermeneutic approach is that meaning is content dependent, tied both to the historical and cultural past and the "present orientation of the interpreter."[3] According to hermeneutics, the "horizon" or "standpoint" of the interpreter, that is, preconceptions based on the interpreter's cultural and historical situation and present orientation, will contribute to the interpretations given to the experience. In the therapeutic approach that Clark used, she sought to fuse her own perspective, that of the occupational scientist, with that of Richardson's narrative about her experience of disability. Both the therapist and the survivor initially have unique but distinct "horizons" of understanding, but as the conversation unfolds, "the horizons of each coparticipate,"[4] and a sense of shared meaning emerges for that time and place. Godamer[5] described this process as one in which a sense of understanding is reached, not simply through the assertion of one's particular perspective, but through a "transformation into a communion, in which we do not remain what we were."[6] Although Clark was immersed first in her own horizon of understanding, through continuing conversations with Richardson, Clark's ideas were transformed. A similar process occurred within Richardson. Richardson made Clark far more sensitive to the experience of disability; Clark, in turn, infused Richardson's standpoint with knowledge about occupation. In the coding process, we identified five techniques that Clark used to build a communal horizon of understanding. These included collaboration with the survivor, development of empathy, inclusion of the ordinary, listening, and reflection.

Collaboration

The first technique is *collaboration with the survivor*. Collaboration is a word with which therapists are familiar and generally think of as working together as equals. In Clark's work with Richardson, *collaboration* occurs as the therapist relinquishes power to control the discourse and the process and the survivor assumes full co-equal status. The following excerpt from the transcript provides an example of how this category encompasses issues of power in the therapeutic relationship. In Clark's first interview with Richardson, after she has told Richardson what she hopes to get out of the session, she is worried that she may seize too much control of the discourse. The dialogue is as follows:

> C: Sometimes, you'll, you know, you'll say something, and I'll want to . . . I'll feel the urge to cut in . . . to redirect it, or something. I . . . I don't want to do that. . . . I want to just sort of get a ball park
> R: Uh huh, uh huh.
> C: You know, we all . . . we can go . . . But what about you? What do you want to get? What do you want to get out of it? I told you what I want to get out of it.
> R: Well . . . Although I do not believe . . . everything happens for a reason, I would personally like . . . for something good to come out of all this awful stuff [that] had happened to me. So if my story can be of use to people in the profession or in their personal lives, then I would feel like, well . . . At least that happened along with all this stuff. So that's what I want to get out of it.

At another point, Clark reinforces the importance of Richardson's perspective to the project and inadvertently illustrates that indeed some good will come out of Richardson's story, thus substantiating how Richardson's purpose was beginning to be realized in their work together.

> C: One of the things I am going to do is, is help therapists to [be sensitive to] the historicity of a person that comes into the clinic; these aren't just entities that somehow materialized one day and have not real personhood.
> R: That's a wonderful idea!
> E: So whenever they see a patient, they won't see a disability; they will think, these 6,000 therapists that hear this talk . . . and to give them ideas of how they can be coaches, for example, [another] one of your ideas.
> R: Uh huh, uh huh.
> C: And, you know, you know more about what their patients really need.

What is important in this passage is that it illustrates how Clark pays homage to Richardson's input. The interview process was not one through which Richardson alone was transformed; so, too, was Clark. This excerpt shows that Clark has begun to adopt Richardson's standpoint on how therapists can help their patients, a perspective that was not part of her horizon of understanding before the interview. Having relinquished control, Clark is able to learn from Richardson just as Richardson is able to benefit from her interactions with Clark.

Development of Empathy

We labeled the second strategy that promoted a communal horizon of understanding *developing empathy*. In this technique, the therapist suspends the self and experiences as closely as possible the world the way the survivor experiences it. Frank[7] writes that empathy, unlike narcissism, "requires the suspension of the self to take the place of the other. It permits a person to leave the self aside for a bit, experience something of another's life as if it were one's own, and conclude with a return to one's own familiar self."[8] For Clark, building empathy often involved self-disclosure, such as confessions about her own experiences of jealousy and fears of never remarrying. The following passage from this first interview illustrates one example of an attempt on Clark's part to be empathetic. Richardson has just disclosed some of her concerns about her potential for dating. She refers to a study that indicated that the prognosis of marriage for women past 40 was something like, "you're more likely to be hit by a truck."

> C: Yeah, that's right. Actually, that's backlash. That's not true.
> R: Or whatever.
> C: Ummm . . . Susan Faludi; she shows [in her book *Backlash*] that that study was erroneous.
> R: Oh good.
> C: Right! Then that affected women's minds, and I think a lot of older women, you know, middle aged women . . . really do feel more affected by that. I was, since I was single at this time when that came out. I thought, oh, well, I'll never marry again. And then when I had somebody that really wanted to marry me . . . my goodness . . . [I thought], it's strange.

In the following passage, Clark attempts to express understanding for what she suspects Richardson feels by discussing her recent loss of teeth. First she reminds Richardson that she is still the same person, though she now has some physical problems.

> C: You are, you're the same Penny. Your mental processing, your personality, your wisdom, it's still there. It is interesting, because in a way it reminds me of aging because I think I told you that I lost my tooth recently?
> R: No, you didn't tell me.
> C: . . . Now I am losing the whole right side of my mouth, so now that I have such a big space I am talking differently, and you probably don't notice it . . . but I notice it and it makes me feel like I am aging, like I have gotten really old in the last 2 or 3 weeks. [Disability] is like aging because you never really grasp [phenomenologically] the person just goes on in the same way, but the internal stuff never ages. . . . Your hair gets grayer . . . your skin wrinkles, . . . but [internally] you don't really feel that something has happened; somebody else has to look to see it. It seems to me disability is that way, that the spirit just keeps on going in the person; the physical self is just kind of separated.

In the previous passage, Clark attempts to feel what she senses Richardson is feeling and does so with much effort, work, and risk. Because Clark was willing to risk self-disclosure in the process, her empathy was real and believable to Richardson.

Inclusion of the Ordinary

Inclusion of the ordinary in the discourse emerged as the third category that fostered the building of a communal horizon of understanding. In the full set of Richardson-Clark transcripts, it is surprising to notice the amount of time devoted to casual interchanges on virtually any subject that normally and spontaneously came up in the conversation. Topics included current events, "girl talk" about male-female relationships, job trivia, fashion, and so on. This excerpt from the seventh interview provides an example of this sort of discourse.

R: My two new vests, I have worn both of them and I like them very much.

C: Vests are very much in style now.

R: Yeah, I like them, they look right on me, it's my look, tailored, but they are both nice patterns and nice material and last night I wore my new dress to . . . an annual event the department has and . . . I felt good in it. I really enjoyed that event because all of us came back for it so it is like a homecoming without football. . . . I enjoyed being in my new style of dress, kind of sweater top and chiffon bottom and a very little sleeveless.

C: Lacy.

R: Silver sweater, so I felt sheer.

C: Sounds nice.

R: Yeah, it was real nice.

C: Sounds real nice.

Such light conversations had the crucial effect of "normalizing" the interaction. They are typical of the way people normally converse, yet sometimes as simple as they appeared at the onset, they could inadvertently generate a climactic moment, one from which a critical insight emerged, as was the case in the following excerpt.

C: There is no limit to what you can do with clothing.

R: Do you think?

C: In fact I have some images of you. Sara just got a top. It's a greenish . . . teal and it's a lacy top.

R: It sounds nice.

C: With short sleeves and lots of pretty lace, but it is not bulky, delicate, and I think you would look real good in a lacy thing of that color and then I would like to see you in suede shoes. What kind of shoes are you wearing?

R: I have about six pairs of the same kind of shoes; these little pumps with a very tiny heel.

C: My first thing would be to get shoes and a cane for you.

R: You think?

C: Really classy, flat suede . . . slightly European. I'd go for something really chic in a flat shoe.

R: Yeah, flat, that is better . . .

C: I think you have to go a bit European. You could do things with a great leather. You know all the power symbols of a sort of British aristocrat!

As reported in the Slagle Lecture,[1] the idea of the British aristocrat eventually became one of the core constructs around which Richardson constructed her new image of herself. Thus, a light conversation, essentially chit-chat, eventually became a key to her recovery. However, even when ordinary interchanges do not lead to climactic insights, they are crucial because they establish a relationship in which disability does not exist at the core and permeate every aspect. Giddens[9] pointed out that in everyday life, normalcy "is managed in fine detail within the textures of social activity."[10] Interludes of normalcy seen in the transcipts provide a foundation for trust that is needed to allow disclosure.

Listening

Listening was the next category of action that we coded essential to building the communal horizon of understanding. Kern[11] reported that Heidegger was especially concerned with how people communicated to one another. In authentic discourse, "listening to or 'being open' to others in a caring exchange" was essential.[12] In coding the transcripts, it was evident that Clark listened actively to Richardson. While engaged in this process, she conveyed attentiveness, appreciation, and sometimes delight. She would ask questions or probe to elicit progressively more detail in the account. In this excerpt from the sixth interview and in numerous other places, Richardson expresses how much she appreciates having someone who will listen.

> R: But you're wonderful, because I can talk and talk about it [the stroke experience] and that is what this is for, so it is great, very therapeutic from that point of view.
> C: Besides, it would be good for people in this situation to have somebody available to do this kind of process.
> R: Absolutely.
> C: Separate from their usual life. . . . This is very important. This is something that I can recommend that occupational therapists put into practice.
> R: Exactly.
> C: . . . They could be providing this as occupational therapy, an hour or two to really talk about daily activity, negotiation, problems, their social world . . . then imaging their whole process of reconstructing life.

The transcripts convey that whether Richardson was giving a detailed account of how she obtained her driver's license, discussing her intimate friendships, telling tales of heroic accomplishments, or simply telling stories of work and play, Clark was responsive, analytic, and engaged in active listening.

Reflection

The last technique that Clark used to build a common horizon of understanding we have labeled *reflection*. In this technique, the therapist verbally reflects on the survivor's statements. She may paraphrase the survivor to make certain she is grasping what the survivor has said or provide an alternative interpretation of the survivor's discourse. A segment from the third interview graphically illustrates this process.

> R: The fact that I really do have this, even if it doesn't work, this desire to get better physically and to be able to walk again and hike again, and all that. That's something else to, to combat for. . . . I, I do well when I'm battling for something that matters.
> C: Let's talk about that battling. Battling means . . . what?
> R: Um . . . It means . . . taking joy in fighting a good fight.
> C: A good fight?
> R: Yeah.

C: The right fight?

R: The right fight, and . . . it gives me energy so that um, I don't really need it. But sometimes it really helps. If I have a feeling that there are forces, be they bureaucratic forces, or people forces, or . . . administrative lethargy forces. These are the forces.

C: These forces are evil?

R: Yeah, forces of evil!

C: In a mythical sense.

R: Right! And here I . . . my sword or whatever!!

One senses that as Clark probes what Richardson calls combat, Richardson's energy level elevates, and her motivation seems to be tapped. She becomes more empowered to fight against the obstacles she has encountered in her world of daily activity.

In the end, Clark and Richardson are transformed. Clark perceives the limitations in traditional occupational therapy and begins to gain a sense of how it can be reforged; in turn, Richardson feels that she can take greater control of her personal destiny through occupation. This communal horizon of understanding was detailed in the Slagle Lecture;[1] here we have detailed the techniques that made it emerge.

Occupational Storytelling

A communal horizon of understanding can be developed in any dyadic relationship, but for it to happen within the context of occupational therapy nurtured by occupational science, the "horizon" must be immersed in a sense of the survivor as an occupational being. Thus, the therapeutic process we are describing begins with probing the history of the survivor in the world of activity, while the therapist remains open to any direction the discourse may take. The therapist possesses the knowledge that humans are constituted in everyday practices. To understand the survivor today, he or she must understand his or her history as an occupational being. In her Slagle lecture,[1] Clark referred to this facet of therapy as occupational storytelling. While the Slagle lecture presented a detailed account of Richardson's childhood occupations and how they shaped her character, it did not explicitly describe the process by which the story was elicited and constructed.

Evocation of Stories of Occupation

Occupational storytelling begins with the therapist evoking *stories of occupation*. The therapist asks the survivor to tell stories of childhood and adult occupations prior to the injury or illness and right up to the time of the interview. Checklists or preconstructed interview schedules are not used, because the content should emerge spontaneously and naturally so that what matters most to the survivor is recounted and given emphasis. General questions are asked, such as "What sort of things did you like to do in childhood?" "What were the themes that guided these activities?" "With whom did you do these occupations?" "How did you feel when you did them?" "Are there products or keepsakes that you still have that were generated or associated with these occupations?" "What were the most memorable activities in which you engaged during this period of your life?" The focus of the interview is not simply on what the survivor did, but on what the activities meant to him or her. The survivors also should be asked what they are doing right now, what a typical day is like, and what kind of losses, in an occupational sense, they are experiencing.

Story Analysis and Synthesis

It is likely that the interview data will not be presented in the form of a coherent narrative. The therapist will need to piece the story together in collaboration with the survivor so that it makes sense, appears accurate to both, and *reflects analysis and synthesis of the occupations in relation to time and value*. The distinguished novelist E. M. Forster[13] saw daily life as actually comprised of two kinds of lives— "the life in time and the life by values."[14] He believed our conduct illustrates this "double allegiance. 'I only saw her five minutes but it was worth it.' "[15] Forster states, "and what the story does is to narrate the life in time. And what the entire novel does—if it is a good novel is to include the life by values as well."[15]

When analyzing and constructing stories about their patients as occupational beings from interview data, therapists need to attend to the historical (chronological) and value-laden aspects of the person's experience of occupation.

Occupation in Time

The chronological aspect can simply be constructed by ordering the events of significance and occupations in time. This is essentially a recording function and should not be particularly difficult. Techniques such as *building a timeline* can be used to expedite the process. To begin to gain a sense of whether or not the occupations had a negative or positive effect on the person, the "turnings" method described by Mandelbaum[16] can be used. Here the survivor would be asked not only to list the significant events of her life, but also to rate them as positive or negative. Clark used this technique in one facet of her work with Richardson to clarify the chronology of the events Richardson recounted.

Occupation by Value

The more difficult and complex aspect of constructing stories of survivors as occupational beings involves interpreting and giving meaning to the survivor's story (the occupation by value). The novelist Milan Kundera[17] stated that "behind all those amusing tales, we can make out this conviction: It is through action that man steps forth from the repetitive universe of the everyday where each person resembles every other person; it is through action that he distinguishes himself from others and becomes an individual."[18] To create a picture of how the survivor's history of occupations can be meaningfully interpreted, the therapist must uncover how engagement in occupations shaped the survivor's character, contributed to who he or she is today, and gave to him or her resources that can be recycled for recovery. Kundera wrote that "making a character 'alive' means getting to the bottom of his existential problem."[19] This involves "getting to the bottom of some situations, some motifs, even some words that shape him."[19] The story must have a forward moving plot, illustrating coherently how the survivor's history of occupational involvement is impacting on his or her ability to cope with the current crisis for which he or she has been referred to therapy. For instance, experience in camping may have helped a person practically and psychologically adapt to homelessness; in Richardson's case, her history of horseback riding revealed that she was fiercely independent. It is particularly important that the story reveal in what activities the survivor has engaged and whether he or she thought the investment was worth it, how occupations shaped the personhood of the survivor, what matters to him or her, and what occupations can be harnessed in the recovery process. The story that is so constructed provides a complex view of the survivor as an occupational being and becomes the starting point for the next step in this form of occupational therapy: occupational story making.

Occupational Story Making

Having identified the survivor's values, having culled a sense of his or her character and how it was shaped in occupation, and having gained a fully realized sense of the person as an occupational being, the occupational therapist now collaborates with the survivor to construct a meaningful future. Occupational story making, as defined in Clark's Slagle lecture, is the process of creating a story involving the therapist and the survivor that will be enacted in the future and focused on further development of the survivor as an occupational being (Fig. 34-2).

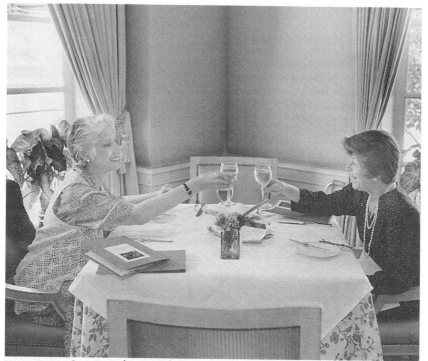

Figure 34–2. Occupational story making involves excursions into the community in which the therapist connects with the survivor as an occupational being and the survivor reexperiences occupations in his or her cultural niche. (Photo by Irene Fertik.)

Mattingly[20] suggests "that in each new clinical situation . . . the therapist must answer the question, What story am I in?"[21] However, in the approach we are describing, the key question must be, "Do I find myself in a story about the survivor as an occupational being?" Such stories would not, for example, emphasize postural responses, diagnostic symptoms, or psychodynamic processes. They would be concerned with how the survivor is functioning in his or her work and social world, whether he or she feels empowered to take control over his or her time and destiny, and how the survivor is using occupation in the process of recovery. It also would include a future image of the survivor immersed in activity, despite the presence of disability. Through the coding process, once again we were able to identify the techniques that Clark used to ensure that the story in which Richardson and she found themselves led to further assertion of Richardson's self as an occupational being.

Occupational Coaching

In the Slagle lecture, Clark described the process by which she gradually began to function as Richardson's therapist-coach.[1] *Occupational coaching* is the first category we coded for this aspect of the therapeutic process. It involved several components, each of which was coded as a subcategory of occupational coaching.

Giving Encouragement and Making Positive Remarks

The first component was *giving encouragement and making positive remarks.* The use of this technique is illustrated in this excerpt from the seventh interview. Richardson has just told Clark that she plans to buy season tickets for the opera next year and invite friends to come along as a way of building a social life.

> C: People would love that. That is a fabulous idea. Who wouldn't want to do that?
> R: Well, there are a few people who don't like opera.
> C: But most people do, and this is really great; this is a great occupational strategy. It is a jewel because it is very upscale, and it puts you in a position of dignity and authority. I mean, being the one who is doing the inviting. It is really great.
> R: I like it.
> C: See, what you are doing is you're constructing this persona. It is really interesting, you are taking charge. That is fabulous, that is one of those gems!

In this sequence, not only is Clark encouraging, but she also simultaneously reflects back to Richardson her interpretation of why she thinks this is such a superb strategy further building their communal horizon of understanding. Moreover, she appropriates credit where it belongs, to Richardson who is orchestrating her recovery.

Teaching Occupational Strategies

Similar to the coach of an Olympian gymnast who offers his or her protégés instruction in techniques to build flexibility, strength, coordination, and skill to improve the larger goal of a routine, an occupational therapy coach teaches strategies that can lead to a more productive and satisfying life. *Occupational strategies* were coded as the second subcategory of occupational coaching. In Clark's work with Richardson, she recommended that Richardson join support groups; use particular occupational contexts, such as card games or dining, as settings for bridging social relationships; and begin to engage in particular occupations that would improve her possibilities of attaining the future she wanted. In teaching occupational strategies, however, one cannot maintain an impartial distance. The coach is often involved in selected excursions into the world of activity. In this excerpt from the fifth interview, Clark suggests that she and Richardson go shopping; the discourse takes on the quality of coaching because Clark begins to offer detailed advice on the style of clothes Richardson might consider purchasing to improve her future. The dialogue begins when Clark tells Richardson that Richardson could exercise a lot of autonomy in the area of personal dress and costume.

> C: This is an area that does not require tremendous physical fitness. This an area that requires some artistic sense and design sense and I think it is a good area for you to express your creativity, to make a personal statement.
> R: I am ready now.
> C: If I'm around, I'll go with you if you would like me to.
> R: Yeah, I would.
> C: Would you like me to? If you go with me, it will be less conservative, but maybe we can come up with a reasonable middle ground. You know, I think you should take a little more freedom [in your style of dress] because you're young.
> R: Young.
> C: 50, what are you, 50?
> R: 51.
> C: You're young enough to have a little freedom, to take some risks.
> R: Yeah.
> C: And I think tailored is nice, except that you need something that you could feel fun and freer in. I don't know. This is a time when you can . . . I think this is a really good occupational therapy project . . . going shopping.

Teaching About Occupation's Role in Recovery

Coaches also spend a good deal of time teaching their protégés about their sport; similarly another role of the occupational coach is to *teach the survivor about the role that occupation can play in recovery*, the third subcategory of occupational coaching. During their project, Clark gave Richardson at least six books to read that dealt with this theme. Later in interview sessions, they would discuss the books. She also invited Richardson to attend Occupational Science Symposia so that Richardson could hear papers on occupation given by scholars. Often, however, Clark would spontaneously insert in the discourse a sort of minilecture on some facet of occupation. The purpose of these efforts was to provide a framework for the survivor to understand herself as an occupational being and to become empowered to use occupation in the recovery process. In the following excerpt from the fourth interview, Clark gives a minilecture. Richardson has just confided that a friend to whom she had been close has become distant but does visit her every so often to play Scrabble. She is confused and wants to understand this situation. Clark then responds:

> C: I want to bring it [our conversation] back to what I call occupational therapy, and this [our discourse] becomes occupational therapy again because we are getting more

layered into the whole meaning of the Scrabble game. The Scrabble game is the bridge. I mean it is serving as a bridge, [the games] are keeping you two connected through a period of time when the readiness was not there to deal with the issue of the Big A [the aneurysm], so it was just maintenance, but I think that through our progress here, you are more ready to talk about this. She [your friend] has not had anybody to really talk to about this, but the fact that she does continue to play tells me she does not want to give you up.

The interpretation that Clark provides is based on her knowledge about how occupations can mediate social interactions. It relies on Clark's understanding of the symbolic vehicle that is present in human occupation. Instead of viewing the Scrabble games on a simplistic concrete level, Clark provides symbolic interpretation that gives Penny hope of rekindling a relationship about which she cares deeply. This information-sharing process becomes possible because of Clark's knowledge about human occupation, which she shares with Richardson and Richardson's willingness to share her concerns about this friendship with Clark.

Marking and Affirming Progress

As a coach therapist, Clark also *marks and affirms the progress* that Richardson is making in her recovery, the last subcategory of occupational coaching. Intermittently, she acts as a kind of mirror reminding Richardson of where she had been and of all that she has accomplished. The following excerpt taken from the third interview provides an example:

R: I'm at a plateau now. I've been on a walker for God knows how long and . . . so enough of that. So we will see.
C: Ummm. But you . . . you are a lot different . . . on the walker now than you were last year on the walker.
R: Am I?
C: Yes.
F: For example?
C: Well, for example, well, I mean . . . in the sense that you're still using the walker, but you're not as dependent on it. . . . You are much more stable on the walker. I remember when you were very unstable on the walker. . . .
R: Well, thanks for that.
C: . . . Do you remember . . . when . . . if we went on grass or something. I think you were really nervous. I remember that, like when we went on grass from . . . Marks Trojan Hall to the Faculty Center or something.
R: Ummmm.
C: . . . uneven surfaces really frightened you even when you were on the walker.
P: Oh, nervous frightening from Norman Topping Student Activity Center.
C: Yeah, see . . . but I remember that. And now . . . the walker's no problem for you. I mean as you said the walker's . . . too easy; it's not a challenge. But I remember when the walker was a challenge. . . .
R: See, that's hard for me to remember . . . but . . . thank you for telling me that because I'm glad.

In the sixth interview, Clark tells Richardson the following:

C: In the last 4 months, I think you have really changed [since the date they began the project].
R: How?

C: You're just a more assertive person. You are much more self-confident. You are re-claiming things that had been taken from you through the rehabilitation process. I think you are rejecting, you know, the status of being disabled. I mean that makes all the difference in the world. You are more empowered, you said that yourself. Your physical appearance looks a lot better, your voice is stronger. It manifests itself in your carriage and your bearing. . . .

Evoking Insights

In addition to occupational coaching, Clark facilitated the occupational story making process by helping the survivor (Richardson) gain insight into the "problematiques" of her life and their solutions. We called this category *evoking insights*. In the Slagle lecture,[1] Clark defined problematiques, borrowing from Foucault (cited in Rabinow[22]), as the things in relation to which Richardson felt threatened. The subplots of the story in which Richardson and Clark found themselves evolved as Richardson confronted the set of problematiques about which she wanted to do something. As it turned out, the story that Richardson and Clark created and lived out had to do with using occupation to fight against consignment to a disability role, building an image that bridged Richardson's old and new self, and taking command of her social world. The plot of the stories each therapist and survivor dyad enacts will be unique to their situation and communal horizon of understanding, but in all cases, it should be about the search for and enactment of solutions to problematiques through occupation. One can never know, although one may have hunches, how the story to be made will unfold. In this excerpt from the sixth transcript, Richardson finally puts into words one of the major themes with which she has been struggling:

C: Are there things about last week that we left hanging?
R: I know I did lot of thinking about it.
C: Oh, did you?
R: . . . One thing I thought was that I really felt empowered. I felt that I can see some new ways that I could behave that would be more in charge of all this, and that was good.
C: What were some of the ways?
R: Well, like we ended up by saying that I have a decision about how I define my-self. I can decide . . . I have been struggling with that? Am I disabled now? Am I handicapped now? Am I denying, if I don't accept that I'm handicapped and disabled or am I falling into being disabled and handicapped when I don't need to be? I am allowing the world to sort of lay a stigma on me and I like the idea that I can decide and if I want to be disabled . . . I can do that, but if I decide that I am not disabled or handicapped, I don't have to be. I can take charge of the way that other people define me by how I act. I am not a VICTIM. . . . I have been trying to sort that out, and one of the things that last week sort of got to me was, well, I thought, I can take charge of the situations in the way that other people define me and the way that I define myself and that was a very exciting idea.

A Broadened View of Activities of Daily Living

We labeled the third facet of occupational story making *a broadened view of activities of daily living*. Within the occupational therapy profession, the emphasis has been on the most concrete functional aspects of occupation; that is, dressing is viewed as a mechanical skill to be taught rather than also as a personal statement about one's self-image or a vehicle for creating a persona. Similarly, "feeding" is seen as a skill to be taught for food injection, rather than as an important means of establishing and furthering social contacts when nested within the context of "dining." Likewise, occupational therapists have traditionally emphasized management of the physical environment by teaching energy conservation and spatial organization and through the use of adaptive equipment. They have not, however, been particularly focused on assisting survivors of disability to handle the social environment with which they inevitably collide following hospitalization, as they return to the world from which they came.

Emotion Handling

The following example illustrates how Richardson began to take control of her social world through the technique we call *handling others' emotions in occupational contexts*:

> R: ... this kind of conversation is helping to raise my consciousness. ... It is very empowering because it seems that I don't have to sit and take what the world does. I can create the reaction, I can manage it.
> C: Have you been managing that in . . . you know, have you been managing people better in daily activities?
> R: I have been trying out different things.
> C: . . . It's a game. You can sit back and play it.
> R: One thing that I did last week quite consciously; I started using my cane.
> C: I saw you at the [homeowners] meeting with your cane.
> R: And went around telling people, hey, look at me, I have made a breakthrough, I have put aside my walker, temporarily anyway, and I am trying to use the cane, and I am happy about it. Then, by my putting the message out, then all of a sudden they praised me, they carried on, they were happy. Since I mentioned it, it was okay to mention it. Meanwhile, they may not have even noticed, but a lot of them probably had noticed, but hadn't wanted to mention it because they felt self-conscious, but once I raised it, I could then have this little conversation where people praised me. Well, it was sort of fun, but it was an experience, an insight. . . . Now I am very proud of myself in some ways, but it was just finding out. I was saying to myself, let's try this one out and it worked.
> C: . . . See managing other people's emotions, I think becomes the essential wish of a person who is breaking with convention. . . . Most occupational therapists never think of helping a person develop [in this area]; they teach managing the toothbrush, but not managing other people's emotions so that they [the survivor] can be in command and not victimized.

If individuals with disability feel walled off and rejected from the able-bodied world, as did Richardson initially, they will refrain from participating in everyday activity to avoid feelings of rejection. As a pattern over time, this can lead to illness and depression. Unless an occupation is solitary, it will have a social component. Importantly, in the above sequence from the sixth transcript, Richardson is able to feel good about her attendance at a homeowners meeting because she was successful in managing the emotions of others. Such triumphs are likely to encourage further risk taking and therefore development of the survivor as an occupational being.

Friendships and Intimacy

Our broadened view of activities of daily living also included *dealing with intimacy and friendships*, particularly in relation to how friends can become part of a support system to encourage further participation in occupation and vice versa how occupation can be used to enhance and even rekindle or repair friendships. In the following excerpt from the fourth transcript, Clark instructs Richardson on how she might use occupation to repair a friendship from which Richardson is experiencing considerable pain. She has just encouraged Richardson to invite the friend to lunch.

R: As I said, food for thought.
C: I would try to do it. . . . This is an occupational thing, an occupational therapy thing. I think that in occupation science, we think about the context, the occupational context, so if you are going to have this honest conversation with [the friend's name], it is important to have this conversation in the right context.

As the conversation unfolds, Clark implies that a setting such as the Four Seasons Hotel would be ideal. As an occupational therapist, Clark is guiding Richardson to use a particular kind of occupational context to handle a difficult social situation. Not only does she explain to Richardson why "the dining context" would be helpful, she also gets specific on the quality and ambience of the restaurant in which this reunion could take place. Eventually, Richardson does find the courage to invite the friend to lunch.

Emotional and Symbolic Dimensions of Occupation

When the survivor does take a risk in an area of activities of daily living, it is crucial that the occupational therapist try to tap how the survivor felt about the experience. Much of Clark's work with Richardson focused on the *emotional and symbolic dimensions of occupation* that Richardson held. For example, in this excerpt from the third transcript, Richardson describes how she felt when, for the first time, she independently took a bus to the Embassy Hotel, a location about 2 miles from her home.

R: I feel excited when I do something risky and it works out. Like that time I took the trip to Embassy.
C: Right, that's right. That was another trip.
R: It was thrilling. I felt so pleased because here I was on a bus. It was night and I managed to get from campus to Embassy. People helped me, helped me get my walker on, helped me get my walker off, gave me directions. I felt very, like a real . . . hot shot. Because I had done something out of the ordinary, and that was a brand new thing. And I had done it successfully, and I had not had any help at all. I just did it.
C: When you were a kid, did you do that? Did you . . .
R: Yeah.

What this dialogue illustrates is that phenomenologically, ordinary activities of daily living can be experienced as triumphs, adventures, and even heroic acts to the survivor. Such experiences unfortunately are sometimes taken for granted by the therapist. Clark demonstrates that she has vicariously experienced Richardson's adventures when she links it to what she knows, having heard Richardson's tales of her childhood occupations and her history of spiritedness.

Image Reconstruction

At one point in the fifth transcript, Richardson states that "you feel a certain way about yourself when you're dressed up and put together, that you don't feel when you aren't . . . and I decided it was time to start caring." What we have coded as *image reconstruction* constituted another subcategory of our broadened view of activities of daily living. Image reconstruction is defined as the process by which the survivor begins to imagine himself or herself as taking on a persona with which he or she will feel comfortable and empowered in the future. Richardson's image reconstruction was focused around the notion of a female British scholar and aristocrat. Because she was a professor, this image was particularly suiting, and the image reconstruction process dealt with her mental picture of herself. She chose words to describe herself, the style of clothes she would wear, the accessories with which she accented her image, her posture, her demeanor, and reshaped her views on disability. The following excerpt from the seventh transcript illustrates how choice of words takes on significance in the image reconstruction process. Richardson has just told Clark that she prefers the word "lame" to disabled or handicapped:

> C: Interesting, why do you like "lame"?
>
> R: I like lame because it says . . . it has a sort of connotation of people, say, he is real lame. You don't mean physically, you mean sort of out of it, so it has that kind of double entendre, and I myself feel that I am sort of lame sometimes the way I handle this . . . I like it that it has a sort of double meaning. On the other hand, I don't like crippled. That is too cruel and negative, so lame in a humorous way is kind of just right. It doesn't have a sort of sense of shoving something under the rug; it is not a very modern term. . . . It brings to mind . . . little Tiny Tim who was lame, and although it was [used] back when people did not have terms like physically handicapped, it was a nice straight forward word for this kind of condition.

Having embraced this term, Richardson then began to use a British-style cane with a quartz handle and was launched on a powerful trajectory of image reconstruction, which gave expression to her humor, wit, and creativity.

Cultural Place

Finally, occupational story making, that is, the process of collaborating with the survivor to help him or her flourish as an occupational being, involves *taking the survivor's cultural place into account*. Cultural place has been defined by Weisner, in relation to children, as "the place in which development occurs, the ecology and locally adapted environment"[23] which includes "meanings, beliefs, values and conventional practices learned and shared by members of a community."[23] We believe that this concept can be applied to the settings to which the survivor returns after hospitalization and in which their recovery will take place. Occupational therapy nurtured by occupational science cannot be divorced from the real world in which the survivor lives. Ideally, therapists using the methods described previously should experience as much of the survivor's world as possible. Caretakers and other significant players in the survivor's world can be interviewed, and the home setting should be studied for its physical characteristics and the values it seems to celebrate. Available resources, technology, adaptive systems, and family support must be assessed. As an example, in Richardson's story, neighbors were converted into an image of "condo comrades," which evolved into a powerful support group for her. Infinite possibilities exist from a survivor's cultural place that can be harnessed for the recovery process.

Inopportune Moments

The reader should not conclude that the process described flowed easily from start to finish. There were several occasions in which Clark's suggestions were not well received by Richardson. In the following excerpt, Clark has offered Richardson strategies that she did not use.

> R: I have never talked to another disabled person. . . . That is something that I have not done, to be more in contact with people. You have given me names and I haven't gone through that at all because I am busy.
> C: The timing is not right.
> R: Maybe not.
> C: I think right now you are re-entering your own world. Your project is to re-enter your old world, to re-established yourself in your School of Education, in your teaching, in yourself and in your appearance. I see you're really putting a lot into that. I think that is great.

This excerpt illustrates Clark's recognition that her idea to Richardson was not useful and appropriate at that time. Despite the inopportune suggestion, Clark seizes the opportunity to provide encouragement and further affirm Richardson's progress. Thus, an error on the part of the therapist (which is a natural part of this process) does not have to remain as such.

Conclusions

In Clark's Eleanor Clarke Slagle lecture,[1] occupational therapists were urged to place occupational storytelling and occupational story making at the core of clinical reasoning to "nurture the human spirit to act." This paper provides a framework for doing so. Beginning with a conception of survivors as occupational beings, we enter into a dialogue seeking to fuse our perspective with that of a survivor to create a communal horizon of understanding. From this vantage point, we can analyze the history of the survivor as an occupational being in the process of occupational storytelling. Through occupational storytelling, we begin to glean a significant understanding of the meaning the survivor holds for certain activities and can use this information in the next step of occupational story making. We create with the survivor a future of immersion in activity through occupational story making, which continues the survivor's life as an occupational being. Thus, we have come full circle. We started with a conception of an occupational being and ended with an occupational being (the survivor) as a reality. It is our belief that all survivors deserve such a reality.

Discussion Questions

1. What were the grounds on which Clark and Richardson built their communal bridge of understanding, and why was this bridge ultimately so fruitful?
2. How might the methods of occupational storytelling and occupational story making be adapted in the interest of helping patients or clients who lack the cognitive abilities and intellectual sophistication of an individual such as Penny Richardson?
3. What strategies might practitioners use within traditional medical settings that could promote a broadened view of activities of daily living as described in this chapter?

References

1. Clark, FA: Occupation embedded in a real life: Interweaving occupational science and occupational therapy. Am J Occup Ther 47:1069, 1993.
2. Chessick RD: Hermeneutics for psychotherapists. Am J Psychother 44:256, 1990.
3. Chessick, p 257.
4. Godamer, H: Truth and Method. Barden, G, and Cumming, J, Trans. Crossroad, NY, 1982, p 262.
5. Godamer, p 341.
6. Godamer, p 341.
7. Frank G: "Becoming the other": Empathy and biographical interpretation. Biography 8:189, 1985.
8. Frank, p 191.
9. Giddens, A: Modernity and Self-identity: Self and Society in the Late Modern Age. Stanford University Press, Palo Alto, CA, 1991.
10. Giddens, p 126.
11. Kern, S: The Culture of Love: Victorians to Moderns. Harvard University Press, Cambridge, England, 1992.
12. Kern, p 119.
13. Forster, EM: Aspects of the Novel. Harcourt Brace Jovanovich, Publishers, New York, 1927.
14. Forster, p 28.
15. Forster, p 29.
16. Mandelbaum, DG: The study of life history: Ghandi. Anthropology 14:177, 1973.
17. Kundera, M: The Art of the Novel. Harper & Row Publishers, New York, 1988.
18. Kundera, p 23.
19. Kundera, p 35.
20. Mattingly, C: The narrative nature of clinical reasoning. Am J Occup Ther 46:998, 1991.
21. Mattingly, p 1001.
22. Rabinow, P: Foucault Reader. Pantheon, New York, 1984.
23. Weisner, TS: Ethnographic and ecocultural perspectives on sibling relationships. In Stoneman, Z, and Berman, P (eds): The Effects of Mental Retardation, Disability, and Illness on Sibling Relationships: Research Issues and Challenges. Paul H. Brookes Publishing, Baltimore, 1993, p 53.

by Jerry A. Johnson, EdD, OTR/L, FAOTA

35

Occupational Science and Occupational Therapy: An Emphasis on Meaning

Applications in Occupation Therapy

The early Occupational Science Symposia generated an enthusiasm for the concepts, values, and practical applications associated with occupational science. Researchers and practitioners presented several common themes inherent in the trajectory of human occupation from neural pathways to symbolic meaning of activities. The greater our understanding of occupations and how they maintain, enhance, and promote health and well-being, the greater will be our ability to link this knowledge with practice and education of future therapists.

The first theme that can be identified is the vision derived from the roots of occupational science. While that vision allows for diversity in the approaches that therapists may take, it also leads to a defined end: the development, creation, testing, and expansion of a body of knowledge now known as occupational science.

Second, by focusing on a common goal and by discussing concepts and ideals and their many avenues for achievement, a feeling of power that encompasses energy and synergy arises. This force empowers occupational scientists who commit to a common goal and vision; it captivates their imagination and stimulates an enthusiasm for generating new ideas. Furthermore, this power differs from the power of politics, economics, or achievement of quotas that promote individual gain and may therefore only enrich one life. In contrast, the power inherent in goals of occupational science that engage vision and idealism encompasses mind, body, and spirit; the subjective and objective cognition and feelings; and human good and the enrichment of all life.

Third, by joining in a valuable cause to enrich all people's lives, occupational scientists and therapists are experiencing a new sense of meaning derived from challenges and the commitment to meet the demands of such challenges. Ultimately, joy comes from testing themselves and learning that the experience of challenge and commitment, rather than the accomplishment of an external goal, brings satisfaction. The reward is in the experience rather than in the product.[1]

Fourth, by promoting content and methodologies that address meaning and outcome, occupational scientists are working to be certain that the meaning of occupational therapy and the relevance of meaningful outcomes for each patient are not lost. It is difficult for the individual therapist to balance subjective meaning against a system that values objective outcomes. However, by committing to the meaningfulness of therapy to the patient and the importance of outcomes that have physical and psychosocial value, the therapist's task will become easier, and the patient will be more satisfied.

On one hand, we can think about what we have learned from occupational science, and we can explore ways to incorporate what we have learned into our own treatment programs. On the other hand, we also can examine the process by which occupational science emerged and is evolving and use this process as a model to enrich our professional lives and the lives of our clients. Thus, occupational science has provided the opportunity to acquire new applicable knowledge. Equally or more important, it has given the opportunity to learn from exceedingly good role models. More specifically, pioneers in occupational science have provided new intellectual leadership for the profession of occupational therapy. Research is the foundation of the educational program known as occupational science, and faculty, students, and faculty-student collaborations contribute to this emerging body of knowledge. Also characteristic of occupational science is the emergence and acceptance of research methodologies (ethnographic and qualitative) in which the subject of research also is a contributor to and a collaborator in the research.

Applications in Occupational Therapy

Some examples from experience in practice may better illustrate these two points. Two patient-occupational therapist interactions with patients following heart attacks will illustrate the importance of a holistic view of an individual's illness or disability.

One of my responsibilities as part of my practice in health and wellness is that of working with clients on the cardiac intensive care unit of a local hospital. My role is to help them identify stressors in their lives and to examine ways in which they might more effectively handle these stressors.

On this unit, I quickly found that although I had to help patients understand the perceived connections between stress and heart disease, it was equally as important to understand and talk with them about their own lives and situations that were difficult for them to manage.

After introducing myself and explaining why I was there, I described the physiologic reactions to stress and the perceived relationship between stress and cardiac disease. I learned then to ask patients if there was anything that had been different or unusual in their lives for the past 3 to 5 (or even 10) years. Almost invariably, the result was a very thoughtful response, often expressed in stories of great pain and even beauty that provided insight into the meaning and purpose of their lives and occupations. At other times, the physical illness seemed to be a metaphor for the emotional pain, which often preceded the physical illness and had not been resolved.

In the first example, the patient was a man who had had a serious heart attack. When I entered the room, he was lying on his bed. His wife was seated in a chair, facing him, near the foot of the bed. I sat between the two of them so I could observe and converse with each of them. After introducing myself, I told them why I was there, at which point his wife turned her chair around and sat with her back to both of us. As I talked with him about stress, its impact on the body, and perceived relationship to heart diseases, his face was strained, and his hands formed tight fists. He started to tremble and then seemed to be straining to say something. Finally, he said, "It's my son." After waiting for a short time, I asked. "What about your son?" To this he said, "Well, he's dead." I waited a bit and finally said, "Is that something you would like to talk about?" to which he responded, "Yes."

Another long silence followed, after which I said, "When did he die?" Again there was silence, after which he said "Ten years ago." Slowly he began to relax, and finally he started to tell me that he and his wife had had only one child, this son, and that he had been the light and life of their lives. They did everything together as a family from his birth until he was in his late 20s. Then the son met a girl, whom his parents did not like, and conflict arose. Finally, the son married the girl. This created a fracture in the family, resulting in much disagreement, discomfort, and unpleasantness. When he was 30, the son committed suicide, without any opportunities for healing the rift between parents and son.

The parents spent the succeeding 10-year period buying a house, moving in, selling it, taking a trip, coming back home, buying another house, and repeating the cycle. Not once had they talked to each other about their son's death; each one was afraid of upsetting the other. During this period, two young men, close friends of their son, tried to show this couple love and affection. However, the couple was so enveloped in their loss and mourning that they failed to see the meaning of these caring acts. They had never spoken of this before with anyone. Their most cherished, and perhaps only, major occupations had been those of parenting, which was negated by their son's suicide.

This experience provides a powerful lesson about the importance of treating people with physical illnesses holistically, without neglecting emotional components or consequences of those illnesses. If we fail to learn to address our own feelings and emotions, we may avoid dealing with the sadness and pain of our patients' experiences. In reality, people are holistic beings who have physical and emotional experiences that are related to one another. We must address the mind-body relationship. When we fail to do so, meaning is often lost from therapy. The question we must address is, "Of what value is a measurable physical outcome if life has no meaning to the patient?"

The second example describes an experience with an 85-year-old woman from the west coast who had had a heart attack while visiting her daughter in Colorado. When I went in to see her, she was highly agitated. The nutritionist had been in to see her earlier, and the patient reported that she couldn't continue life if she had to follow the dietary rules she had been given. It was impossible to change the subject, so I asked what was so upsetting to her. She said, "She told me I've got to change the way I eat. I can't eat out any more. I've got to stay home and cook all those good foods." I knew that I could not discuss the nutritionist's advice and recommendations with her but did let her continue to talk until she calmed down so that I was able to pursue an agenda that was not contradictory to that of the nutritionist.

After telling her about stress and its physiological implications, I asked her about unusual events in her life in recent years. She immediately said, "Well, if I can't go out to eat, I can't keep being a foster grandparent." (Being a foster grandparent was her prized occupation.) I asked how the two were related, and she said that she only had so much energy, and if she had to cook for herself, there would be no energy to be a foster grandparent. I then asked her what it was like to be a foster grandparent and what that experience meant to her.

She responded with a story. "I went to work [as a volunteer foster grandparent] in a home for children with developmental disabilities. One day I walked on the ward and saw this little boy who was about 8 years old sitting along the wall. I started to go over to him, and an attendant ran over and said to me, 'You can't work with him. You must stay away from him. He is nothing but danger. He'll just get you in trouble, and he's liable to hurt you. He's a very difficult child.'"

After a pause, she said, "I knew that I was going to work with him. So I did. I started reading to him as he had both visual and hearing problems. I would read to him and talk to him, and you know, I even got him to the point where he'd tie his shoes, dress himself, and then he'd feed himself." She talked more about the little boy, about what good times they had, and what changes she brought about in his life. As she talked and reflected on their time together, it was obvious that the experience had profound meaning for her.

Then she said, "One day I went on the ward and he wasn't there. When I asked the attendants about him, they said he had gone into a coma and was in the hospital in an intensive care unit. I decided right then and there that I was going over to be with him because I knew that his parents lived down south and wouldn't be here for 8 hours or so. I couldn't bear the thought that he might die alone. The attendants told me I couldn't see him. But I went anyway. When I got to the hospital, the nurse said I couldn't see him, and then the doctor tried to stop me. He said that even if I went in, the boy wouldn't recognize me or know that I was there. But I said, 'I don't care, and I am going in.'"

When she got to the room, she looked at him lying there—so tiny and small on the bed—so "I took his hand and I held it like I did on the ward, and wrote on his palm with my finger as I said the Lord's Prayer and the 23rd Psalm. When I finished," she said, "He gripped my hand, and he smiled, and he died." Tears were flowing down my face, but her expression conveyed only her joy in having shared his life and death so that he did not have to die alone.

This woman was so invested in her occupation that her wish was to recover from her heart attack and get back to "her grandchildren." The cost of conforming to a diet that she perceived as irrelevant could not compare with the meaning and relevance she found in working with children as a foster grandparent.

The point of both of these stories and their relation to occupational science and occupational therapy is that we must listen to our patients to find out what is relevant and irrelevant to them, to use their stories to inform us, and to collaborate with them. Occupational science has validated the importance of stories, of meaning, and of feelings as equal partners with physical illnesses. We are now challenged to examine our practice, our approach to education, and our research so that we include what is meaningful and relevant to our patients in the treatment plans and programs that we, patients and therapists together, develop. In summary, the more we collaborate, the more our efforts are directed toward shared goals and shared visions and the more powerful and productive our endeavors will be. In so doing, we also can contribute to the continuing evolution and development of occupational science and occupational therapy.

Discussion Questions

1. How have practitioners traditionally sought or avoided understanding and communicating with patients concerning the emotional dimensions of disability and illness?
2. What is Johnson's vision of occupational science?

Reference

1. Csikszentmihalyi, M: Flow: The Psychology of Optimal Experience. Harper & Row, Publishers, New York, 1990.

Section VIII

Wilma West Lectures

There have been and will continue to be many contributors to the development of occupational science. As we have seen, many individuals in disciplines outside occupational science and occupational therapy have concepts, foci, and research that may illuminate questions of interest to occupational scientists. However, some of the most priceless contributors will be those within the field of occupational therapy. They may be contributing from behind the scenes, assisting in the endless search for research grant support or helping agencies become aware of the need for research and training reflecting the questions of occupational therapy and occupational science. They may be scholars and clinicians whose primary focus is not the occupational science development project but who nevertheless have been stimulated by the ideas presented in the symposia or publications regarding occupational science. They provide a rich source of issues and ideas with which we all can grapple and for which we all can be grateful.

In her lifetime of leadership within occupational therapy, Wilma West has had unmeasurable influence on many aspects of our development: clinical, educational, in research, and in our philosophy. The development of a background of support for the ideas and processes of occupational science occurred, in part, because of her extensive contributions. The first Wilma West lecture, presented by Nedra Gillette in Santa Monica, California, at the 1988 Occupational Science Symposium, traced Miss West's history, finding predictors of her later contributions in her earlier development. Her role as a mentor and model to many reminds all of us that it is not only what we accomplish individually that benefits our field, but how we help each other grow and develop that leads to the greatest levels of accomplishment. The message is clear that as educators, clinicians, theoreticians, and scientists, we can build for the future of our profession through supporting the development of our newer professionals.

Burke's paper, presented at the 1989 Occupational Science Symposium in Los Angeles, California, focuses on play, a major category of occupation. She raises some challenging topics for occupational science study of play, growing from Burke's practice experiences, research, and theoretical interests. Identifying the unique qualities of play may help us all identify playfulness in our lives, not only in the lives of children, and improve our quality of life by the addition of play (perhaps occasionally even within our work). The occupational nature of play is closely related to one's views about the purposefulness of play. Is it a lingering biological survival mechanism, a pleasurable activity for childhood or leisure times when excused from more productive occupations, a preliminary practice of core skills to be later assembled according to cultural scripts, a means of practicing adult behavior without serious danger, or some combination of all of the above? We cannot be sure, but each perspective has proponents and needs to be considered. Occupational scientists are further encouraged to consider questions about how to support play experiences for children with chronic disease or disability.

In the next paper, presented by Linda Florey at the 1991 Occupational Science Symposium in Philadelphia, Pennsylvania, addresses the ordinariness of occupations and the devaluation of their importance that has often occurred as a result. A similar devaluing and potential loss to our practice is recognized by Florey in the area of social and emotional aspects of pediatric practice. Sounding an alarm, she cites professional literature that appears to ignore these vital developmental areas, while still intending to represent the range of developmental milestones or comprehensive occupational therapy evaluation tools. In response, she suggests that we must value the ordinary, including the social aspect of children, to reflect accurately an occupational focus for our therapy because without this element, we cannot truly see occupation.

The last paper in this section was presented by Charles Christiansen at the 1992 Occupational Science Symposium in Chicago, Illinois. Christiansen addresses a core issue in occupational therapy and occupational science: What is a balance of occupations? Many of us go through life feeling that less time is spent on the things that are important to us, and more time is spent on work, studies, or routine activities that are less interesting and rewarding. What is the elusive balance that we are seeking? Christiansen reviews three potential concepts of balance.

The first concept of balance in occupation is measured by perceived or actual time use. Students in Occupational Science review the time use studies and decide, as does Christiansen, that a balance of occupation means more than just an equal number of hours in work, play, rest, or sleep. People acknowledge the impact of our perception of time in the commonplace remark "How time flies when we're having fun" (frequently stated with a rueful tone when people are *not* having fun).

A second concept of balance in occupation arises from the study of routines in daily patterns of occupation. In Ludwig's[1] Occupational Science dissertation, focused on routines in older women, the participants frequently planned physical activities for morning hours when their energy level was still high. This finding supports work reviewed by Christiansen and depends on underlying chronobiological rhythms. The term "zeitgeber" (literally "time giver"), an environmental factor that calibrates our internal clocks, relates clearly to Pierce's (this book) discussion of the importance of the innate rhythm of occupations, especially the writing work of scholars. The clock does not control that work, nor do biological or environmental factors alone. As the editors of this book found, the work of writing sets its own timetable, and scholars involved in this entrancing occupation may ignore social signals, such as ordinary work hours, or biosocial ones, such as their family's dinner hours. This occupatiotemporality, ordering time by the flow of our occupations, is an important element of orchestration of one's day.

A third view of occupational balance suggests that the compatibility of each individual's unique configuration or pattern of occupations may provide the balance. That is, people have a number of occupations in which they participate, but there are differences in the amount of value which each has for the individual. The conflict or agreement between the amount of time one can allocate to occupations of varying value may be the key to feelings of occupational balance or imbalance in our daily life. One can easily imagine using this literature, shared in Christiansen's paper, as a starting point for research that may provide occupational science support for one of occupational therapy's earliest and key propositions: a balance of occupations promotes a healthy and satisfying life.

Reference

1. Ludwig, A: The Use and Meaning of Routine in Women over 70 Years of Age. Unpublished doctoral dissertation in occupational science, University of Southern California, Los Angeles, 1995.

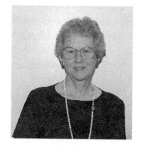

by *Nedra P. Gillette, MEd, OTR, FAOTA*

36

Tribute to Wilma L. West

Wilma West is one of the foremost individuals in the profession of occupational therapy today. Her contributions have been vigorous, dynamic, and philosophical. Collectively, they have made an impact on the field that is perhaps more broad and significantly deeper than those made by any other occupational therapist of her time.

It is fitting that Miss West should be honored by University of Southern California (USC), where she was awarded the first graduate degree ever given in occupational therapy. It is equally fitting that she be honored by an annual scholarly lecture. I have chosen, however, to set the stage for such lectures by telling you about Wilma herself, as I have come to know her over the last 30 years. Because most occupational therapists subscribe to developmental history, we should examine the past to see how it predicts the present and the future. I am in the process of collecting interview data for an oral history of the women who have been leaders in occupational therapy. Much of what follows was obtained through an interview with Wilma: although other material was solicited from her friends and colleagues.

Who Is She?

Wilma Louise West (Willie) (Fig. 36–1) was born in upstate New York 73 years ago, just outside Rochester. Her father and his brothers owned a nursery and truck farm, a successful small business that often involved many members of the family.

One brother's family lived across town, but another lived just next door, and Wilma was raised in a warm extended family, where the sharing of affection and support for each other was continuously in evidence. Here we have predictor number one: Willie has a most unusual ability to work in harmony with others, providing support and challenge just at the time one needs it most. Always offered gently with no hint of intrusion or directiveness, her affectionate guidance has helped many achieve well beyond their expectations for themselves.

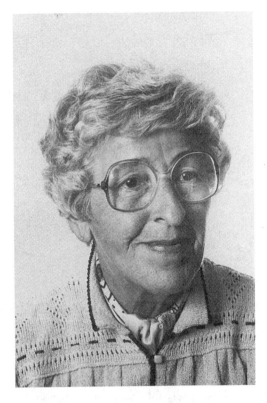

Figure 36–1. Wilma West. (Photograph courtesy of the American Occupational Therapy Foundation, Bethesda, Maryland.)

Willie says as a child, she was a tom-boy. With the cousins and neighbor children, there were many hours of outdoor games and activities. Sports were a part of her life, and horses were her dearest love. Work and play helped to balance her life at an early age. Often she worked in the greenhouses, but her favorite way to help in the family business was to go with her father on Saturdays to the market in Rochester to sell vegetables and flowers. She liked the excitement of the market and particularly enjoyed watching and meeting the many different kinds of people who shopped and worked there. Here is predictor number two: Wilma is drawn to the heart of any affair, and it's important to her to know all the players. Her sensitivity to each person she meets was perhaps cultivated through these early experiences at the market and through the family's other activities.

In the household next door, there was a maiden aunt, who was a school teacher. This aunt was a strong positive influence on Willie as she grew up, and she was a competitive lady. The cousins next door were going to Wellesley College, and Willie's aunt argued that she should go to Mt. Holyoke, which she believed was more intellectually stimulating and exciting than Wellesley. This is predictor number three: Miss West has one of the keenest minds in the profession, the clear product of a liberal arts program where she developed the classic traits of critical thinking, judgment, ethics, and social conscience. She remains, of course, one of the profession's best advocates for a liberal arts background prior to an education in occupational therapy.

During her senior year in college, her roommate's mother urged them to attend a career day on occupational therapy. The roommate chose not to attend, but Wilma and another friend did go. The charismatic speaker of the day was none other than Marjorie Fish, then a faculty member at the Boston School of Occupational Therapy (BSOT). (She later became the executive director of the American Occupational Therapy Association [AOTA] and the occupational therapy consultant for the Rehabilitation Services Administration.) Marge immediately had two recruits. Wilma received her BA degree from Mt. Holyoke in 1939 and went directly to BSOT.

Education

At BSOT, her classmates included such lifelong friends and occupational therapy heroines as Mary Reilly and Carlotta Welles. She found the program to be stimulating and was particularly drawn to the medical aspects of the instruction. In those years, many were the hours spent in perfecting the required skills as artisan-therapist: weaving and bookbinding, leather work and ceramics, needlecrafts and sewing, woodworking and jewelry making. All of these were "known" to be essential parts of the therapist's repertoire. Arts and crafts, however, while enjoyable to Willie from the perspective of viewer and appreciator, proved to be neither terribly manageable nor satisfying to her as a student. The predictor number four: Wilma West is one of those occupational therapists whom we recognize as thinkers, not just as doers.

The director of BSOT was Marjorie Greene. It is to her that Wilma attributes her own standards for professionalism and her belief that one must support AOTA as a means of enhancing the viability and strength of the profession. Mrs. Greene, who was not an occupational therapist, was one of the greatest entrepreneurs of the field. BSOT was a small private school and as such, was always in need of funds. Mrs. Greene organized the "Boston Musicales," a weekly morning performance of the Boston Pops Orchestra. One of the beneficiaries of these concerts was BSOT, and one of the socialization processes used at the school was to "reward" students by allowing them to attend the Musicales. The foresight and ability to establish such an institution on behalf of her commitment to the profession leads us to predictor number five: When circumstances suggested the need, Miss West saw to it that the AOTA established the American Occupational Therapy Foundation. This is discussed later in this paper.

Employment

Physical disabilities had been of particular interest to Willie throughout school, and when she completed her certificate in occupational therapy in 1941, she took her first position at the Robert Breck Brigham Hospital in Boston on an arthritis service. Extensive research was under way on the disease in those years, and she was quickly caught up in the latest in treatment and rehabilitation. She remained in this job from July 1941 until February 1943 and was prompted to leave it only because she encountered another of the profession's most influential people, Winifred Conrick Kahman.

Miss Conrick was the remarkable individual who established occupational therapy in the U.S. Army. She worked in the Office of the Surgeon General as a civilian consultant and determined the standards for selection and recruitment of occupational therapy personnel and for occupational therapy practice in U.S. Army facilities everywhere.

Recognizing an outstanding young clinician, she urged Willie to resign her position in Boston and to go to Walter Reed Army Hospital in Washington, D.C., which she did. She served there until sometime in 1944 on the orthopaedics unit, with special concern for the rehabilitation of amputees. In 1944, Miss Conrick added Miss West to her staff in the Office of the Surgeon General, where she became the assistant chief of the Occupational Therapy Branch, a position she held until the end of the war. Another colleague in that office was Elizabeth Messick, later the director of the School of Occupational Therapy at Richmond Professional Institute (now Virginia Commonwealth University).

These three, Conrick, Messick, and West, were legendary among the therapists in Army facilities for their ability to inspire the bureaucracy and to see that much-needed supplies and personnel were provided, somehow magically making the Army red tape dissolve! Winifred Conrick's commanding presence and her imaginative and highly successful administrative abilities in the male worlds of medicine and Army helped shape Wilma West's career in a most powerful fashion. This is predictor number six: Leadership, coupled with clarity of vision and commitment to the highest standards, would become synonymous with Wilma L. West.

After leaving the Army, Willie came to USC, where Margaret Rood had begun the first graduate program in occupational therapy. She had been given the first Bernard Baruch Fellowship for graduate study in rehabilitation and chose to apply the fellowship at USC. This is predictor number seven: The Baruch Fellowship was to be the first in a long series of awards and professional recognitions that she received during and after her working career, and in 1946, she also received the Meritorious Civilian Service award for her work in the office of the surgeon general.

Her master's degree was completed in August 1947, and she went immediately to AOTA to assume the newly created position of educational field secretary. This position was established through a grant from the Kellogg Foundation, providing an opportunity for AOTA to promote uniform standards of education and the expansion of programs to prepare occupational therapists. She remained in this position only 1 year when she was promoted by the board to become the executive secretary of AOTA (now known as executive director). In both positions, Wilma consolidated her commitment to occupational therapy education, a theme that continues to hold her interest today.

A major accomplishment of the Conrick, Messick, and West trio had been the decision of the U.S. Army to commission occupational therapists. Previously and all during World War II, these individuals worked as civilian employees of the Army, a status that held some advantages but greater disadvantages. With the onset of the Korean war in 1950, Captain Wilma West found herself drawn to return to the Army. Resigning her position as executive secretary at AOTA, she became the chief, Occupational Therapy Section, Medical Field Service School, Fort Sam Houston, Texas. Here she had the opportunity to try out her beliefs about occupational therapy education, because the Army trained its own occupational therapists in this setting. Her experiences as a beginning teacher, under the stern and watchful eye of a rigid old army general, make for wonderful entertainment. Using the core beliefs and skills of occupational therapy, one can maneuver safely through the obstacles inherent in most systems and effect constructive change. Captain Wilma West prevailed!

After leaving the Army in 1953, Miss West entered a 10-year period in which her career was tempered by the long illness of her mother and her need to be near home much of the time. During this period, she assumed several part-time jobs for AOTA, the best known of which is perhaps with the curriculum study; she was a member of the study team from 1960 to 1961, and director of the study from 1961 to 1963, when it ended. Also funded by the Kellogg Foundation, the curriculum study provided a thorough evaluation of the present state of education in occupational therapy and established goals and directions for the education of the future. It required and benefitted from the long-time commitment of Wilma West to the finest in education. During this same time, she was further honored by being named consultant to the Surgeon General from 1958 to 1964.

Move to Washington, D.C.

In 1964, a new position became available, and Miss West was determined to have it. She saw this as an opportunity to speak for occupational therapy at a national level, to make an impact on one branch of the national health program by demonstrating the efficacy of occupational therapy. She applied for the position of consultant in occupational therapy at the Bureau of Maternal and Child Health (MCH), although she had never held a job working with children. Although history does not record the names of any competitors she might have had for the position, it seems clear that there were none who could have so effectively and imaginatively accomplished what Wilma West has done for the children of America. She remained with the bureau until her retirement in 1975, becoming Chief of the Health Services Training Branch in July 1973. Her colleague, friend, successor, and admirer is Jim Papai.

She used her role at MCH to provide support for higher education in occupational and physical therapy. Some examples of this follow: Willie was instrumental in providing support for the beginning of the master's program at Boston University (BU). Later, she provided a year of planning time in 1978 for the BU doctoral program, which led to a commitment of University support. As Dr. Anne Henderson says, "The program would never have been funded without her." Many know of her early support for graduate study at USC through their University Affiliated Program. The Occupational Science Symposia are one of the long-term outcomes of her earlier vision and the support she laid down for occupational therapy and physical therapy education while she was in the Bureau.

Throughout her career, she has been interested in the development of the minds of occupational therapists. In 1958, her leadership produced the Allenberry Conference, an interdisciplinary study of the use of activities in psychiatric occupational therapy. *Changing Concepts in Practice in Psychiatric Occupational Therapy* was the resulting publication.[1]

Within 1 year of going to MCH, she had organized and funded the first of many conferences about children and occupational therapy. The proceedings of this conference were published in 1965 as *Occcupational Therapy for the Multiply Handicapped Child*.[2] Books available to us at that time for use as teaching materials were Willard and Spackman and Fidler and Fidler. With these two publications, Willie doubled our access to available texts.

Other Honors

Predictor number seven suggested that many honors would follow the Bernard Baruch Fellowship received in 1946. Let me mention just a few other honors bestowed on Wilma West, before moving on to share with you some memories and special tributes from other colleagues and friends.

In 1972, she received the Superior Service Award for Health Services and Mental Health Administration (U.S. Department of Health, Education and Welfare). She is the only occupational therapist ever to receive this award. In 1981, she was awarded the Certificate of Appreciation by the U.S. Army Surgeon General.

A number of honors have come to her through her own professional organizations:

1948 to 1951	AOTA Executive Secretary
1951	AOTA Award of Merit
1961 to 1964	AOTA President
1967	Eleanor Clarke Slagle Lecture, on the occasion of AOTA's 50th Anniversary
1973	Charter Fellow of AOTA
1972–82	President, American Occupational Therapy Foundation (AOTF)

| 1982 | Testimony of Appreciation, and Honorary Life Membership, AOTF |
| 1985 | Dedication of the Wilma L. West Library of Occupational Therapy |

American Occupational Therapy Association

Wilma West's tenure as President of AOTA was marked by several outstanding achievements. A management consulting firm was hired to study the relationship between the volunteer sector, the national office staff, and the membership at large. New bylaws resulted, and new structures were implemented for conducting AOTA's business. The delegate assembly became the representative assembly; four Councils were established, providing for the first time equal voices for the important functions of practice, finance, education, and development (conference, publications, and awards). Perhaps the most enlightened decision of all was to establish AOTF, which had particular appeal to Willie, because as predictor number five suggests, her long-range vision for the profession activated her entrepreneurial leadership, and an important milestone was accomplished.

Predictor number three, concerned with her commitment to the best in education, is also influential here. AOTF represents Wilma's conviction that learning must be the heart of any profession. AOTF has assumed a mission of providing support for education, research, and scholarly publications. True to form, she saw to it that AOTA and AOTF would always be partners in providing service and leadership to the profession.

Bureau of Maternal and Child Health and the University-Affiliated Facilities

Knowing that Wilma considers the University Affiliated Facilities (UAFs) to be one of the most important links in the pediatric health care system, I inquired of colleagues about her role in developing them. Here are some of their views.

- *Dr. Anne Henderson.* It was through her (Willie's) sponsorship that occupational therapy was established in the UAF. Willie fought some heavy-duty battles to see that rules were established that would require each UAF to include occupational therapy; then, of course, she continued to be there to provide support for the UAF people as the new programs developed.
- *Dr. Wylda Hammond.* She (Wilma West) was active in creating a good basic philosophy and guidelines for the UAFs, and much of her energy was focused on ensuring the development of a truly interdisciplinary process.
- *Martha Moersch.* In helping to shape these new facilities, her (Willie's) influence was strongly evident in several ways: establishing training programs for UAF personnel toward increased professionalism; conceptualizing training programs that would lead to interdisciplinary collaboration; demonstrating through her own administrative abilities her understanding of the services and programs needed by developmentally disabled children and their families.

Martha also recalls President John F. Kennedy's remarks concerning the needs of the country's retarded citizens, which led to the development of the UAFs. Martha suspects that his speech was inspired by the vision of Wilma L. West, somehow subtlely conveyed to him across Washington bureaucracy.

Mrs. Moersch also notes that the MCH-supported pediatric conference on the multiply handicapped child, Chicago, 1965, marked the beginning of occupational therapy services to these children *and* paved the way for occupational therapists to be ready to respond to PL 94-142, The Education for All Handicapped Children Act. At the present time, nearly one-third of the total AOTA membership works with children or in the public school system. It is fortunate that we were ready to provide these services when the opportunity was created.

Ideas

Do you remember predictions number three and number four? Wilma West is a thinker. No tribute to her would be complete without acknowledging some of the ideas that guide the profession today. Her Eleanor Clarke Slagle lectureship was published in January 1968.[3] It represents another of her efforts to bring others along with her in their commitments to and understanding of occupational therapy in the future. In this lecture, she stated her challenge in the form of five "shoulds" directed toward therapists individually and collectively.

Because occupational therapists are committed to serving the occupational needs of people rather than attending only to problems and deficits, we *should*:

1. Identify with the field of health services, broadening our concerns to include more than medicine
2. Enlarge our concept of ourselves from being therapists to becoming health agents concerned with normal growth and development
3. Think more about our roles in prevention as well as those in treatment and rehabilitation
4. Think more about socioeconomic, cultural, and biologic causes of disease and dysfunction
5. Think more about serving health needs of people in many other settings than the hospital

These challenges are now 20 years old. I think we are still struggling to meet them.

In a paper 2 years later, she told the story of the fishermen who suddenly found children floating down the river and began frantically to try to save them. Suddenly, one said to the other, "Where are you going?" And his companion replied, "You stay here and save as many as you can. I'm going upstream and try and find the so-and-so who's throwing them in!"

She went on to say, "Our failure as a group to concern ourselves more broadly and dynamically with prevention and with the maintenance and promotion of health would constitute a dereliction of professional responsibility, equal to that of forsaking those who have already fallen or been pushed into the main stream of medical care."[4] In other words, we must address our responsibilities in prevention and continue to meet our obligations to provide treatment.

In 1981 she received another honor as the graduating class at the University of Texas-Galveston selected her as their class mentor. In her address to them, she made the following points:

1. Occupational therapy's special contribution to health care is made through "accent on fulfillment in human occupation and to understanding the significance and worth of human enterprise."
2. Occupational therapy is concerned with "all factors, intrinsic and extrinsic, that affect the health of the individual's functions and interactions" with others. This is a view of health centered on occupational performance, not on the absence of pathology. It "implies an awareness of occupation as a human trait, a human need, and a natural mode of influencing health." (This latter quote is attributed to Dr. Mary Reilly.)
3. We have a focus on the patient's remaining physical and mental capacities, not on those that have been lost; our rehabilitation goal is to regain maximum possible function, relative to the ways in which those gains can enhance self-care and independent living skills.[5]

Tributes to Wilma West

Friends and colleagues have provided tributes of various kinds, some of which I have included.

Martha Moersch, who first knew Willie through a UAF in Michigan and who later succeeded her as President of AOTF, says, "Willie just does what she has to do most of the time and she doesn't have any *mishaps* the way the rest of us do!"

Another tribute states, "She recognized ability in young occupational therapists, and fostered their development; then she'd stand back and let the younger person reap the rewards of professional involvement and leadership. . . . She pushes your sights!"

Lela Llorens recalls similar experiences: "So often, there was the behind-the-scene support, things that might really further your career, like an invitation to do a joint presentation." Lela also says that in her own pioneering work with adolescents in the community (another MCH-sponsored program), she always felt she was putting into practice what Wilma West had been preaching.

Anne Henderson says, "She's *always* been there to help."

Marge Fish says, "She could do anything and do it perfectly . . . ever so many different kinds of things." Their mutual friend Marie-Louise Franciscus says, "I have truly deep admiration for her. . . . She's really brilliant."

Wylda Hammond recalls that she was always more than helpful, making herself "available to us even at peculiar hours; always willing to try new ways to do things . . . and then would get involved in developing ideas that would make them work."

Jim Papai remembers her boundless energy and unlimited ideas, "that sometimes made it hard to keep up with her! And she has to be the most warm-blooded individual there ever was: her office was always around zero degrees! But her constant professionalism was always accompanied by her great warmth."

Research

Finally, I must mention the program through which Willie has had the most direct influence on my own life. As AOTF president, she hired me to open the Office of Professional Research Services. It became my immediate privilege to have her as "boss" yet to be treated with that sensitivity referred to in predictor number two and by Martha Moersch and Lela Llorens. Predictor number one was in evidence as well. Her support was constant; her guidance was gentle and affectionately offered.

She always met with the Research Advisory Council during its formative years and continued for several years after that as an active member of the Research Development Committee, the foundation's think tank for research. She was always ahead of us! Her ideas had been brewing, and her knowledge and use of strategies to help us achieve our goals were critical to the success the research program has enjoyed.

As for her many contributions to research, I think one perhaps outshines all the others. In April 1976, using her support through MCH, Wilma West assembled the best minds in occupational therapy at a research symposium held in St. Louis. Betty Yerxa and Ellie Gilfoyle chaired the symposium and collaborated on writing the report, which was published in the *American Journal of Occupational Therapy* in September 1976.[6] This remarkable meeting and the ensuing document were created under Wilma West's quiet monitoring. Ten years after establishing the Research Advisory Council and opening the AOTA-AOTF research program, we are still working toward the goals established by this group. This is an appropriate testimony to her genius, for genius she is. I call her occupational therapy's national treasure.

References

1. West, WL (ed): Changing Concepts and Practice in Psychiatric Occupational Therapy. American Occupational Therapy Association, New York, 1958.
2. West, WL (ed): Occupational Therapy for the Multiply Handicapped Child. University of Illinois, Chicago, 1965.
3. West, WL: 1967 Eleanor Clarke Slagle lecture: Professional responsibility in time of change. Am J Occup Ther 22:9–15, 1968.
4. West, WL: The growing importance of prevention. Am J Occup Ther 23:226–231, 1969.
5. West, WL: The Challenge of Practice. Talk to first OT graduates of the College of Allied Health Sciences, Thomas Jefferson University, Philadelphia, PA, June 6, 1985.
6. Yerxa, ES, and Gilfoyle, E: The foundation: Research seminar. Am J Occup Ther 30:509–514, 1976.

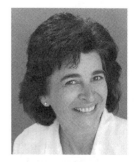

by Janice Posatery Burke, MA,
OTR/L, FAOTA

3 7

Variations in Childhood Occupations: Play in the Presence of Chronic Disability

Identifying Play

Play as Purposeful Activity

Purposeful to Competent: Interactions Within the
Environment

Play and Chronicity

Summary

An occupational science perspective of play requires an examination of three congruent issues: What about play makes it such a unique phenomenon (the magic of play, the sense of well-being that is derived from playful activity)? What about that phenomenon is related to what we know about occupation (the purposefulness of play, its goal-directed quality, the meaning of play activity)? How can the physical, cognitive, and psychosocial variations that are present in children with disabilities or chronic disease be shaped to ensure that they yield equally magical experiences in play?

Identifying Play

Play is a way for children to find out about and put meaning to their worlds. Through their manipulations of objects and actions, children create an image of the world and an understanding of the ways that all parts fit together.

Traditionally, society has viewed play as the "work of children," but within an occupational science perspective, that view is far too limiting. Play is more than a role that is assumed; it is more than a job to be completed. Play has an open-endedness. Because of its self-initiated, self-directed, almost limitless quality, play offers the player a flexibility that is not typically found in work or self-maintenance activities. It is a purely pleasurable phenomenon. In play, children are able to create a world that includes all that they need or want—what Bruner calls the combinational richness of play.[1]

Sylva[2] described the potential biological significance of playful, curious animal behaviors as having survival value. Indeed, the playful manipulations of seemingly useless novel objects lead to a store of information that can be used when need arises. Lorenz found the following:

> Through this process of learning the properties attached to things, independently of the momentary physiological condition and requirements of the organism, curiosity behavior has an objectivating function in the most literal and important sense of the word. It is only through curiosity behavior that objects come to exist in the environment of an animal as in that of [the human].[2]

Through this process of curious playful exploration, young humans and primates come to know their worlds.

Play is the first learning in which members of our species engage. The importance and attention given to it vary greatly across cultural groups.[3] For many, play represents a time of preparation for future role behavior, including the later childhood roles associated with doing chores, part-time work, assuming apprenticeship roles, and ultimately fulfilling worker roles.

Perhaps the greatest contribution to our study about play will be in our discovery of the nature of play: how we know when we are playing and how we can incorporate the pleasure of the play experience into some yet unconnected behaviors traditionally thought to lack a quality of play (that is, therapy). In addition, we need to learn to what extent we are able to teach play, the kind of play and the kinds of settings that encourage development, and other similar information. Questions to ask in the study of play include:

- What is the function of play?
- Who plays with whom?
  How are playmate preferences made?
  What do play-based sociograms look like?
- Why do kids play?
- What are the cultural, gender, and ethnic variations in play?
- What are human play signals?
- What does the individual look like and act like when there has been play deprivation?
- What is play in adulthood?
- How do play patterns vary in children's play?

What are the different strategies for approaching, withdrawing, and briefly engaging in play?

How are strategies used for different types of play (that is, contact, rough and tumble play, solitary play)?[4]

Play as Purposeful Activity

In 1972, the American Occupational Therapy Association's Council on Standards defined occupational therapy as "the art and science of directing man's participation in selected tasks to restore, reinforce and enhance performance, facilitate learning of those skills and functions essential for adaptation and productivity, diminish or correct pathology, and to promote and maintain health."[5] This definition was later refined as follows:

> OT is the use of purposeful activity with individuals who are limited by physical injury or illness, psychosocial dysfunction, developmental or learning disabilities, poverty and cultural differences or the aging process in order to maximize independence, prevent disability and maintain health.[6]

This inclusive definition highlights the important role of purposeful activity as a vehicle for transforming nonfunctional behavior to a functional state. The concept of purposeful activity, in which the individual directs attention to the task itself rather than to the internal processes required to achieve the task, leads one to consider the critical variable of engagement, the factor that ensures a person will be involved or invested in a given activity, such as play.

Purposeful activity is product-oriented activity. When the literature on purposeful activity is examined and lined up next to that on play, the compatibility inherent in the two concepts is striking. Set in the arena of occupational therapy, purposeful activity is the product of a well-designed process in which the therapist has come to know the child, and together they have found activities that have purpose and meaning while they also address physical, emotional, and cognitive needs. Accordingly,

> purpose or purposeful action cannot be defined in terms of tools with which, or activities in which, therapists engage their patients. Purposeful activity must be defined in terms of the unique directions of individual patients and the enabling of patients toward enhanced growth and development, and by involvement and organization of self and environment.[7]

Purposeful play activities can achieve such an effect. Investigators, including Heck and Kircher, have studied the effect of purposeful activity on pain tolerance and perception of workload.[8,9] Findings indicated that engagement in purposeful activities enabled individuals to perform longer, even in the presence of pain. Activity not only provides an intrinsically motivating experience, it also is a distraction from pain.

Fidler and Fidler conceptualized purposefulness as "doing." They used this word to "convey the sense of performing, producing or causing."[10] Doing was concerned with a multidimensional perspective of the person, other people, and the nonhuman environment. In this view, doing was visualized as "enabling the development and integration of the sensory, motor, cognitive and psychological systems; serving as a socializing agent and verifying one's efficacy as a competent, contributing member of one's society."[10] Doing also was credited with feeding on and into an inner assurance.

Purposeful to Competent: Interactions Within the Environment

Fidler and Fidler further discuss doing as a mediation point between one's inner and outer world. Doing can "nurture the capacity to invest, teach realistic responses to success and failure, provide concrete evidence of one's capabilities and limitations, test the reality base of fantasy and perceptions, and validate the ability to achieve and influence one's environment."[11] If play is considered the doing of children, then by engaging in play, children can learn about themselves in relation to the outer world.

White's discussion of the critical importance of the environment as a motivator provides a further link to the value of purposeful activity. Using the concept of "an urge toward competence," White described how such a behavior emerges. "A sense of competence arises basically out of having exerted an influence upon the environment."[12] This sense of competence and efficacy emerge from direct encounters with and mastery of the environment, and in stressful situations, competence is what drives the coping mechanism. In assessing the strong evidence that associates stress and life-style as related factors affecting immunocompetence, Clark and Jackson[13] suggested that what we do each day, that is, our participation in daily occupation, may be crucial in modulating stress levels and shaping lifestyles. Engagement in purposeful activities can enable people to cope more effectively with environmental demands. For children, involvement in the purposeful activity of play may be their most effective coping strategy for dealing with the demands of chronic illness, disability, and poverty.

"Play, a child's most valued form of purposeful activity, is a medium for assembling and reassembling behavior sequences for skilled action."[14] It is a neutralizer, reducing the pressure of goal-directed action. It is a way to resist frustration because play with materials improves later problem solving that recalls important materials and actions. In addition, more inventive, exploratory behavior leads to more creativity and originality.[15] Indeed, interesting and fulfilling lives often are characterized by a sense of playfulness. However, does the play of children with chronic disabilities include these qualities of play and playfulness, or does the nature of the specific disabling problem and the daily occupations that are in place to address them in some way prevent sufficient involvement in the world of play?

Play and Chronicity

In the child with a chronic disability, individual abilities and disabilities may be confined to one domain (physical, cognitive, psychosocial) but more likely will touch several or all domains of performance. Each child presents a unique profile of strengths and deficits even when they share the same diagnosis. It is not uncommon to see contrasting patterns, characteristics, and difference in children with the same type of disability.

Play is a behavior that may or may not be part of the everyday repertoire of the child with a disability and his or her family. For this child, greater agendas—therapeutic, medical, surgical priorities—take the time and energy that would otherwise be directed toward play. Researchers and health professionals become concerned when illness, disability, and their concomitant intervention regimens interfere with play and in a sense, trigger the potential of an iatrogenic influence on development. According to Garvey, "the failure of a child to engage in play behavior that displays progression, complexity and elaboration is often regarded as a symptom of cognitive, social, physical or emotional disability."[16] The inability to play due to chronic illness or disability presents some special considerations and is an appropriate area for research and treatment attention in occupational therapy:

- How do we know when we are playing?
- What about the playful experience opens more channels for learning?
- Are there specific conditions that must be present to ensure that play will be experienced (adult models, mood, time, materials)?
- Do children need maximum use of all their biological, cognitive, and psychosocial systems to attain the bliss of play?
- Is there a way to provide play experiences that include special play environments, physical influences, and human influences to affect play positively?

In play among children with special needs, the opportunities to explore and interact with the environment are significantly altered. Most typically, the difficulties of a given child are compound and rob the child of opportunities to learn, practice skills, and find ways around handicapping barriers. Disabilities often delay independent exploration of the environment; failure and frustration lead to passivity and decreased drive and interest. Most significantly, the societal attitudes we hold about people with disabilities color the values and goals we impart to parents, families, and children. Television, contemporary movies, and fiction are testimonials to the distorted, deficient, and demoralized view of disability that continues to prosper in our everyday lives.

In children with mental retardation, we see less spontaneous play; the most marked differences in play are in preference for play materials. Children with mental retardation prefer more structured materials (pegboards, scrapbooks, puzzles). They appear to need a model of the finished product to initiate their play, demonstrating what might be thought of as a more narrow, inflexible method for exploration. Additionally, children with mental retardation are seen as lacking sustained attention; engaging in rougher, more destructive play; and showing inappropriate use of objects. In some situations, the child has certain behavior patterns, such as lack of eye contact, that alter patterns of interaction, that is, nonverbal positive encouragement; these patterns in turn affect further play emergence.

Summary

By studying, observing, and reflecting on the play of children, we acquire more than a catalog of activities and interests of ages and stages of growth and development. We come to know more than how children learn physical, cognitive, and social-emotional strategies that will provide them with the skill needed to propel them into a satisfying, well-balanced adulthood. Our study of play identifies the unique biopsychosocial core behaviors that are called on in play and that satisfy and further the nature of skills acquired and the methods of skill acquisition.

Think back on your own youth. Remember your own play. Your memories may rest on a familiar play place, play object, play activity, or playmate. Go beyond that point to your feeling state—the excitement, pleasure, feeling of contentment, of not wanting or needing anything more; there was a timelessness where food and sleep and drink were inconsequential. That state is what we seek to evoke in children. I suggest that we focus our attention on play and play behaviors as the measures of dysfunction prior to intervention and as measures of efficacy at the close of treatment.

Discussion Questions

1. What are the qualities Burke describes that identify play as a major occupation?
2. How might you proceed to find the answers to some of Burke's questions about play and the child with a chronic disease or disability in a research study? How might you try to answer them in a therapy session?

References

1. Bruner, JS: Nature and uses of immaturity. In Bruner, JS, Jolly, A, and Sylva, K (eds): Play: Its Role in Development of Evolution. Basic Books, New York, 1976.
2. Sylva, K: Play and learning. In Tizard, B, and Harvey, D (eds): Biology of Play. J.B. Lippincott, Philadelphia, PA, 1977.
3. Lorenz, K: Psychology and phylogeny. In Bruner, JS, Jolly, A, and Sylva, K (eds): Play: Its Role in Development of Evolution. Basic Books, New York, 1976, pp 88–89.
4. White, L: Play in animals. In Tizard, B, and Harvey, D (eds): Biology of Play. J.B. Lippincott, Philadelphia, PA, 1977.
5. American Occupation Therapy Association: Council on Standards: Occupational therapy: Definition and functions. Am J Occup Ther 26:204, 1972.
6. American Occupational Therapy Association: Representative assembly minutes. Am J Occup Ther 35:792, 798, 1981.
7. Breines, E: The issue is—An attempt to define purposeful activity. Am J Occup Ther 38:543–544, 1984.
8. Heck, SA: The effect of purposeful activity on pain tolerance. Am J Occup Ther 42:577, 1988.
9. Kircher, MA: Motivation as a factor of perceived exertion in purposeful versus non-purposeful activity. Am J Occup Ther 38:165, 1984.
10. Fidler, G, and Fidler, J: Doing and becoming: Purposeful action and self-actualization. Am J Occup Ther 32:305, 1978.
11. Fidler and Fidler, p 306.
12. White, R: The urge towards competence. Am J Occup Ther 25:271, 305, 1971.
13. Clark, FA, and Jackson, J: The application of the occupational science negative heuristic in the treatment of persons with human immunodeficiency infection. Occup Ther in Health Care 6:69, 1989.
14. Bruner, Jolly, and Sylva, p i.
15. Hutt, C: Exploration and play in children. In Bruner, JS, Jolly, A, and Sylva, K (eds): Play: Its Role in Development of Evolution. Basic Books, New York, 1976.
16. Garvey, C: Play with language. In Tizard, B, and Harvey, D (eds): Biology of Play. J.B. Lippincott, Philadelphia, PA, 1977, p 74.

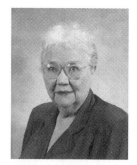

by Anne Henderson, PhD,
OTR, FAOTA

The Scope of Occupational Science

Occupational Science and the Environment

As occupational therapists, we want to provide services that improve the abilities and the lives of our patients. In serving our patients, we rely on clinical judgments based on our values, our personal experience, and the knowledge that has accumulated throughout our history of practice. This leads to good occupational therapy. However, we are all aware that we do not have strongly tested theory to support our practice, and we need a stronger scientific base for our methodologies.

The framework of occupational science has been developed by the University of Southern California's (USC) Department of Occupational Therapy in response to this need for a basic science to support the practice of occupational therapy and to affirm the value of occupation in human life. Faculty and students in occupational therapy at USC have organized knowledge during the last 30 years loosely framed by the concept of occupational behavior. These years of scholarship have identified new areas of knowledge of occupation from which has grown the concept of occupational science. The establishment of doctoral education in occupational science is a landmark in the development of occupational therapy as an academic discipline. The annual conference celebrates the movement of the growth of knowledge into a new and exciting phase.

This paper discusses the scope of occupational science. Several comprehensive descriptions of occupational science have been recently published by the USC faculty. I have read them with great interest, and my paper draws heavily on them. Of particular importance to me is that these recent publications make it clear that the concept of occupational science is broad; it is of sufficient scope to incorporate many streams of research that are ongoing elsewhere. To speak personally, the scope of occupational science is large enough to include the study of occupation in which I have a particular interest: how a child develops occupational competency in his or her physical-spatial environment. Therefore, this paper focuses on occupational science and activity in the physical-spatial sphere.

Evidence of the intended scope of occupational science is found in the inclusion of the work of A. J. Ayres in the research of faculty members and in statements, such as, "Occupational science, however, must also include studies on the neurobiological substrates of skills and occupation such as those of eye-hand coordination or praxis."[1] Theoretical identification of the scope of occupational science is found in the centrality of the systems approach to the study of occupation. All levels of the human system contribute to the output of occupation. The human systems identified include the physical, biological, information processing, sociocultural, symbolic evaluative, and transcendental systems.[1] These systems and the connection among them provide the framework for understanding occupation at different levels. The three lower systems (the physical, biological, and information processing systems) provide the framework for understanding competency in the physical-spatial environment. The physical subsystem, including the anatomic-motor subsystems, supports the enactment of occupation. The biological subsystems directly relate to biological adaptation and become manifest, for example, in the drive for competence or in exploratory behavior. The information processing system encompasses perceptual and conceptual systems and abilities such as learning and memory.

When we consider these lower systems, we also are considering lower levels of occupation, smaller units of action, smaller units of time, and smaller environmental contexts.

Occupation is described as chunks or units of culturally and personally meaningful activity within the stream of human behavior.[2] Each level of occupation can be divided into smaller units, and each can be nested into larger units. Occupation is most often defined as work, play, leisure, and self-maintenance. Each of these abstract units can be divided into concrete occupations. Concrete units also can be broken down into progressively smaller units. Thus, the occupation of housekeeping involves meal preparation, which could involve making a pudding, which involves stirring, which involves grasping and manipulating a spoon and stabilizing a bowl.

Occupational therapy has a long history of this process of activity analysis, consisting of the identification of levels of occupation, of discovering the level at which intervention should occur, of further analysis to determine the need for practice in subroutines or to alter the context of the occupation. However, we have not yet agreed on a vocabulary to classify all the units of occupation in which we are interested. We do not agree as to the extent to which occupation can be unitized and still be considered occupation. To some of us, the term occupation is used only for larger chunks of activity. Teaching school and playing golf are occupations. To others, the term is equated to purposeful activity, as that term is defined in occupational therapy. Then grading papers, learning to write, and putting pegs in a board also are occupations. I do not have the answers, but progress in understanding the inter-relationship between larger and smaller chunks of activity in the physical-spatial world will require that each level be precisely defined and differentiated.

Occupational Science and the Environment

A basic tenet in writings on occupational science is an emphasis on the environmental context of activity. Individuals are studied in purposeful, meaningful interaction with their environments, not as decontextualized beings.[2] Occupation is seen as action *on* the environment but requiring the interaction of an active human being with a particular environmental context. An important form of such interaction is with the physical-spatial world. We need to develop a vocabulary for describing the more immediate, more proximal environments in which we interact with objects in the physical-spatial world.

Bronfenbrenner and Crouter provide an example of a vocabulary describing environmental levels in Bronfenbrenner's[3] proposal for an ecological approach to the understanding of human social-emotional development. His approach provides a viewpoint and a vocabulary for describing environmental contexts at different levels. He uses the terms microsystem, mesosystem, exosystem, and macrosystem to define contexts ranging from the home environment to the cultural environment.

I mention Bronfenbrenner only as an example of defining larger and smaller environmental contexts. His viewpoint does have relevance to higher levels of occupation, but what he calls a microsystem includes, for example, the school environment, which is a large system in the physical-spatial world. The classification for the physical-spatial environment needs to include the most proximal environment, the chair on which you are sitting, the utensils on the table in front of you. Competency in the physical-spatial world requires action using these environmental artifacts that make up your immediate environment.

Two areas of research in psychology and neuropsychology are focusing on a more immediate environment. Classification has begun in the study of space and action systems theory. There have been many studies of how humans perceive and act in the spatial environment and how perceptions and actions are altered by cerebral lesions. As Ratcliff[4] noted, progress in understanding factors that limit performance has been hampered by the inclusion of various deficits in a general category of spatial orientation. Therefore, a number of researchers have begun to classify spatial functions on several different dimensions. For example, whereas Ratcliff[4] differentiates sensory analysis from perceptual integration, Semmes[5] et al. differentiate personal space from extrapersonal space. The differentiation between object-focused perception and environment-focused perception is widely accepted.[6,9] A classification developed by Kolb and Whishaw[10] combines some of these, and I like their classification because it describes spatial abilities in terms of action on the environment.

Kolb and Whishaw[10] have defined three levels of the spatial environment: body space, grasping space, and distal space. Body space includes perceptual factors, such as tactile localization, body knowledge, and unilateral neglect. Grasping space is the immediate, most proximal environment, defined as the physical space that is within arms' reach of the person. Distal space is that in which we move our bodies, the space into which we go. Distal space could be further divided into the space in which we move and the space we can know but not directly perceive, for example, route finding or map reading.

The three levels of spatial environment with which we directly interact have relevance to occupational science because the classification has been developed from studies of spatial dysfunction observed in people with brain damage. One patient's dysfunction is often only in distal space, as in a topographic disorder. Another patient might only demonstrate misreaching. Studies of disorders within each space and of inter-relations among the levels can help us better understand neural mechanisms of recovery and how therapy can impact recovery of occupational performance.

Body, grasping, and distal spatial environments also have relevance in studies of the development of a child. The motor, cognitive-perceptual, and motivational subsystems that guide activity in infancy occur primarily within grasping space. Spatial development appears to occur in the direction of increasing size of the environment.

Another area of research that is studying the physical environment is action systems research. Reed's associates[11, 12] defined such research as the study of actions as they unfold in the natural context. These researchers have studied common activities, such as mixing a cup of instant coffee and buttering a slice of bread; an important aspect of their study of such routine action skills is attention to what the environment affords. Actions performed in an activities of daily living (ADL) task are situated; that is, they make extensive use of the immediate environment and what it affords for action. These descriptive studies focus on the information processing aspects of the ADL tasks.

Reed's associates[11,12] make use of a multilevel coding system for describing disorganization in ADL activities in patients with brain injury. The ADL task is the goal; A2 actions are subroutines that accomplish subgoals and are, in turn, made up of A1 acts. The A1 acts are the smallest units of analysis and are possessing, relinquishing, moving, and altering the state of an object or, in occupational therapy terminology, grasping, releasing, transporting, and manipulating. The research methodologies being developed in action system research show promise for research in occupation.

When one considers the scope of occupational science and looks at the ends of the continuum of occupation in human life experiences, they seem distant. At the higher levels, concepts are illustrated by the valuing of time and resources, the relationship of work and leisure to health, happiness, and the quality of life, and how cultural differences in the customary round of activities of children shape their adult work habits. It is not immediately apparent how questions such as "What are the perceptual and motor antecedents of manipulating a pencil?" fit with such high level concepts.

The relationship is found in the systems approach conceptualized by the founders of occupational science, which governs the process of nesting small chunks of activity in larger contexts and supports occupational therapy's traditional activity analysis. A second commonality lies in the constructs about occupation that are integral to occupational science. Many aspects of occupation are the same whether investigating a person's work or a single action. Both occupations and the simple acts that make up occupations are most effective when they:

1. Have meaning for the individual
2. Are intrinsically motivated and fired by a drive for competence
3. Are self-initiated, active, a result of an act of the will

4. Are goal-directed, purposeful for the individual
5. Are the ordinary activity of everyday living

I believe that research in occupational science needs to address its full scope. To understand how a highly specific injury impacts on occupational function, molecular variables, and how they affect occupational behavior needs to be studied. At the same time, molar variables must be studied to understand the behavior itself and how it impacts on human life experiences. By embracing the full scope of occupation, the science developing at USC can provide a framework for unifying research and theory development in support of the practice of occupational therapy.

Discussion Questions

1. Henderson supports the use of a systems model for guiding research in occupational science because she believes it allows a broad and a detailed examination of occupational engagement within diverse environmental contexts. Do you agree with this point of view?
2. How does a systems approach fit with occupational therapy's traditional investment in activity analyses?
3. How has Henderson's application of a systems approach illuminated the inter-relationships between salient levels of the spatial environment during engagement in activity?

References

1. Clark, F, Parham, D, Carlson, M, Frank, G, Jackson, J, Pierce, D, Wolfe, R, and Zemke, R: Occupational science: Academic innovation in the service of occupational therapy. Am J Occup Ther 45:300–310, 1991.
2. Yerxa, EJ, Clark, F, Frank, G, Jackson, J, Parham, D, Pierce, D, Stein, C, and Zemke R: An introduction to occupational science, a foundation for occupational therapy in the 21st century. Occup Ther Health Care 6:1–17, 1990.
3. Bronfenbrenner, U, and Crouter, A: The evolution of environmental models in developmental research. In Mussen, P (ed): Handbook of Child Psychology. Wiley, New York, 1983.
4. Ratcliff, G: Disturbances of spatial orientation associated with cerebral lesions. In Potegal, M (ed): Spatial Abilities: Development and Physiological Foundations. Academic, New York, 1982.
5. Semmes, J, Weinstein, LG, and Teuber, HJ: Correlates of impaired orientation in personal and extra-personal space. Brain 86:742–772, 1963.
6. Elliot, J: Models of Psychological Space. Springer-Verlag, New York, 1987.
7. Benton, A: Visuo perceptual, visuo spatial and visuo constructive disorders. In Heilman, K, and Valenstein, E (eds): Clinical Neuropsychology (2nd ed). Oxford University Press, New York, 1985.
8. Trevarthen, C: Two mechanisms of vision in primates. Psychologische Forschung 31:299–337, 1968.
9. Mishkin, M, Ungerleider, L, and Macko, K: Object vision and spatial vision: Two cortical pathways. Trends in Neurosciences 6:414–417, 1983.
10. Kolb, B, and Whishaw, I: Fundamentals of Human Neuropsychology (3rd ed). W. H. Freeman, New York, 1990.

11. Mayer, N, Reed, E, Schartz, M, Montgomery, M, and Palmer, C: Buttering a hot cup of coffee: An approach to the study of errors of action in patients with brain damage. In Tupper, D, and Cicereno, K (eds): The Neuropsychology of Everyday Life: Assessment and Basic Competencies. Kluwer Academic, Boston, 1990.
12. Schwartz, MF, Reed, E, Montgomery, M, Palmer, C, and Mayer, N: The quantitative description of action disorganization after brain damage: A case study. Cognitive Neuropsychology 8:381, 1991.

by Linda L. Florey, MA, OTR, FAOTA

39

Valuing the Ordinary

Teilhard de Chardin was a French priest, scientist, and philosopher who began his work in the early part of the 20th century.[1] He might have had the newly emerging profession of occupational therapy in mind when he wrote, "What matters is not to do remarkable things, but to do ordinary things with the conviction that their value is enormous" (see endnote).

Occupational therapy has always celebrated the ordinary everyday activities that bind people to society. These activities have been labeled differently throughout history as functional or diversional activities; employment; activities of daily living; work, play, or leisure; and recently, occupations. Clark et al. have stated "We have come to call the ordinary and familiar things that people do everyday *occupations*, and we believe that humans are most true to their humanity when they are engaged in occupations."[2] There is a challenge to occupational therapy embedded in the Teilhardian quote, and that is that one must do the ordinary things with conviction of their value. Occupational therapy must value what it does.

When we, as occupational therapists, have wavered in our conviction of the importance of the ordinary activities in which we engage our patients, we have abandoned those activities subtly but surely. At one time, we nearly dropped play from our repertoire because we did not like being called "playladies." The worst case scenario for occupational therapy was articulated by Mary Reilly in a videotaped interview from the American Occupational Therapy Association (AOTA) archives at the University of Texas at Galveston. In discussing whether occupational therapy would be a part of the 21st century, Reilly said, "We won't be put out of business by any budget change or any malice from any other group or any kind of neglect on the part of society. It will be because we who are out practicing in the field fail to realize the enormous nature of the work that we do. Our failure to appreciate what we do for patients will be the cause of our disappearance." Reilly was describing a lack of conviction in valuing what we do and who we are.

As occupational therapists have abandoned different media or chunks of activities, they have been picked up by others. Whole professions have been constituted on what occupational therapy has discarded. We have dropped most of the creative arts from our practice, such as dance, art, music, and sports. Now we work with colleagues from the professions of dance therapy, art therapy, music therapy, and recreation therapy. The lesson is that engagement in activities has an intrinsic worth that contributes to productive living. If we drop our focus on engagement in activity and daily occupation, in all probability, another group will be constituted to carry out this important work with our patients.

One critical component within practice may be at risk for abandonment by occupational therapists. The critical component that is slipping from practice is the social and emotional development and behavior of children. In 1988, I was asked to contribute to a series of Nationally Speaking articles in the *American Journal of Occupational Therapy* focusing on specialty areas of practice in occupational therapy and the knowledge and skills needed to practice within them. The specialty areas under focus were gerontology, hand rehabilitation, management, home health, child psychiatry, and occupational therapy for infants, toddlers, and their families. I was asked to write the Nationally Speaking article on child psychiatry. After reviewing the literature in our field, I titled the article "Treating the Whole Child: Rhetoric or Reality?"[3] The title reflects my concern with the rich rhetoric in occupational therapy regarding treating the whole person and how that rhetoric is measured in practice as reflected in our journals and textbooks of the last 10 years. It was not surprising to me that there were few articles or chapters dealing specifically with children with emotional problems. What was surprising and distressing was that concerns for the social and emotional realm of all children may be slipping from pediatric practice.

Let me cite a few examples. In the pediatric sections of the 1983 and 1988 editions of the premier textbook in occupational therapy, blatant omissions existed in the social and emotional area of development. One author[4,5] developed a chart that identified developmental expectations from infancy through 12 years, including general reflex development, sensory development, body scheme, equilibrium, bilateral integration, visual perception, eye-hand coordination, and language. Milestones of children's relationships with others were not included. However, the author stated, "the chart is intended to promote continual awareness in the mind of the therapist of all the goals established for each child, and their interrelationship."[6] If the milestones of social and emotional development are not listed, how can they become an arena for intervention by occupational therapy? They cannot, and therefore they do not become a focus for treatment.

In another chapter of this basic occupational therapy text, a comprehensive pediatric evaluation tool was presented. Its categories included neuromuscular reflex and gross motor development; physical findings related to posture, muscle tone, range of motion, and adaptive appliances; activities of daily living, including feeding, dressing, grooming, and written communication; upper extremity functional activities; and sensory integration. Again, how children relate to others was not included. The absence of a social and emotional focus was particularly evident in a discussion of abused children. Although the author advocated that these children receive a complete evaluation, the recommended assessment for children younger than 4 years included only neurodevelopmental reflex maturation levels, gross motor development, fine motor development, activities of daily living skills development, and sensory integration.[9,10] There was no focus on social and emotional concerns for children who have suffered at the hands of another. This is not only an incomplete assessment for abused or neglected children, it is an incomplete assessment for *any* child.

In the school system, children with emotional disturbances form the fourth largest handicapped group,[11] although one fifth of the full-time work force in occupational therapy work within the school system.[12] Few of these children are seen by occupational therapists. The Robert Wood Johnson Foundation published findings of a 5-year collaborative study of children with special needs in five large metropolitan school districts throughout the country.[13] The overall purpose of the study was to identify the extent to which the procedural guarantees of Public Law 94-142 were in place. With regard to therapeutic services, the investigators concluded that "nearly half of all children in special education receive speech or hearing therapy, whereas physical and occupational therapy are concentrated on children with physical, vision/hearing, or health impairments, as well as on the mentally retarded."[14] This is not surprising. The AOTA guidelines for occupational therapy in the school system recommend that if the results of evaluation indicate possible deficits in the psychosocial area, the student be referred to the appropriate services. This suggests that we have no role in the psychosocial domain. Colleagues working in the school propose that occupational therapists are concerned with the psychosocial area but only at a sensory motor processing level. Sensory motor processing is viewed as a substratum of the child's social, emotional, and psychological state.[16] This theme is evident in the AOTA role and function paper for early childhood intervention. Occupational therapy was described as the use of purposeful activities to promote normal development and coping behaviors. It also stated that "treatment stems from a scientifically based neurophysiological framework."[17] Clearly sensory-motor, neurodevelopmental, and neurophysiological frameworks are valuable bases for practice. When used alone, these frameworks are too narrowly focused to support the claim that we treat the whole child or that we engage the child in purposeful, productive activity. The interactive and engagement processes in human behavior use an additional knowledge base.

All is not doom and gloom. Recent textbooks in pediatrics include the social and emotional concerns of children, and past texts and articles have paid attention to this area.[18,19] However, the knowledge base in pediatric occupational therapy is weighted far too heavily in the areas of neuromotor and sensory motor concerns. The emphasis placed on these systems has overwhelmed and overshadowed the social and emotional realms of behavior.[3] Occupational therapy cannot ignore, forget, or pay lip service to this area. As occupational therapists, we know that purposeful activity is done within a social context. We know that discourse and negotiation are embedded within the commonplace occupations of play, work, leisure, and self-care. We must always pay attention to relatedness and relationships because they are part and parcel of everyday activities and events. Engagement in occupation may require sharing, cooperating, competing, talking, listening, agreeing, or disagreeing and may evoke laughter, tears, anger, frustration, or joy.

We must imbue the social emotional realm with value, because we have never promoted decontextualized learning nor the development of splinter skills. We must give equal time to this "softer," more ambiguous domain of behavior in our practice, education, and research. We have always prided ourselves on treating the whole person within a context that has relevance and meaning to our patients.

Children with medical and educational diagnoses also have problems in the ordinary activities of daily life. Children with sensory integrative dysfunction, neurological impairments, musculoskeletal dysfunction, conduct disorders, and attention deficit disorders also have "cub scout disorders," "playmate disorders," "kicking the soccer ball disorders," "getting dressed in gym class disorders," "best friend disorders," "no one to eat lunch with disorders." These are the important disorders. These are the ones with which we must ultimately concern ourselves. We must not lose our commitment to ordinary activities nor to the interpersonal context in which they occur. Their value to our patients is enormous.

Discussion Questions

1. Florey, in quoting Mary Reilly, asserts that the greatest threat to occupational therapy comes not from outside sources, but from our own failure to value the "enormous nature of the work" that we do. How might educational programs better instill in students an appreciation of the enormous nature of occupational therapy that can withstand the power of an often philosophically incompatible medical culture?
2. Can, and if so how, pediatric treatment approaches currently predominating in occupational therapy be adapted in the interest of addressing children's social and emotional development in an effective and substantive manner?

Endnote

The work of Teilhard de Chardin has been translated from French to English and quotations vary according to translations. Alison M. Williams, Hon Secretary to the Teilhard Centre in London, was not able to find the exact source of this quotation, which is attributed to de Chardin. She writes on May 29, 1991, "You would find somewhat similar thinking in 'Writings in Time of War' pp. 42–3 and in 'The Divine Milieu' pp. 38–49 and 45–6, but not with the incisiveness of your quotation."

References

1. Leroy, P: Teilhard de Chardin: The man. In Teilhard de Chardin, The Divine Milieu (William Collins Sons, London, Trans). Harper & Row, New York, 1960, pp 13–42. (Original work published 1957.)
2. Clark, F, Parham, D, Carlson, M, Frank, G, Jackson, J, Pierce, D, Wolfe, R, and Zemke, R: Occupational science: Academic innovation in the services of occupational therapy's future. Am J Occup Ther 45:300, 1990.
3. Florey, L: Treating the whole child: Rhetoric or reality? Am J Occup Ther 43(6): 365, 1989.
4. Kauffman, N: Occupational therapy with children—The school setting. In Hopkins, HL, and Smith, HD (eds): Willard and Spackman's Occupational Therapy (6th ed). J. B. Lippincott, Philadelphia, 1983, pp 683–719.
5. Kauffman, N: Occupational therapy in the school system. In Hopkins, HL, and Smith, HD (eds): Willard and Spackman's Occupational Therapy (7th ed). J. B. Lippincott, Philadelphia, 1988, 707–714.
6. Kauffman, pp 714–720.
7. Ramm, P: Pediatric occupational therapy. In Hopkins, HL, and Smith, HD (eds): Willard and Spackman's Occupational Therapy (6th ed). J. B. Lippincott, Philadelphia, 1983b, pp 573–587.
8. Ramm, P: Pediatric occupational therapy. In Hopkins, HL, and Smith, HD (eds): Willard and Spackman's occupational therapy (7th ed). J. B. Lippincott, Philadelphia, 1988b, pp 601–627.

9. Ramm, P: The occupational process in specific pediatric conditions. In Hopkins, HL, and Smith, HD (eds): Willard and Spackman's Occupational Therapy (6th ed). J. B. Lippincott, Philadelphia, 1983a, pp 589–641.

10. Ramm, P: The occupational process in specific pediatric conditions. In Hopkins, HL, and Smith, HD (eds): Willard and Spackman's Occupational Therapy (7th ed). J. B. Lippincott, Philadelphia, 1988a, pp 589–641.

11. U.S. Department of Education: Ninth annual report to Congress on implementation of Public Law 94–142: The education of All Handicapped Children Act. Government Printing Office, Washington, D.C., 1987.

12. American Occupational Therapy Association. Occupational Therapy Manpower: A Plan for Progress. AOTA, Rockville, MD, 1985.

13. Robert Wood Johnson Foundation. Serving Handicapped Children: A Special Report (No. 1). RWJF, Princeton, NJ, 1988.

14. RWJF, p 4.

15. American Occupational Therapy Association. Guidelines for Occupational Therapy Services in School Systems. AOTA, Rockville, MD, 1986a.

16. Royeen, C, and Marsh, D: Promoting occupational therapy in the schools. Am J Occup Ther 42:713–717, 1988.

17. American Occupational Therapy Association. Roles and functions of occupational therapy in early childhood intervention. Am J Occup Ther 40:835, 1985.

18. Dunn, W (ed): Pediatric Occupational Therapy. Slack, New Jersey, 1991.

19. Pratt, P, and Allen, A (eds): Occupational Therapy for Children (2nd ed). C. V. Mosby, St. Louis, 1989.

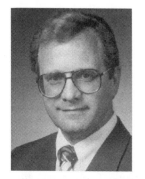

by Charles H. Christiansen,
EdD, OTR, OT(C), FAOTA

40

Three Perspectives on Balance in Occupation

Social Zeitgebers

Balance as the Relationship Among Life Tasks

Summary

One of the most widely cited philosophical beliefs in occupational therapy is that a balance of occupations is beneficial to health and well-being. Despite the widespread acceptance of this tenet, the meaning of balance has not been satisfactorily defined in an operational sense, nor has its validity been systematically examined. Recognizing the need to understand better the dimensions that underlie and are affected by patterns of daily time use, Clark et al.[1] identified "an exploration of what constitutes a healthful balance of work, rest, and leisure within the daily round of occupations" as an example of a potential research topic that would be appropriate for the emerging discipline of occupational science.

In this paper, I first introduce the origin of the belief in occupational therapy in occupational balance and trace its significant developments in the last 25 years. Then I examine current views of balance in light of studies of time use from the social sciences literature, which raise questions about its legitimacy. Finally, I identify concepts from biology and psychology that may hold promise as alternatives for considering balance as a characteristic of activity patterns.

History of the Concept of Balance in Occupational Therapy

Origins of the Concept of Balance

The neuropsychiatrist Adolph Meyer[2] was among the first to speculate that the organization of daily activity should be a consideration when planning occupational therapy. Reed[3] noted that other early proponents of occupational therapy (e.g., Sawyer,[4] Hall[5]) had emphasized that there was an optimal range of activity engagement for each individual; too little or too much could be problematic. Meyer[2] emphasized a view of human beings as deriving meaning and maintaining well-being through their organization of time. He identified four areas of daily activity—work, play, rest, and sleep—as interacting to determine overall adaptation to the requirements of daily life. His paper suggested that through the opportunities for engagement provided by the normal routines of living, especially work, the individual should be able to fulfill personal interests and meet needs for physical and psychological well-being.

This philosophy formed the basis for the habit training program developed by Eleanor Clarke Slagle at Rochester State Hospital in 1901. In this program, the lives of mental patients were organized into 24-hour schedules, during which caregivers attempted, through structured and graded tasks, to entrain daily rhythms of occupation, which included work, rest, and play.[6] The philosophy underlying the program, according to Slagle,[7] was that:

> for the most part, our lives are made up of habit reactions. Occupation used remedially serves to overcome some habits, to modify others, and construct new

ones to the end that habit reaction will be favorable to the restoration and maintenance of health.

Mary Reilly[8] embraced the concept of incorporating a daily pattern of work, play, and rest in the lives of mental patients at the Neuropsychiatric Institute (NPI) at UCLA during the 1960s. Her treatment program, based on principles of the occupational behavior model, was designed to restore a patient's life skills within a balanced pattern of daily living. Drawing its definitions from economics, the NPI program grouped daily occupation into *existence* (tasks related to personal maintenance, including eating, sleeping, and hygiene), *subsistence* (working for an income), and *choosing time* (life space left over or discretionary time for the individual to choose recreation and leisure). Reilly emphasized differing functions of leisure and recreation and the relationship of each to work. Recreation was viewed as relaxation in preparation for work; whereas leisure, she suggested, was a period made possible as a result of a satisfying work experience.

Because of the centrality of work in defining the purposes of recreation and leisure, work was posited to be the integrating focus of rehabilitation within the occupational behavior framework. Shannon[9] suggested that occupational therapy prepares the individual for work through recreation or play and serves recreation and play needs. He described a psychiatric program for soldiers that was based on several assumptions surrounding the work-play model, one of which was that a balance in the work-play relationship must be maintained for positive mental health.

More Recent Concepts of Balance

Influenced by the writings of Meyer, Slagle, and Reilly, Kielhofner[10] proposed a conceptual model of occupational therapy he labeled *temporal adaptation*. The central premise underlying temporal adaptation is that one's use and organization of time is an indicator of successful adjustment to the demands of living. Kielhofner asserted that there is a natural temporal order to daily living organized around the life space activities of self-maintenance, work, and play. He equated health with a proper balance of the life spaces that is satisfying and appropriate to an individual's roles. This implied that from a clinical standpoint, the occupational patterns that constituted balance would be variable from one person to the next. Kielhofner noted that balance would represent more than a certain amount of work, play, or rest. Rather, balance would reflect a dynamic interdependence of these life spaces and their relationship to internal values, interests, and goals and to the external demands of the environment (see endnote 1).

More recently, Kielhofner and Burke[11] incorporated concepts from temporal adaptation within the habituation subsystem of the model of human occupation. As guides to performance, this model viewed habits as images guiding the routine and typical ways in which an individual performs the tasks and roles of daily living by organizing skills into larger purposeful routines. One index of the adaptive value of a habit, according to Kielhofner and Burke, is its degree of organization. This was defined as the extent to which time is used by the individual in a manner that supports competent performance in a variety of settings and roles and provides for a balance of activity. The authors noted that it was *not* doing the same thing every day that reflected organization in habits, but an individual's ability to respond to a range of typical demands that might be encountered during daily role performance.

Addressing the concept of balance and rhythm in their model, Kielhofner and Burke[11] proposed that habits organize behavior to enable needs for rest, recreation, self-maintenance, and productivity to be met. A person's failure to allocate discretionary time, they suggested, would reflect a disorganized habitual subsystem. Kielhofner and Burke speculated that meeting needs over time was more important than having a daily pattern of engagement in specific categories of occupation.

A closely related concept within the human occupation model is *role balance*, which is defined as an integration of an optimal number of appropriate roles into one's life. A balance of roles, as suggested by Kielhofner and Burke, provides some rhythm and change between different modes of doing. Role balance exists when roles are not conflicting or competing for time and when there are adequate roles to structure one's use of time. Role loss, which occurs naturally during the life trajectory (ontogenesis), can result in role imbalance. The relationship between role balance and balance in occupation is not addressed in writings about the model of human occupation. Viewed as a whole, the human occupation model indicates that a balanced pattern of daily living takes into account individual interests and abilities and tailors daily events to age, sex, and occupational role; it is guided by an understanding of the objectives of each subdivision of daily life space.

Patterns of Time Use and Individual Characteristics

How people organize and perceive time has been recognized as an important dimension in understanding human behavior. Nearly 2 decades ago, Wesman[12] suggested that research supported the view that "characteristic ways of experiencing and utilizing time vary greatly among individuals along dimensions that can be assessed and measured, and that these differences are meaningfully related to personality characteristics." Since that time, literature has shown that time perspective and structure are related to a host of individual attributes, which besides personality traits, include such psychological dimensions as motivation, purpose, and self-esteem.[13-14] Demographic and sociocultural factors also are important, so age, employment, ethnicity, marital status, and sex are related to perspectives about time and how it is organized.[5,15] Finally, studies have suggested a relationship between perceptions and use of time and psychological dysfunction.[16,17]

Balance as Perceived or Actual Time Use

We live in a temporal world where time and activity form the sides of a rolling coin. Philosophers, sociologists, and phenomenologists, including Ricouer,[18] Young,[19] and Kerby,[20] agree that we experience time not as so many minutes, days, and years, but as activities in which we have participated and that have meaning. Times gone by have meaning only in terms of recollected experiences, and our perceptions of the past are constantly revised as we accumulate new experiences. Who we are is very much a product of what we have done, what we expect to do, and how we spend our time. To consider activity patterns is to contemplate how we allocate or "budget" time.

In occupational therapy, the concept of balance in occupation has most often been viewed from a time budget perspective. This concept springs from a belief that health and well-being are related to a life-style where time spent in productive, recreational, and rest activities is relatively equivalent. Although Kielhofner[10] observed that balance "refers to more than just so much work, play, and rest," the only study of balance and well-being found within the occupational therapy literature adopted a time-use perspective.

In this study, Marino-Schorn[21] sought to determine whether the amount of time spent by retired subjects in work, rest or sleep, and leisure was related to well-being. Balance was operationalized as the extent to which hours of time spent within these three categories were equal. Although the method of statistical analysis was not explicit, the investigator reported that subjects who spend most of their time in rest or sleep and leisure activities with very little work had lower morale as measured by the *Philadelphia Geriatric Center Morale Scale*. The subjects who had low morale averaged 3 hours of work, 10 hours of leisure, and 11 hours of rest or sleep and other activity per day. In comparison, subjects who had higher morale averaged 6 hours of work, 8 hours of leisure, and 9 hours of rest, sleep, and "other" activity. The author concluded that the greater "balance" among subjects in the group composed of those with higher morale scores confirmed the hypothesis that balance in time use across the categories of work, leisure, and rest or sleep was related to morale. However, if equivalence in the amount of time allocated to different categories of engagement is of theoretical importance, then one would expect to find a negative correlation between the extent of deviation from a measure of equivalence and some measure of well-being. This was not reported.

One study showed wide disparity among subjects as to the classification of a given activity. For example, yard work, general shopping, and sewing were each classified as work activities by some subjects and leisure by others. Because data on time use were analyzed according to the subject's classification, the balance hypothesis cannot be explained on the basis of *how* people spent their time; the classification of activities was not uniform across subjects.

Setting these concerns aside for the moment, one must ask whether it is plausible that allocating equivalent amounts of time to activity categories can actually explain increased well-being. Certainly, it can be argued that the meaning, impact, or benefit of an activity is not always proportionate to the time spent on it. Compare, for example, watching a 20-minute sunset at a scenic spot on the Pacific coast and having 20 minutes elapse in a dental chair (with or without earphones and a television screen). For most people, the two periods, although equivalent in length, would have a different impact.

Is it possible then that how people *perceive* their distribution of time use is important to their well-being? One study would suggest that this is so. Seleen[22] investigated the degree of perceived congruence between the actual and desired time allocated to 10 categories of activity in a sample of 205 older adults. Subjects expressed most dissatisfaction with time use related to sleep and personal care, although 69% were satisfied with their overall pattern of time use. Perceived discrepancies between desired and actual time use were inversely related to life satisfaction.

Unfortunately, the few studies completed to date fall considerably short of providing increased theoretical insight into *how* the perceived and actual use of time may be related to health and well-being. A systematic inquiry into the meaning of occupational balance as time use would begin with an examination of how people typically organize their days.

General Patterns of Time Use

Because time is a universal measure having ratio scale properties, comparison among studies is easier. Because we know that each day has 24 hours, we can make reasonable inferences about the amount of time allocated for some categories of activity by knowing how much is given to others. Thus, as a person spends more time sleeping, for example, we know that the time available for other activities is reduced.

Much of the current information on time use has been provided by consumer research, although gerontologic and leisure-related studies during the past 2 decades also have made useful contributions to our general understanding of how people organize their lives. Unfortunately, the lack of consistent approaches to classifying activities has made detailed comparisons among these various studies difficult. However, one approach that permits cross-study comparisons involves distinguishing between *obligatory* activities (such as work and self-care) and *discretionary* activities (typically classified as leisure).

Using this classification approach, a summary of research on time use seen in Figure 40-1 suggests that on average, for adults in the United States, approximately 30% of a typical 24-hour day is spent sleeping, 10% is allocated to self-care activities (including eating), and another 10% is allocated to instrumental activities of daily living such as cooking, laundry, housecleaning, and marketing. For those who are employed, approximately 25% of daily time is spent on actual

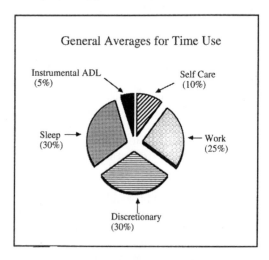

Figure 40–1. Approximate average percentages on a 24-hour day, spent in various categories of occupation for employed adults in the United States (based on time use data from several studies).

work time (excluding breaks). Thus, for a typically employed adult, nearly 60% of the *waking* day is devoted to obligatory or required activities, including employment. This proportion of obligatory activity also has been found for adolescents.[23]

These general patterns of time allocation for subjects in the United States are consistent with data collected in other countries. Information on Swedish subjects reported by Sjoberg and Magneberg,[24] and analyses of time use among Australians by Mercer[25] and Germans by Baltes et al.[26] show remarkably similar proportions of time allocation for obligatory and discretionary categories of time use. This also was true, as well in more specific activities, such as those devoted to self-care and household maintenance.

Frequency Versus Duration of Activity

While the classification of time use into discretionary and obligatory categories is useful for determining general patterns of activity, it is less practical as a guide to what people specifically do during their waking hours it also does not provide information on the level or intensity of activity. Studies have shown that the frequency of activities performed during any given time segment varies across and within subjects. Consequently, caution should be used when generalizing time use from frequency data.

For example, although Baltes[26] and colleagues found a 2:1 ratio between the frequency of obligatory and leisure activities, the corresponding ratio for *duration* of time spent in those categories was only 1.2:1. The phrase "doing things in a leisurely way" has empirical relevance because data show that discretionary tasks, which would include leisure pursuits, tend to be undertaken for longer periods when compared with obligatory activities. This relationship also is illustrated by the finding that people who report engaging in more obligatory activities also engage in a greater number of discretionary activities. This suggests that active people tend to be busy in all aspects of their lives, not just in a single category.

Stones and Kozma[27–28] have studied the possibility that there is a propensity or latent tendency for some people to be active, just as there may be a propensity for some people to be happy. They question traditional views in social gerontology, which suggest that happiness is a function of activity, speculating that the propensity to be happy is independent of the latent tendency to be active. They have found that activity and happiness are characteristics of individuals that remain stable and are moderately overlapping but not bonded in coexistence as suggested by the disengagement and activity theories.

Influences on Time Use

Besides the propensity to be active, which influences the frequency of activity, what else has been learned about influences on how people spend their days? Despite conventional beliefs to the contrary, data suggest that the region of the country in which one lives, the time of the year, and the climate do not seem to influence patterns of time use.[29] However, studies have shown a correspondence between physical well-being and patterns of time allocation. For example, Moss[30] and Lawton studied the time budgets of four groups of older people who were living in various settings and required differing levels of support. As might be expected, the groups who were more functionally independent spent more time away from home, less time in personal and sick care, and more time in travel, shopping, housework, and cooking. The overall proportion of the waking day spent in obligatory activities among these groups ranged from 18% for independent residents to 21% for impaired residents living in the community. The only major difference found between the groups in their discretionary behavior was the higher level of inactivity (rest and relaxation) among those impaired. Despite these differences in activity during waking hours, the average time spent sleeping was the same for both groups.[31]

Other studies of the influence of impairment on time use have reported similar findings. For example, in a study of the actual and perceived differences in activity patterns of men with and without disabilities, Brown[32] found that while patterns of activity were similar, there was greater diversity and frequency in the activities of the able-bodied group. Other studies have confirmed that increasing disability is related to activity patterns characterized by diminished diversity and frequency and slower tempo, with greater proportions of time spent on personal care and fewer activities outside the home (e.g., Brown & Gordon,[33] and Stenager, Knudsen, and Jensen[34]).

Because activity provides a context for socialization, its frequency and location have implications for the acquisition of rules, skills, and competencies necessary for role development and social maturation. One recent study found that the number of different activities and the frequency of activities in the home were related to the size of the social networks of adults with severe developmental disabilities.[35] Studies of children with disabilities have shown that their activity patterns are impoverished compared with those of able-bodied peers with respect to characteristics that have a positive impact on the development of socialization skills.[33,36]

Collectively, studies of time use have suggested that there are remarkable similarities in the manner in which people allocate time to discretionary and obligatory activities. When variations in general patterns of time use have been found, these differences seem to be related to role differences or diminished functional ability.

A recent study by Bird and Fremont[37] is relevant. They sought to understand why women live longer than men but experience more morbidity than men during their lives. They hypothesized that social role differences explain this paradox and compared time spent by men and women in various role-related activities, such as paid work, housework, child care, helping others, sleep, and active and passive leisure. Relationships between time spent in these activities and self-rated health and other demographic variables were examined. Among many interesting findings was the observation that men and women *do not* differ in the amount of sleep or in the time allocated to passive leisure activities. However, the researchers found important differences in the amount of time, on average, spent by men and women in paid work and housework. Men spent twice as much time in paid employment, whereas women spent three and one-half times as many hours per week in household labor than men. While paid employment is consistently found to be related positively to improved health and well-being (see also Ray and Heppe[38] and Gregory[39]), household labor has been found to be associated negatively with health. Aside from its provocative findings regarding the association between various specific activities and rated health, this study is notable for its association of time use with social roles and its view of activity patterns as being influenced significantly by role expectations.

Perceived Versus Actual Time Structure

Another important dimension of time use is the extent to which individuals *perceive* their daily activity to be structured and purposeful.[13] The concept of perceived time structure emanated from studies of groups whose typical pattern of daily activity had been disrupted—people who were unemployed. It has been suggested that one reason for the remarkable consistency of time use patterns across groups of adults can be explained by the time structure imposed by employment and the daily routines into which we are socialized during childhood. It seems reasonable to assume that these structures are learned and become routine in the socialization process embedded within the daily lives of working families.

Jahoda[40] suggested that regular activity and the imposition of time structures are among five categories of experience that have become psychological requirements in modern life and that unemployed people must meet these regular activity and time structure needs in other ways, or diminished well-being will result. Research has shown that unemployed people often have difficulty filling their days and may spend long periods sitting, sleeping, or watching television.[41,42] These deficits in the perceived use of time may be linked to a lack of purpose and a reduced structure in daily activities.

Feather and Bond[43] found that an unemployed group had lower time structure scores than an employed group on a *Time Structure Questionnaire*, which they developed to measure perceptions of structure and purpose in everyday life. They found that diminished time structure was related to lower self-esteem and higher levels of depression. The factor structure derived from analysis of their 26-item measure suggests that sense of purpose, structure, routine, present orientation, effective organization, and persistence are dimensions of perceived time use. These factors correlated with various dimensions of subjective well-being, including purpose in life, self-esteem, neuroticism, optimism, and reported health.

On the basis of their work over several years, Bond and Feather[13] concluded that time structure is related to role demands and personality variables. They speculated that when role changes occur during the lifespan, there are accompanying changes in perceived time structure and in sense of purpose. Consequently, individuals must accommodate these changes with the development or acquisition of new roles or interests that provide purpose and a framework for structuring time. This is similar to the notions expressed by Kielhofner and Burke[11] when describing role balance, which was addressed previously.

Chonobiological Balance

Routines

Thus far, we have reviewed studies that have provided information about how people use time characteristically and how their perceptions of the structure and purpose of time use are related to well-being. One dimension of time use identified by Bond and Feather is the extent to which daily activities fall into a structured routine. A routine, they write, "has a stability about it that extends over time and pertains to a particular set of activities within a defined situation."[44] They suggest that the imposition of an orderly structure on daily activities may have healthful consequences.

To the extent that the term "routine" implies regular and recurring patterns of time use, the concept of activity rhythms comes to mind. It is clear that Adolph Meyer held the view that the beneficial aspects of occupation were related to recurring patterns of time use, or rhythms, as suggested in the following excerpt:

> The whole of human organization has its shape in a kind of rhythm. It is not enough that our hearts should beat in a useful rhythm, always kept up to a standard at which it can meet rest as well as wholesome strain without upset. There are many other rhythms which we must be attuned to: the larger rhythms of night and day, of sleep and waking hours, of hunger and its gratification, and finally the big four—work and play and rest and sleep, which our organism must be able to balance even under difficulty.[45]

The temporal order in which Meyer identified work, play, rest, and sleep as important categories of activity suggests that he recognized a correspondence between the time of day and the nature of the activities that tend to predominate during those periods in human beings. When discussing their study of the daily lives of older adults in Germany, Baltes[26] and colleagues observed a clear association between the type of activity and the time of day. In their subjects, work and self-maintenance activities tended to predominate in the morning and early afternoon, whereas leisure and restful activities tended to be associated temporally with late afternoon and evening period. Similar activity rhythms have been found in studies of higher order social primates, such as mountain gorillas.[46]

Some empirical support for the benefits of rhythm in the everyday activity of humans can be found in the literature. A study of bereavement among 87 widows and widowers who had recently lost their spouses examined social patterns in the context of daily routines.[47] Among their findings was the observation that the presence of emotional distress was associated with a decrease in the number of *regular* activities experienced each day. The investigators realized that a possible confound existed between cause and effect in this study, but they remained convinced that regular routines were important in maintaining mental health in the population studied. They hypothesized that routine daily activities play an important role in synchronizing biologic rhythms. To understand fully the implications of this hypothesis requires a brief review of recent developments in chronobiology.

Biological Rhythms

It has been well established that the behavior of humans and other animals is influenced significantly by biological rhythms. Figure 40-2 illustrates hypothesized influences on biological rhythms. It is known that there are many physiological rhythms, and these are classified according to the duration of their cycles. Perhaps the best known are those following an approximate 24-hour period of oscillation, which were first termed circadian rhythms by Franz Halberg[48] and his colleagues. An important example of a circadian rhythm is the sleep-wake or rest-activity cycle. Among other biological rhythms are those evident in blood pressure, core body temperature, hormonal fluctuations, and sexual activity. Cycles with a duration of less than 24 hours (frequency greater than one in 24) are termed *ultradian* rhythms, while those with longer periods (and lower frequency) are known as *infradian* rhythms.

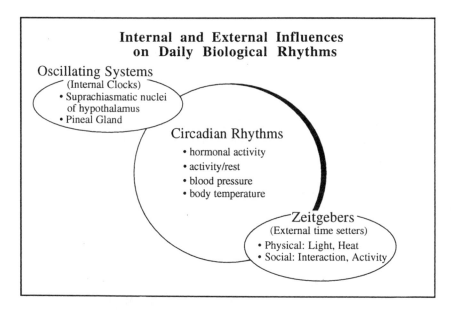

Figure 40–2. Hypothesized influences on circadian rhythms.

Although the mechanisms that govern the timing of biological rhythms are not completely understood, it is generally accepted that many internal clocks (known as oscillating systems) may operate at the cellular level to maintain the regular cycles of physiological events. Currently, various structures in the central nervous system are suspected of serving important functions in these timing mechanisms, including the pineal gland, which secretes the light-influenced hormone melatonin, and the suprachiasmatic nuclei of the hypothalamus (e.g., Wever[49]).

Zeitgebers

Our internal clocks have natural free-running rhythms that are highly consistent when they are not influenced by outside factors. Because we are normally exposed to environmental factors, such as light and temperature changes, our internal clocks are affected, with the result that they entrain or synchronize themselves according to these external factors. The term "zeitgeber" (meaning *time giver*) has been given to these outside influences on our internal clocks; zeitgebers are classified as physical or social.[50] Daylight and noise are examples of physical zeitgebers, while mealtimes and bedtime rituals constitute social zeitgebers, all of which influence circadian rhythms by entraining them to a 24-hour day. It is now well accepted that an ongoing interaction with the physical and social environment is an important factor in maintaining synchrony between rhythms within the individual and between the individual and the environment.[50]

In humans, the circadian sleep-wake or rest-activity rhythm has a free-running cycle of approximately 25 hours. This means that under ordinary circumstances, natural zeitgebers act to set our internal clocks back nearly an hour each day in order to be in phase with the diurnal clock. Some studies have been conducted to determine what occurs when the influences of natural zeitgebers are removed. In some of these studies, subjects have been isolated from all environmental time cues, including noise, which would ordinarily entrain their sleep cycle to correspond to a 24-hour day. Under such free-running conditions, subjects shift progressively to later retiring and awakening hours. Since the free-running cycle is 25 hours, they tend to go to sleep about an hour later in each 24-hour period.

In other isolation studies, artificial zeitgebers (such as bright light) were manipulated experimentally to determine the extent to which rhythms can be entrained to different cycles and to ascertain what occurs when cycles are out of phase or desynchronized with the environment. Desynchronization is experienced commonly in everyday life by airline workers and passengers who cross time zones and by shiftworkers. In chronobiology, this type of desynchronization is technically called a phase shift. Studies of the effects of phase shifts have provided some insights into individual differences in circadian rhythms, the effects of desynchronization, and the influences of zeitgebers.

Desynchronization

When physiologic rhythms are not in synchrony with the environment, sleep displacement occurs. In other words, activity takes place when the individual would normally be sleeping. This desynchronization often results in various types of symptoms that affect alertness and general feelings of well-being. Studies of shift workers, who must place themselves in situations where performance requirements are desynchronized with their circadian rhythms, have shown that total sleep time is decreased and that performance on various dimensions is decreased. For example, Folkard[51] et al. showed that under controlled laboratory conditions, performance efficiency on tasks of logical reasoning and reaction time followed a 21-hour (ultradian) cycle, even though physiological rhythms remained entrained to a 24-hour period. In one study, subjects who experienced internal desynchronization were more likely to score higher on measures of neuroticism and to complain of more somatic problems than did other subjects.[52] There also is growing evidence that certain mental conditions, including bipolar depression and seasonal affective disorder, are associated with desynchronized internal rhythms in physiological function.[53,54]

Diurnal Type: Morningness and Eveningness

One finding from phase shift studies is that some people have endogenous or free-running circadian rest-activity cycles that are significantly shorter or longer than average. Since the 1930s, it has been known that people can be distinguished by their tendency to function better either earlier or later in the waking period; people with these diurnal characteristics have been referred to as morning and evening types.[55] Numerous studies have provided evidence of the validity of these diurnal types (e.g., Kerkhoff[56]).

Various self-report questionnaires have been developed to measure diurnal types, with the intent of selecting people who would be more suitable for shift work (e.g., Smith, Reilly, and Midkiff[57]). It is presumed that because of the characteristics of their circadian rhythms, morning types are better able to adjust to phase shifts than are evening types. Subsequent studies have confirmed that there are measurable physiological, psychological, and performance-related differences related to time of day between these two types (see Kerkhoff[56]).

For example, Thayer, Takahashi, and Pauli[58,59] found that differences in the energetic arousal states of the two types explained up to one third of the variation in optimism, problem perception, self-esteem, and interpersonal affect on an hour-by-hour basis. The implications of these findings for interpersonal relationships have been pursued by Hoskins[60] and Adams and Cromwell,[61] who have studied the extent to which differences in diurnal rest and activity cycles influence conflict and stress in married couples. Findings from these studies show clearly that differences in diurnal types affect the overall quality of interaction between spouses.

Given what we know about diurnal types and performance, it is clear that some differences in activity patterns between individuals can be explained by differences in their circadian activity-rest cycles. These differences would likely be revealed, not in the duration or frequency of activities, but in the times at which they were performed. Although apparently few studies have examined diurnal type and performance in everyday activities, it would be interesting to note if circadian rhythms explain any of the variation in performance among students in evening classes or patients in early morning therapy programs.

Social Zeitgebers

Recall that zeitgebers are the mechanisms that keep our internal clocks synchronized with the 24-hour day. The importance of social factors, such as human interaction and daily routines, represents an important class of zeitgebers that is gaining renewed attention in the literature. These social zeitgebers, which occur as part of the regular patterns of behavior that characterize daily life, are ubiquitous and begin almost at birth when parents attempt to synchronize the sleep and activity rhythms of infants to the domestic routine of the family. The plausibility of social routines (such as meals or daily rituals) influencing physiological rhythms is made more probable when one considers the body of evidence from studies of animals. These show that social factors result in the synchronization, desynchronization, and disruption of biological rhythms in a wide range of organisms (e.g., Regal and Connolly[62]).

Some theorists believe that the function of social routines as synchronizers of internal clocks is so important that it may explain some types of depression. For example, Hofer[63] postulated that bereavement may be the result of desynchronization of internal clocks that results from an interruption in the normal daily routine when one experiences a significant loss. Hofer's hypothesis suggests that interruption reduces exposure to social zeitgebers and diminishes their effectiveness as synchronizers of the internal oscillators. The specific mechanisms through which internal oscillators are synchronized through daily routine are not known. These mechanisms were first hypothesized, however, when laboratory studies showed that physical zeitgebers, such as light and noise, could not alone account for observed changes in the circadian rhythms of subjects under study.

Individuals living together tend to adopt patterns of behavior that reflect a compromise between their natural rhythms. Significant life events, such as divorce or the birth of a child, disrupt daily patterns and influence the entrainment of biological rhythms. For example, Cartwright[64] showed that half of a group of women coping with divorce proceedings manifested symptoms of phase-relation disorders, such as disturbed rapid eye movement sleep. The extent of disruption was thought to be related to the degree to which a particular activity routine had been established as a social zeitgeber.

Ehlers, Frank, and Kupfer[65] have proposed a theoretical model that describes a chain of events leading from a change in social zeitgebers and a consequent instability of biological rhythms to a condition of pathological entrainment characterized by major depression. This model (Figure 40-3) is seen as sufficiently plausible to warrant the development of an instrument to measure recurring social rhythms. Consequently, the *Social Rhythm Metric* has been developed by researchers in Pittsburgh and Chicago.[66] This instrument is designed to assign a numeric value to the average regularity with which 15 daily activities, ranging from having breakfast to going to bed, occur within a one-week interval, and offers a satisfactory approach to quantifying the rhythmic character of daily activities.

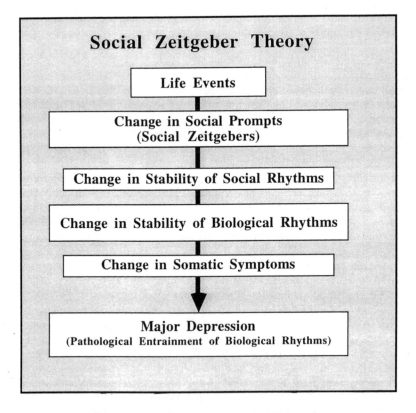

Figure 40–3. Sequence of events hypothesized in a social Zeitgeber theory of depression. (Adapted from Ehlers, et al.[65])

Although the *Social Rhythm Metric* was not used in their research, Minors et al.[67] studied the activity patterns of a large sample of older adults (ages 50 to 92 years) to determine if aging was associated with changes in life-style (social zeitgebers), which could affect circadian rhythms. They found that increasing age was associated with less variation in activity routines, but differences between subjects increased with age.

Although much additional work is needed before we fully understand the importance of activity rhythms in daily life, there is a link between our physiological rhythms, what we do, and the regularity with which our daily routines take place. Considering this, an alternative view of balance in occupation may be represented by our patterns of activity and how they maintain synchrony in our physiological rhythms. More attention should be given to chronobiological explanations when performance and satisfaction fall short of expectations. While being out of balance with our internal rhythms is seldom considered as a performance factor in occupational therapy, it may well be substantially more important than we realize.

Balance as the Relationship Among Life Tasks

This paper now addresses a view of balance that is derived from a social ecological perspective. In this view, the unique activity patterns of individuals are examined for their collective compatibility.

During our daily lives, much of our activity, whether of an obligatory or discretionary nature, is organized into sets of goal-directed acts that are logically connected and extend over time. These sets of activities were labeled "personal projects" by Little[68] and were the basis for an extended series of studies at Carleton University in Ottawa, Canada. Examples of personal projects might include cleaning the garage, getting in shape, or becoming more actively involved in family activities.

At any one time, a person typically has many projects under way, and each individual's unique group of projects can be considered a personal project system. Studies examining personal project systems have revealed a relationship between life satisfaction and the amount of time an individual allocates to projects viewed as personally important.[69] Conversely, people who reported spending a greater amount of time on projects they viewed as difficult showed lower life satisfaction.[70]

One characteristic of personal project systems that seems particularly germane to the issue of balance in occupation is the extent to which one's activities are complementary or discordant. Little and his colleagues[71] devised a means to examine the degree of harmony or conflict within personal project systems, called the cross impact matrix. Using this matrix, individuals compare each of their personal projects with every other project to determine the impact each has on the other.

Subjects are asked to start with their first project and determine whether carrying out that project will have a positive, negative, ambivalent, or neutral impact on the second project. The process continues until a pair-wise analysis has been completed for every project listed. These comparisons yield positive, negative, or neutral values.

For example, consider an analysis of several projects that might be typical of a high school adolescent, such as that seen in Figure 40-4. The impact of a project

Personal Project Impact Matrix

Project	A	B	C
A Getting better marks in school.	■	+	+
B Getting Jill to like me.	–	■	–
C Earning a place on the varsity basketball team.	–	+	■

Figure 40–4. Example of a portion of a personal project system impact matrix. For a typical individual, 15 to 20 projects would be analyzed using pairwise comparisons of the positive or negative impact of one project on another. (From Little, Lecci, and Watkinson,[71] with permission.)

labeled "getting high marks in school" would be compared with other projects, such as "getting Jill to like me" or "earning a place on the starting line up for the varsity basketball team." It is possible that the impact of project A is slightly positive on project B and neutral or slightly positive on project C. These values assume that Jill admires people with good grades, and the varsity team has academic standards that must be met. On the other hand, "getting Jill to like me" may have a negative impact on getting good grades and earning a starting place on the basketball team because of the time and attention typically required for success in those tasks.

Thus, a completed matrix reflects the impact received and given between each pair-wise comparison within a given project system. Viewed as a whole, each project system can be assigned a total score by summing the values assigned to each comparison. This total impact score can reflect either a degree of internal cohesion and overall harmony or a state of conflict, wherein each project seems to frustrate others.

As might be expected, studies have shown that people with less overall conflict within their project systems tend to have a greater sense of well-being. Beyond this linear relationship, however, Little[68] has suggested that the absence of conflict may suggest a degree of organization in one's life pursuits that offers a sense of coherence in the manner defined by Antonovsky.[72] That is, to the extent that one's array of personal projects are less characterized by conflict, they are likely to influence a general perspective that "things are under control,"[73] and that assuming favorable conditions, outcomes will turn out as one expects.

Although personal project systems can be evaluated along several other dimensions that relate to indicators of successful adaptation, the use of impact scores illustrates a possible approach to viewing balance in occupation that seems more conceptually meaningful than simply determining how one allocates time across general categories of work, play, or rest. Project system analysis does not make *a priori* assumptions about the meaning or benefit of a given activity but examines the individual and collective impact of activities within an individual's unique array of current endeavors.

Summary

Three views of balance in occupation have been considered in this paper. The most common perspective, a time budget approach to balance in occupation, is based on the assumption that daily activities can be classified according to intrinsic characteristics and that equivalent time spent among these categories will result in improved well-being. This view of balance may represent a misinterpretation of the early writings of Adolph Meyer and seems to lack a theoretical justification.

In the second view, balance can be considered from the perspective of chronobiology, suggesting that well-being results when internal clocks and external behaviors are synchronized. Although this view could have important implications for occupational science and occupational therapy, the linking of biological rhythms and activity patterns has not been studied within the field.

The third perspective offers a view of balance that considers the degree of complementarity among an individual's unique array of goal-oriented and time-extended endeavors or personal projects. Although this third approach derives from social ecology and action psychology, it offers a promising methodology that combines qualitative and quantitative dimensions and may represent a productive line of inquiry for researchers interested in occupation.

Available evidence suggests that there is great consistency and stability in patterns of time use; daily occupations are influenced by sociocultural patterns, psychological dispositions, and physiological rhythms and by physical and mental capacities. With regard to activity patterns and well-being, however, we have much less empirical evidence on which to rely. We can speculate that biological and social rhythms may be more important to occupational adaptation than previously thought. Moreover, by examining our perceptions about time and the degrees of harmony or conflict in our unique configuration of goal-directed activities, we may be able to increase our understanding of the relationship between human occupation and general well-being.

It may be fair to conclude that because of the many dimensions influencing activity patterns in daily life and the difficulties associated with explaining well-being, simplistic views regarding relationships between the two must be questioned. At the same time, alternative approaches to viewing patterns of personal enterprise must be identified and studied if we are to come to terms with the idea that occupation can be balanced.

Endnotes

1. Influenced by Kielhofner, Neville suggested that future time perspective could be used as an indicator of a person's ability to adapt to his or her environment.[17] She reported on studies of this variable among psychiatric patients.
2. One of the few attempts to operationalize balance among work, leisure, and self-care for clinical purposes was proposed by Kaplan and Kielhofner.[74] Based on earlier work by Cubie and Kaplan,[75] an item on the occupational case analysis rating scale form rates habits according to a continuum that ranged from failure to describe a schedule of activities to describing a very well-organized daily schedule of valued activities. The item is scored according to the degree to which the evaluator feels the patient's response indicates a balance among work, leisure, and self-maintenance activities. As such, the rating is based on the subjective impression of the evaluator.

Acknowledgments

I acknowledge with appreciation the assistance, encouragement, and comments provided by Pamela Christiansen, Gary Kielhofner, Margaret McCuaig, Gregory McGann, Melinda Suto, and Brian Little in preparing this paper, which was given on the occasion of the Wilma West lecture, Occupational Science Symposium V, Chicago, IL, September 1992. Appreciation also is extended to Florence Clark, Sarah Skinner, and Robert deVito, who organized and sponsored the symposium.

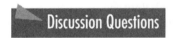

Discussion Questions

1. Christiansen has presented an overview of three perspectives pertaining to occupational therapy's historic concern with the balance of work, rest, play, and sleep: a time budget perspective, a chronobiologic perspective, and a perspective that addresses relationships among life tasks. What limitations are suggested by the time budget perspective? How might they be ameliorated?
2. How might occupational therapists begin to integrate chronobiologic research concerning biologic rhythms and daily activity into practice? What research questions are suggested by this approach that could shed further light on the inter-relationships of biology to activity performance?
3. How might occupational therapists begin to integrate knowledge generated from the third perspective, which focuses on relationships among goal-oriented and time-extended personal projects, into practice? How might research from this perspective use quantitative and qualitative dimensions to generate knowledge concerning the temporal dimensions of occupation?

References

1. Clark, F, Parham, D, Carlson, ME, Frank, G, Jackson, J, Pierce, D, Wolfe, R, and Zemke, R: Occupational science: Academic innovation in the service of occupational therapy's future. Am J Occup Ther 45:303, 1991.
2. Meyer, A: The philosophy of occupational therapy. Arch Occup Ther 1:1, 1922.
3. Reed, K: Models of Practice in Occupational Therapy. Williams & Wilkins, Baltimore, 1994.
4. Sawyer, CW: Occupation for mental cases during institutional care. Mod Hosp 5:85, 1915.
5. Hall, HJ: Neurasthenia. A study of etiology. Treatment by occupation. Boston Med Surg J 152:29, 1905.
6. Slagle, EC: Training aids for mental patients. Arch Occup Ther 1:11, 1922.
7. Slagle, p 15.
8. Reilly, M: A psychiatric occupational therapy program as a teaching model. Am J Occup Ther 22:61, 1966.
9. Shannon, PD: The work-play model: A basis for occupational therapy programming in psychiatry. Am J Occup Ther 24(3):215, 1970.
10. Kielhofner, G: Temporal adaptation: A conceptual framework for occupational therapy. Am J Occup Ther 31:238, 1977.
11. Kielhofner, G, and Burke, JP: Components and determinants of human occupation. In Kielhofner G (ed): A Model of Human Occupation: Theory and Application. Williams & Wilkins, Baltimore, 1985, p 12.
12. Wesman, AE: Personality and the subjective experience of time. J Pers Assess 37:103, 1973.
13. Bond, MJ, and Feather, NT: Some correlates of structure and purpose in the use of time. J Pers Soc Psychol 55(2):321, 1988.
14. Van Calster, K, Lens, W and Nuttin, JR: Affective attitude toward the personal future: Impact on motivating in high school boys. Am J Psychol 100:13, 1987.
15. Robinson, JP, and Nicosia, FM: Of time, activity, and consumer behavior: An essay on findings, interpretations and needed research. J Bus Res 22:171, 1991.
16. Melges, FT: Time and the Inner Future: A Temporal Approach to Psychiatric Disorders. Wiley, New York, 1982.
17. Neville, A: Temporal adaptation: Application with short term psychiatric patients. Am J Occup Ther 34:328, 1980.
18. Ricouer, P: Time and narrative (Vol. 1) (Translated by K McLaughlin & D Pellauer). University of Chicago Press, Chicago, 1984.
19. Young, M: The Metronomic Society. Harvard University Press, Cambridge, 1988.
20. Kerby, AP: Narrative and the Self. Indiana University Press, Bloomington, IN, 1991.
21. Marino-Schorn, JA: Morale, work and leisure in retirement. Phys Occup Ther Geri 4(2):49, 1986.
22. Seleen, D: The congruence between actual and desired use of time by older adults: A predictor of life satisfaction. The Gerontol 22(6):95–99, 1982.
23. Csikzentmihalyi, M and Larson, R: Being Adolescent: Conflict and Growth with the Teenage Years. Basic Books, New York, 1984.
24. Sjoberg, L, and Magneberg, R: Action and emotion in everyday life. Scand J Psychol 31:9–27, 1990.
25. Mercer, D: Australians' time use in work, homework, and leisure: Changing profiles. Australian and New Zealand Journal of Sociology 21:371, 1985.
26. Baltes, MM, Wahl, HW, and Schmid-Furstoss, U: The daily life of elderly Germans: Activity patterns, personal control, and functional health. J Gerontol 45(4):173, 1990.
27. Stones, MJ, and Kozma, A: Happiness and activities as propensities. J Gerontol 41(1):85, 1986.
28. Stones, MJ, and Kozma, A: (1989). Happiness and activities in later life: A propensity formulation. Can J Psychol 30(3):526, 1989.
29. Robinson, JP: The arts in America. Amer Demograph 434–437, 1987.
30. Moss, MS, and Lawton, MP: The time budgets of older people: A window on four lifestyles. J Gerontol 37(1):115, 1982.
31. Lawton, MP: Aging and the performance of home tasks. Human Factors 32(5):527–536, 1990.
32. Brown, M: The consequences of impairment in daily life activities: Beliefs versus reality. Rehabil Psychol 33(3):131, 1988.
33. Brown, M, and Gordon, WA: Impact of impairment on activity patterns of children. Arch Phys Med Rehabil 68:828, 1987.

34. Stenager, E, Knudsen, L, and Jensen, K: Multiple sclerosis: The impact of physical impairment and cognitive dysfunction on social and spare time activities. Psychother Psychosom 56(3):123, 1991.

35. Kennedy, CH, Homer, RH, and Newton, JS: The social networks and activity patterns of adults with severe disabilities: A correlational analysis. J Assoc Pers Severe Handicaps 15(92):86, 1990.

36. Margalit, M: Leisure activities of cerebral palsied children. Israel Journal of Psychiatry and Related Sciences 18:209, 1981.

37. Bird, CE, and Fremont, AM: Gender, time use, and health. Journal of Health and Social Behavior 32:114, 1991.

38. Ray, RO, and Heppe, G: Older adult happiness: The contributions of activity breadth and intensity. Phys Occup Ther Geri 4:31, 1986.

39. Gregory, M: Occupational behavior and life satisfaction among retirees. Am J Occup Ther 37:549, 1983.

40. Jahoda, M: Employment and Unemployment: A Social Psychological Analysis. Cambridge University Press, Cambridge, England, 1982.

41. Fagin, L, and Little, M: The Forsaken Families. The Effects of Unemployment on Family Life. Harmondsworth, England, Penguin, 1984.

42. Kilpatrick, R, and Trew, K: Lifestyles and psychological well-being among unemployed men in Northern Ireland. J Occup Psychol 58:207, 1985.

43. Feather, and Bond, p 327.

44. Bond, and Feather, p 328.

45. Meyer, p 7.

46. Harcourt, AH: Activity periods and patterns of social interaction: A neglected problem. Behaviour 66:122, 1977.

47. Flaherty, JF, Hoskinson, K, Richman, J, and Kupfer, D: Social zeitgebers and bereavement. In 140th Annual Meeting of the American Psychiatric Assoc., Chicago, IL, 1987.

48. Halberg, F, Halberg, E, Barnum, CP, and Bittner, JJ: Physiologic 24 hour periodicity in human beings and mice, the lighting regimen and daily routine. In RD Withrow (ed): Photoperiodicity and Related Phenomena in Plants and Animals. American Association for the Advancement of Science, Washington, DC, 1959.

49. Wever, RA: Man in temporal isolation: Basic principles of the circadian system. In Folkard, S, and Monk, TH (eds): Hours of Work. John Wiley & Sons, Chichester, 1985.

50. Brown, FA: The "clocks" timing biological rhythms. Amer Scient 60:756, 1972.

51. Folkard, S, Marks, Minors, DS, and Waterhouse, JM: Chronobiology and shift work: Current issues and trends. Chronobiologia 12:31, 1985.

52. Lund, R: Personality factors and desynchronization of circadian rhythms. Psychosom Med 36(3):224, 1974.

53. Lewy, AJ, Sack, RL, Fredrickson, RH, Reaves, M, Denney, DD, and Zielske, DR: The use of bright light in the treatment of chronobiologic sleep and mood disorders: The phase-response curve. Psychopharmacol Bull 19:523, 1983.

54. Wehr, TA, and Goodwin, FK: Biological rhythms in manic depressive illness. In Wehr, TA, and Goodwin, FA (eds): Circadian Rhythms in Psychiatry. Boxwood, Pacific Grove, CA, 1983.

55. Kleitman, N: Sleep Characteristics: How They Vary and React to Changing Conditions in the Group and the Individual. University of Chicago Press, Chicago IL, 1937.

56. Kerkhof, GA: Inter-individual differences in the human circadian system: A review. Biol Psychol 20:83, 1985.

57. Smith, CS, Reilly, C, and Midkiff, K: Evaluation of three circadian rhythm questionnaires with suggestions for an improved measure of morningness. J Appl Psychol 74:728, 1989.

58. Thayer, RE: Problem perception, optimism, and related states as a function of time of day (diurnal rhythm) and moderate exercise: Two arousal systems in interaction. Motivation and Emotion 11:19, 1987.

59. Thayer, RE, Takahashi, PJ, and Pauli, JA: Multidimensional arousal states, diurnal rhythms, cognitive and social processes, and extraversion. Personal Indiv Diff 9(1):15, 1988.

60. Hoskins, CN: Activation: A predictor of need fulfillment in couples. Research in Nursing and Health 12:365, 1989.

61. Adams, BN, and Cromwell, RE: Morning and night people in the family: A preliminary study. The Family Coordinator 27:5, 1978.

62. Regal, PJ, and Connolly, MS: Social influences on biological rhythms. Behaviour 72:171, 1979.

63. Hofer, MA: Relationships as regulators: A psychobiological perspective. Psychosom Med 46(3):183, 1984.

64. Cartwright, RD: Rapid eye movement sleep characteristics during and after mood disturbing events. Arch Gen Psychiatry 40:197, 1983.

65. Ehlers, CL, Frank, E, and Kupfer, DJ: Social zeitgeibers and biological rhythms: A unified approach to understanding the etiology of depression. Arch Gen Psychiatry 45:948, 1988.

66. Monk, TH, Flaherty, JF, Frank, E, Hoskinson, K, and Kupfer, DJ: The social rhythm metric: An instrument to quantify the daily rhythms of life. J Nerv Ment Dis 178:120, 1990.

67. Minors, DS, Rabbitt, PMA, Worthington, H, and Waterhouse, JM: Variation in meals and sleep-activity patterns in aged subjects: Its relevance to circadian rhythm studies. Chronobiol Internat 6(2):139, 1989.

68. Little, BR: Personal projects: A rationale and method for investigation. Environ Behav 15:273, 1983.

69. Palys, TS, and Little, BR: Perceived life satisfaction and the organization of personal project systems. J Pers Soc Psychol 44:1221, 1983.

70. Palys, TS: Personal project systems and perceived life satisfaction. Doctoral Dissertation, Carleton University 1979. Dissertation Abstracts International 41:1894B, 1980.

71. Little, BR, Lecci, L, and Watkinson, B: Personality and personal projects: Linking Big Five and PAC units of analysis. J Pers 60:501, 1992.

72. Antonovsky, A: Health, Stress and Coping. Jossey-Bass, San Francisco, 1979.

73. Antonovsky, p 155.

74. Kaplan, KL, and Kielhofner, G: Occupational Case Analysis Interview and Rating Scale. Slack, Thorofare, NJ, 1989.

75. Cubie, S, and Kaplan, K: A case analysis method for the model of human occupation. Am J Occup Ther 36:645, 1982.

Index

Numbers followed by an "f" indicate figures; numbers followed by a "t" indicate tables.

"ABC song" game, 222t
Academic discipline, 325, 419
  development of, 329–330
Academic profession, 329
Acquaintance(s), occasional, in old age,
    357–358
Action space, 116
Action systems theory, 421–422
Action theory, applied to Miles Davis,
    265–267
Activation (psychological state), 186–188
Activities of daily living
  in brain injury, 422
  broadened view of, 387–390
    emotion handling, 388
    emotional and symbolic dimensions of
      occupation, 389
    friendships and intimacy, 389
    image reconstruction, 390
    information processing aspects of, 422
Activity analysis, 420
Activity cycle(s), in band community, 95–106
Activity pattern(s), 440
  in old age, 350–351
Adaptation
  concept as foundation for occupational
    science research, 47–53
  definition of, 43–44, 47–50
  through occupation, 50
  running as cultural adaptation, 278–279
  temporal, 433
Adaptive response(s), 48, 160, 175
  contribution to sensory integration, 173
  sensory input used to elicit, 172
Adaptive skill(s), 256
Adaptive strategy(ies), 44, 51–53
  in old age, 339–360
Adaptive system(s), 48, 51–53

person-oriented, 44, 51–53
Addiction, to running, 283
Adult play, 78
Adultery, 208
Aerobic training, 280
Affective factor(s), in occupational
    perseverance, 149–151, 152
African American(s)
  HIV infection in black women, 322, 326
  jazz musician, 259–272, 260f
Age grade(s), 101–102
Aggression, decrease when work is available,
    178
Aging. See Elder(s); Old age
AIDS, 11, 321–322. See also HIV infection
American Occupational Therapy Association,
    409
Amyotrophic lateral sclerosis, 27–30
Androcentric focus, in social sciences, 44,
    57–58
Androgen(s), 182, 185
"Animal sounds" game, 222t
Annual cycle, 90, 92, 105
  in band community, 99–101
  of scholars, 137
Appreciation of occupation, 149
Arousal level, 75
Arranged marriage, 194, 197–200
"Arrow of time," 307, 317
Artistic creation, 10
Arts and crafts movement, 290
Assistant professor, 137
Assortative characteristic(s), in mate selection,
    196–197
Assortative mating, 195–196
Athletic professionalism, 276
Attractor state(s), 309–310, 319–320
  deep attractor, 310, 319